BIOLOGY OF CARCINOGENESIS

CANCER BIOLOGY AND MEDICINE

Series Editors M. J. Waring and B. A. J. Ponder

BIOLOGY OF CARCINOGENESIS

Edited by

M. J. Waring

Lecturer in Pharmacology
University of Cambridge, UK

and

B. A. J. Ponder

Consultant Physician, Institute of Cancer Research and
Royal Marsden Hospital, Sutton,
Surrey, UK

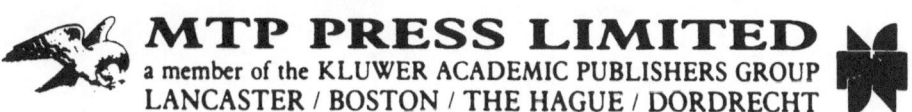

MTP PRESS LIMITED
a member of the KLUWER ACADEMIC PUBLISHERS GROUP
LANCASTER / BOSTON / THE HAGUE / DORDRECHT

Published in the UK and Europe by
MTP Press Limited
Falcon House
Lancaster, England

British Library Cataloguing in Publication Data

Biology of carcinogenesis. — (Cancer
  biology and medicine)
  1. Carcinogenesis
  I. Waring, Michael J.   II. Ponder, B. A. J.
  III. Series
  616.99′4071   RC268.5

  ISBN 0-85200-935-6
  ISBN 0-85200-827-9 Series

Published in the USA by
MTP Press
A division of Kluwer Academic Publishers
101 Philip Drive
Norwell, MA 02061, USA

Library of Congress Cataloging in Publication Data

Biology of carcinogenesis.

  (Cancer biology and medicine)
  Includes bibliographies and index.
  1. Carcinogenesis.   I. Waring, Michael J.
  II. Ponder, B. (Bruce), 1944-   . III. Series.
  [DNLM: 1. Neoplasms—etiology.   QZ 202 B6159]
  RC268.5.B58 1986   616.99′4071   86-21356

ISBN-13: 978-94-010-7942-6   e-ISBN-13: 978-94-009-3213-5
DOI: 10.1007/978-94-009-3213-5

Typeset by Witwell Ltd, Liverpool

Contents

List of Contributors

P. Alexander
Dept. of Medical Oncology
University of Southampton
Southampton General Hospital
Southampton SO9 4XY, UK

D. C. Bennett
St. George's Hospital Medical School
Department of Anatomy
Cranmer Terrace
London SW17 0RE, UK

J. M. Birch
Dept. of Epidemiology and Social Oncology
Christie Hospital and Holt Radium Institute
Withington
Manchester M20 9BX, UK

S. A. Eccles
Institute of Cancer Research
Block X
Clifton Avenue
Belmont, Sutton
Surrey SM2 5PX, UK

W. J. Gullick
Imperial Cancer Research Fund Laboratories
PO Box 123
Lincoln's Inn Fields
London WC2A 3PX, UK

P. D. Lawley
Chester Beatty Laboratories
Institute of Cancer Research
Fulham Road
London SW3 6JB, UK

R. Montesano
International Agency for Research on Cancer
150 Cours Albert Thomas
69008 Lyon
France

D. M. Parkin
International Agency for Research on Cancer
150 Cours Albert Thomas
69008 Lyon
France

B. A. J. Ponder
Institute of Cancer Research and
Royal Marsden Hospital
Sutton
Surrey SM2 5PX, UK

D. Sheer
Imperial Cancer Research Fund Laboratories
PO Box 123
Lincoln's Inn Fields
London WC2A 3PX, UK

E. Solomon
Imperial Cancer Research Fund Laboratories
PO Box 123
Lincoln's Inn Fields
London WC2A 3PX, UK

C. Tickle
Dept. of Anatomy and Biology as applied
   to Medicine
The Middlesex Hospital Medical School
Cleveland St.
London W1P 6DB, UK

L. Tomatis
International Agency for Research on Cancer
150 Cours Albert Thomas
69008 Lyon
France

D. J. Venter
Dept. of Neuropathology
Institute of Psychiatry
Denmark Hill
London SE5 8AF, UK

M. J. Waring
University Department of Pharmacology
Jesus College
University of Cambridge
Cambridge, UK

Preface

There is no shortage of books on cancer. Why publish another? Simply because the subject is important: possibly the most important challenge facing medicine today, and consequently the focus of one of the fastest-growing areas of fundamental biological research. The quest to understand and control cancer is so absorbing that from time to time we really need to pause for a moment and try to take stock of the situation. Given the sheer breadth of cancer-related research that is not an easy task.

This book, together with its planned successors in the series *Cancer Biology and Medicine*, represents our attempt to draw back from the bench or the bedside for a moment and take a slightly longer look at what we are doing, what we are trying to do, and where we stand. It is impossible to be comprehensive or even representative of more than a fraction of relevant knowledge, but that is no excuse for not trying to see things in perspective. Accordingly we set out to persuade a number of our colleagues to join us in writing a book which might admit a little fresh air into the confined atmosphere within which we mostly work: a glimpse, perhaps, of fresh vistas. The result is a book of nine chapters, each written by one or more experts in the field, which are intended to provide the reader with an up-to-date account of an important area of current thinking about cancer. The authors have been encouraged, where possible, to take a deliberately 'sideways' view of their topic so as to present a personal but balanced assessment of where we stand, what we need to know, and how research can be expected to throw light on some fundamental aspect(s) of the cancer problem. It is intended to be read by graduate students, interested clinicians, and scientists who work in related areas but wish to gain a useful perspective of a topic which may be new to them. There is no attempt to provide comprehensive cover of any selected field, but adequate referencing is provided to enable the reader to pursue issues of interest if he or she so wishes. A strong bias towards approaches inspired by modern genetics and cell biology is apparent, reflecting those areas which we as editors have considered most promising among current efforts to comprehend the nature and origins of cancer in man. We have not sought a 'popular' style of writing but one which offers a critical interpretation and assessment of a fairly broad field. Our contributors were warned that this is in many ways the toughest kind of review to write. The measure of their success will lie in what the book can do for the minds of its readers, to whom we respectfully commend it.

M. WARING
B. A. J. PONDER

1
Concepts of carcinogenesis

P.D. LAWLEY

HISTORICAL ORIGINS OF THE CONCEPTS OF INITIATION, PROMOTION AND PROGRESSION

Our present ideas about the biology of carcinogenesis owe much to the classic work of the late Leslie Foulds, the second volume of whose book *Neoplastic Development*[1] was published ten years ago. His principal theme was 'the general concept of neoplasia as a sequential developmental process'. This led to the definition of three groups of lesions. Group A (non-neoplastic) is exemplified by 'freckles and other familiar consequences of over-exposure of skin to sunlight'. Those of group B (often referred to as benign neoplasms) were defined as non-invasive, and are typified in experimental carcinogenesis by papillomas of mouse skin. Malignant tumours were designated as group C; they frequently constitute the sole manifestation of disease, in which case it is assumed that phase B has been 'masked'. Lesions of group B do not inevitably lead to malignancy, and the various possibilities found experimentally are shown in Figure 1.1 which is taken from Foulds' studies (mainly on development of mammary tumours in mice).

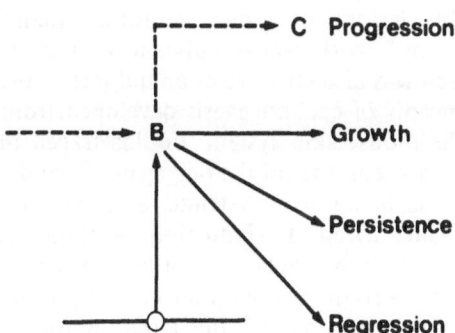

Figure 1.1. Possible fates of Group B ('precancerous') lesions. These may originate from 'regions of incipient neoplasia' (denoted by the circle) or by progression (broken line) from another Group B lesion. From Foulds[1] (part 1, Fig. 40) by permission of Academic Press, London

The first recognition of successive stages in tumour development was attributed by Foulds to Haaland, in a report to the Imperial Cancer Research Fund in 1911 on mammary and pulmonary tumours and leukaemia in mice. A few years later experimental work on the production of cancer began, with the induction of tumours by persistent application of coal tar to rabbits' ears (by Yamagiwa and Ichikawa in 1915) and subsequently to mouse skin (by Tsutsui in 1918). Use of the latter technique led to the isolation of the first pure chemical carcinogen, a polycyclic aromatic hydrocarbon, dibenz(a,h)anthracene, by Kennaway and Hieger[2] in 1930.

Rous and Kidd[3] (1941) noted that limited treatment of skin with tar induced benign tumours ('carcinomatoids') which were subject to spontaneous regression; prolonged treatment was required to yield malignant carcinoma. They therefore introduced the concept of a 'subthreshold neoplastic state' in premalignant carcinogen-treated skin.

At about the same time, Berenblum[4] discovered that croton oil, a noncarcinogen used as solvent for hydrocarbons, had a marked 'cocarcinogenic' effect in reducing the latent period for the appearance of papillomas. Mottram[5] then introduced the simplified classical method of demonstrating 'two-stage carcinogenesis' in mouse skin, by showing that a single application of benzo(a)pyrene, of itself non-tumorigenic, could suffice to elicit formation of papillomas provided prolonged treatments (e.g. three times weekly for over ten weeks) with croton oil were also given.

Mottram's experiments also showed that application of further doses of benzo(a)pyrene to the 'patently benign' papillomas obtained by this procedure markedly enhanced their conversion into carcinomas.

In this way the three stages of carcinogenesis that are now regarded as virtually axiomatic were recognised. The standard terminology was first introduced by Friedewald and Rous[6] in 1944, 'initiation' replacing the former 'subthreshold neoplastic state', and 'promotion' denoting the process by which latent tumour cells were stimulated to proliferate to form visible tumours. 'Progression' denotes the development of malignant tumours (Foulds' group C) from tissues bearing benign neoplasms (group B). As stressed by Foulds, malignant tumours often arise from neoplastic tissues surrounding visible lesions of group B, rather than from the lesions themselves. Mottram's work was significant in that it showed that an initiating carcinogen was also effective as an inducer of progression.

These basic concepts of carcinogenesis developed from work using what may be termed the mouse skin system. Foulds traced the development of another important concept, that of the oncogene, to studies on the induction of thymic lymphoma in mice by systemic, as opposed to local, action of carcinogens. He categorized the induction of thymoma in mice by X-irradiation, much studied by Kaplan and others[7], as an 'indirect' mechanism of carcinogenesis. He also drew attention to the importance of factors other than the overt inducing agent, including murine leukaemia virus, constitutional properties of the lymphoid system of the host animals, and genetic traits which could determine susceptibility[8]. According to Foulds, considerations of this type were instrumental in the development of the concept of the oncogene, attributed to Heubner and Todaro[9].

The essence of the idea is that the genetic information which is present in RNA tumour viruses and is responsible for their tumour-forming ability is also present in normal cells of animals. Neoplastic conversion of cells can result from 'activation by derepression' of these 'cellular oncogenes'.

The RNA tumour viruses replicate by way of a DNA provirus which becomes integrated into cellular DNA. (Viruses of this group are also sometimes called 'retroviruses' because their RNA genome is copied into DNA by the enzyme reverse transcriptase.) One group, the acutely transforming retroviruses, are able to induce tumours after a short latent period in infected animals. The genomes in these viruses which are responsible for transformation are called, as a class, *onc* genes. Some 20 distinct *onc* genes have now been identified and named after the RNA virus in which they were found – e.g. Ha-*ras* from Harvey rat sarcoma virus (Table 2.3, Chapter 2). These oncogenes differ not only in DNA sequence but in the spectrum of tumours which they will induce. Genes closely resembling the viral *onc* genes are widely distributed in the normal cells of many species, including *Drosophila* and even yeast. Their widespread distribution and conservation suggests that they may have important cellular functions. It is probable that the *onc*-containing RNA human viruses are generated by rare recombination events between retrovirus and cellular genes, which result in partial deletion of the retrovirus genome and insertion of a cellular gene which now comes under the influence of the virus promoter (Figure 1.2).

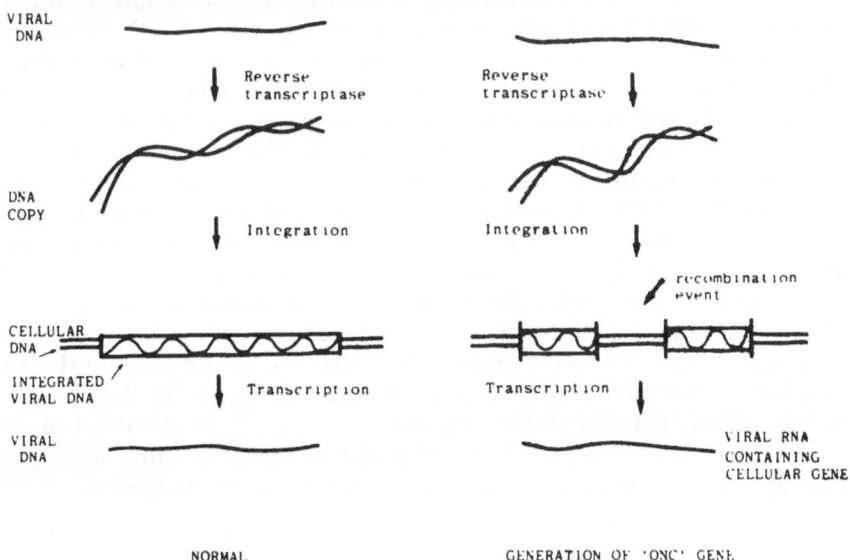

Figure 1.2 Scheme to show generation of viral *onc* gene by recombination between the virus genome and cellular DNA at the site of a cellular 'oncogene'

A possible role in carcinogenesis for the cellular homologues of the viral *onc* genes (c-*onc*) has recently been investigated in two ways: (i) by experiments involving 'transfection' which is the assay of cellular DNA fragments for transforming activity by transfer into an indicator cell culture (Figure 1.3); and (ii) by direct examination of the c-*onc* genes in the tumour cell DNA for rearrangements and increases in copy number ('amplification') which might lead to increased activity (discussed further in Chapter 2).

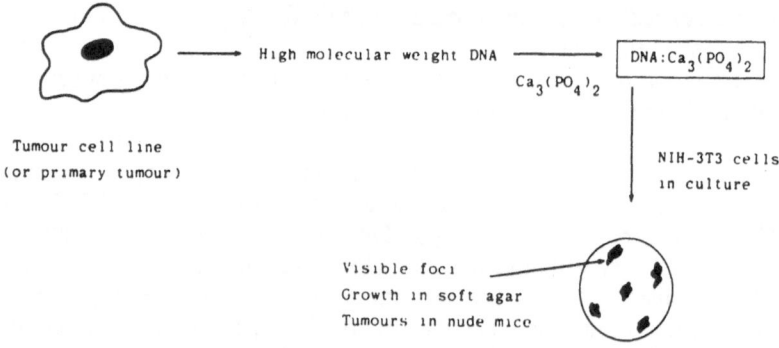

Figure 1.3 Scheme of the transfection assay for transforming sequences in tumour DNA

In most transfection experiments, the indicator cells have been an established line of mouse fibroblasts, NIH-3T3 cells. The results show that tumour cell DNA can indeed display transforming activity[10]. DNA from cell lines derived from a variety of human tumours, and in some cases isolated directly from tumour material, will transform NIH-3T3 cells with an efficiency of approximately one transformant per 0.1 to 1.0 microgram of donor DNA. DNA from normal cells is at least 100-fold less active. Some tumour cells therefore contain a DNA sequence or sequences, absent from normal cells, which can induce transformation in what appears to be a genetically dominant fashion. In most (but not all) cases so far[11], the sequences responsible have turned out to be homologous with one or other of the known viral *onc* genes, indicating that c-*onc* genes may well be important in carcinogenesis. An important outcome of further experiments has been the finding that *ras* oncogenes in tumour DNA (detected by homology to Harvey and Kirsten rat sarcoma virus) differ in base sequence from their normal cellular counterparts by single base-pair substitution[12]. As discussed in the next section, studies on the mode of action of chemical carcinogens had already pointed to the importance of gene mutation in carcinogenesis.

MUTATION AND CARCINOGENESIS

The beginnings of what is often termed the somatic mutation theory of carcinogenesis have been traced to the 1890s and attributed[13] to the observations of von Hansemann and Boveri on abnormalities of mitosis in tumours. However, at first this theory appeared to have little relevance to the mode of action of the classical chemical carcinogens, typified by aromatic

4

hydrocarbons, since no evidence was available for their activity as mutagens. The discovery of the first chemical mutagen, the alkylating agent mustard gas, is generally attributed to Auerbach and Robson[14] in 1939. Studies of the carcinogenic potential of mustard gas and its chemical analogues, the nitrogen mustards, did little to support the somatic mutation theory, since it was not easy to demonstrate their activity by conventional procedures[15] (reviewed[16]). Nevertheless mustard gas subsequently emerged[17] as a very

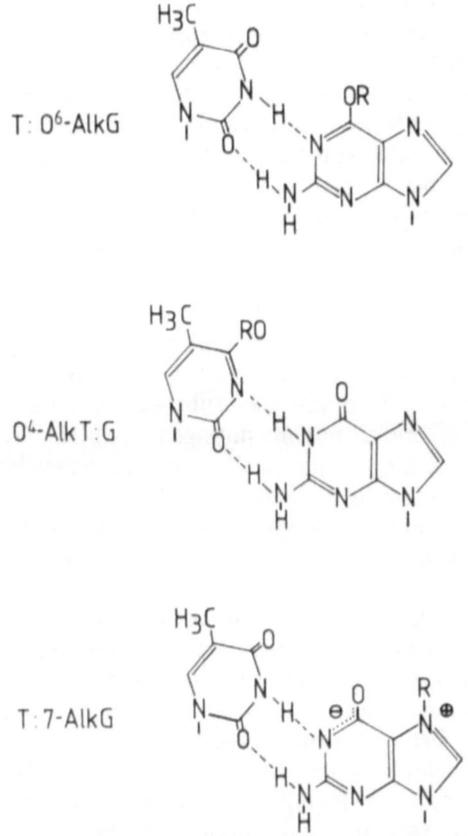

Figure 1.4 Formulae to show suggested mechanisms for miscoding induced by alkylated bases in DNA.

R denotes the alkyl group: corresponding formulae with R = H would represent examples of anomalous tautomers proposed by Watson and Crick[20] to cause spontaneous mutations. Whereas there is evidence for the participation of O^6-alkylguanine and O^4-alkylthymine in alkylation-induced mutagenesis, the earlier suggestion that ionized 7-alkylguanine miscodes has not been verified (reviewed[16]).

Alkylation at O-6 of guanine is expected to cause GC→AT, and at O 4 of thymine, TA→CG transitions. As a proportion of total methylation products formed in DNA by the alkylating carcinogen N-methyl-N-nitrosourea (MNU), about 7% is O^6-methylguanine and about 0.7% is O^4-methylthymine.

So far only GC→AT transition mutations have been detected in oncogenes of tumours induced by MNU (see Table 1.1)

effective carcinogen in man, being a potent inducer of lung cancer in Japanese workers involved in its manufacture for use in the Second World War.

A further significant finding[18] arose from the use of ^{35}S-labelled mustard gas to show that its characteristic reactions with DNA, involving principally alkylation at the N-7 atom of guanine bases, also occurred *in vivo* in mice. It was also found[19] that alkylation at this position caused the corresponding 7-alkyldeoxyguanosines to ionise much more extensively than does unsubstituted deoxyguanosine at neutral pH, and this suggested a possible mechanism of miscoding induced by the alkylated base (Figure 1.4).

This was the first suggestion for a mechanism of induction of mutation by base-pair substitution due to carcinogens, along the lines proposed by Watson and Crick[20] as a corollary of their model for DNA replication, *viz.* that occasional occurrence of bases in abnormal tautomeric forms at the time of DNA replication would cause substitution with an anomalous base as partner to the abnormal tautomer.

In the original suggestion of a mechanism for alkylation-induced mutation, it was recognized that ionization was suppressed by the hydrogen-bonding in the Watson-Crick double helical structure for DNA. A more satisfactory mechanism was provided by the work of Loveless[21], who pointed out that most alkylating agents of the classical type such as dimethyl sulphate or methyl methanesulphonate were comparatively weak mutagens measured in terms of their ability to induce base-pair substitution[22]. He showed that the significant feature of more potent mutagens typified by N-methyl-N-nitrosourea (MNU) was their ability to alkylate the extranuclear O-6 atom of DNA guanine, thus generating a 'fixed' form of miscoding tautomer leading to GC→AT transition mutations (Figure 1.4). Subsequently MNU was shown to react also at O-4 of thymine[23] thus generating a complementary miscoding base leading to TA→CG transitions.

The reactive molecular species which mediates these O-alkylations by MNU is the methyldiazonium ion, $CH_3N_2^+$, and analogous reactive intermediates are generated by oxidative metabolism of dialkylnitrosamines. Thus plausible mechanisms are available by means of which these ubiquitous environmental carcinogens can cause mutations.

For over three decades following their discovery, the polycyclic aromatic hydrocarbons were not convincingly demonstrated to act as mutagens. Boyland[24] in 1951 stressed the 'radiomimetic' nature of carcinogens, and noted from some of his own studies on the metabolism of aromatic hydrocarbons that aralkylating epoxides could be reactive intermediates. Brookes and Lawley[25] showed in 1964 that carcinogenic polycyclic aromatic hydrocarbons could react with DNA of mouse skin *in vivo* and that the extent of reaction paralleled their carcinogenic potency. The formation of the activated metabolites involved was found, perhaps surprisingly, to involve two successive epoxidations, yielding diol-epoxides[26] typified by anti-BPDE (Figure 1.5) which reacts principally at the extranuclear N-atoms of DNA bases (reviewed[27]).

Attachment of relatively bulky aralkyl groups might appear at first sight to contribute a block to the function of DNA as a template, but several lines of evidence suggest that DNA polymerase can bypass these molecular lesions,

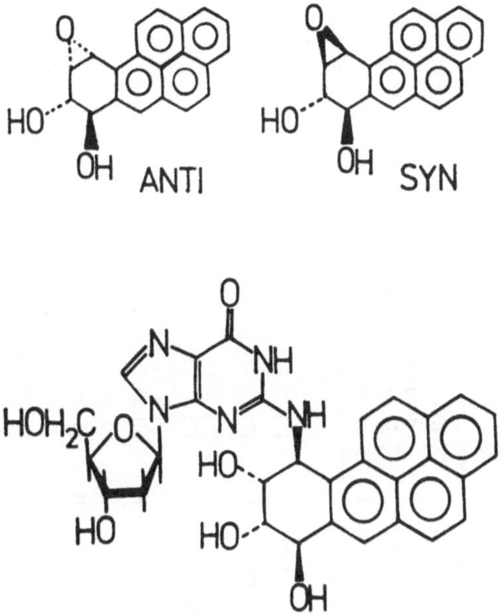

Figure 1.5 Diol-epoxide metabolites of the carcinogenic polycyclic aromatic hydrocarbon benzo(*a*)pyrene and the principal reaction product in DNA, resulting from aralkylation at N-2 of deoxyguanosine by the anti-diol-epoxide (anti-BPDE).

Mutagenesis and carcinogenesis are thought to be mediated mainly by reactions of the anti-isomer (r-7, t-8-dihydroxy-t-9, 10-epoxy-7,8,9,10-tetrahydrobenzo(*a*)pyrene). The principal sites of reaction in DNA are the extranuclear N-atoms of the bases: N-2 of guanine; N-6 of adenine; and (probably) N-4 of cytosine (reviewed[27]). The mutations induced by anti-BPDE in the human oncogene c-Ha-*ras*, which activate it to the form capable of transforming NIH-3T3 cells by transfection, include GC→TA, GC→CG, and AT→TA transversions (Table 1.1)

and that aromatic carcinogens (both hydrocarbons and amines) can act as mutagens by inducing base-substitutions. Thus, in extensive studies of the induction of forward mutations in the *lac I* gene of *Escherichia coli*, J.H. Miller and co-workers[28] found that GC→AT transitions predominated with the aliphatic alkylating agents ethyl methanesulphonate and *N*-methyl-*N'*-nitro-*N*-nitrosoguanidine (which, like MNU, alkylates through $CH_3N_2^+$), while the diol-epoxide (BPDE) derived from benzo(*a*)pyrene yielded mainly GC→TA transversions[29]. Recent studies[30] of the properties of mutants to 8-azaguanine resistance induced in Chinese hamster V79 cells are also consistent with the concept that BPDE can cause base substitutions.

Even more convincing evidence for a causal relationship between aralkylation of DNA and carcinogenesis is the demonstration[31] that treatment of a c-*ras* proto-oncogene *in vitro* with anti-BPDE can lead to its activation, in the sense in which this term is applied to the oncogenes of tumours arising spontaneously (Table 1.1). DNA containing activated *ras* oncogenes was recognized by use of the technique of transfection into NIH-3T3 cells, the same technique which had previously been used to reveal a

Table 1.1 Activation of *ras* oncogenes by base-pair substitution mutations

Source of DNA	Carcinogen	Gene*	Codon (position)	DNA base change	Type of DNA base change	Amino acid change in p21 protein gene product	References
(a) Changes in exonic sequence of normal c-ras gene into that of activated gene of tumour cells							
Human lung carcinoma	cigarette smoke (?)	K-ras	12(1)	GC → CG	transversion	gly → arg	32
Human lung carcinoma (cell line Calu-1)	?	K-ras	12(2)	GC → TA	transversion	gly → val	33
Human colon carcinoma (cell line SW480)	?	K-ras	12(1)	GC → TA	transversion	gly → cys	33
Human lung carcinoma (cell line HS242)	?	H-ras	61(2)	AT → TA	transversion	gln → leu	34
Human bladder carcinoma (cell line T24)	?	H-ras	12(2)	GC → TA	transversion	gly → val	12
Human neuroblastoma (cell line SK-N-SH)	?	N-ras	61(1)	CG → AT	transversion	gln → lys	35
Human acute myelocytic leukaemia (AML)	?	N-ras	13(2)	GC → AT	transition	gly → asp	36
		N-ras	13(2)	GC → TA	transversion	gly → val	36
Rat (Buf/N) mammary carcinoma	MNU	H-ras	12(2)	GC → AT	transition	gly → glu	37,38**
Mouse (AKR × RF/J) thymic lymphoma†	γ rays	K ras	12(2)	GC → AT	transition	gly → asp	39

(b) *Activating mutations of normal c-H-ras gene (human, in pEC plasmid) aralkylated in vitro with anti-BPDE (metabolite of the carcinogen benzo(a)pyrene) detected by transfection into NIH 3T3 cells*

NIH-3T3 cells after transfection with mutagen (anti BPDE)-treated pEC plasmid DNA	anti-BPDE				
	H-ras	61(1)	CG → AT	transversion	gln → lys
	H-ras	61(2)	AT → TA	transversion	gln → leu
	H-ras	61(3)	GC → TA	transversion	gln → his
	H-ras	61(3)	GC → CG	transversion	gln → his

*For amino-acid sequences of human *ras* gene-coded proteins see ref. 41, where other activating mutations induced in H mutagen, at codons 12, 13, 59 and 63, are also listed.

†Ref.42 reports activation of N *ras* in MNU-induced murine thymomas.

**Ref.38 reports activation of H *ras* in 7, 12-dimethylbenz (*a*) anthracene-induced mammary carcinoma at codon 61 po:

9

spectrum of activating mutations in human tumour tissue and cell lines derived from human tumours, or from experimental tumours induced with chemical carcinogens or X-irradiation.

Since chemical mutagens are expected to react in fairly random fashion throughout the base sequence of DNA, it is clear that the apparent 'hot spots' for mutation around codons 12 and 61 of the c-*ras* proto-oncogene (Table 1.1) must reflect the requirement for an activated gene product in which the function has been modified by changes in amino acid composition around either of two limited sites in the protein molecule. This is in accord with observations that the best quantitative correlations between ability to induce mutation in cultured mammalian cells and carcinogenic potency of mutagens have emerged from studies using mutation to ouabain resistance[43], where it is apparent that only limited changes in structure of the gene product can give rise to viable mutants. In this system γ-irradiation cannot induce a detectable level of mutation[44] indicating a feeble ability to cause base-pair substitution[45]. It is somewhat surprising, therefore, that γ-ray-induced murine thymoma exhibits oncogene activation through GC$\rightarrow$AT transitions[39].

So far the system of Marshall *et al.*[31] for activation of oncogenes *in vitro* has not been able to show the mechanism of activation by MNU, although *in vivo* it occurs by GC$\rightarrow$AT transitions[38]. This may be because the small number of DNA base methylations is rapidly removed by a process of DNA repair in 3T3 cells[46]. The existence of such a repair mechanism was first discovered in *Escherichia coli*[47]; repair-deficient strains are several thousand times more susceptible to the mutagenic action of MNU than are wild type bacteria[48]. Repair is 'error-free' and involves transfer of the methyl group from O-6 of DNA guanine to a thiol group of an acceptor protein which is thereby inactivated[49].

Mouse cells other than liver lack such repair proficiency. For example Craddock and Henderson[50] found that the content of the alkyl acceptor protein in a mouse thymus cell was less than about one twentieth of that in a mouse liver cell. Human cells, such as peripheral blood lymphocytes[51] or diploid fibroblasts in culture[52], are generally highly proficient (the maximal proficiency so far found corresponds to a level of around 80000 molecules of alkyl acceptor protein per cell)[53]. However, human cells may be less proficient at removal of mutagenic ethylated, as opposed to methylated, bases, since the ethyl analogue of MNU is a more efficient mutagen than MNU for diploid human fibroblasts known to be proficient at removal of O^6-methylguanine[54].

In summary, therefore, deficiency in ability to remove promutagenic alkylated bases leading to their persistence in the DNA template may well be necessary for the initiation of carcinogenesis, though it is not of itself sufficient.

The further question arises, in view of the requirement for mutagenesis at the stages of both initiation and progression, of the nature of the oncogenes involved at each stage. For example, the data of Table 1.1 do not enable specification of which stage is due to activation of the *ras* oncogenes, and evidence is available to support either alternative. Thus, activation through mutation is indicated to occur at the initiation stage in the induction of skin tumours in mice by hydrocarbons, since both the papillomas and carcinomas induced were found[55] to possess the ras^H gene in the activated form. Furthermore, whereas transformed NIH 3T3 cells with activated ras oncogenes formed only localized non-metastasising tumours when injected into immunocompetent mice, introduction of other genes by transfection conferred metastatic capability on these cells[56].

On the other hand, ras gene activation was found to be associated only with later stages of tumour progression in certain mouse lymphoma cell lines[57]. Comparative studies of premalignant and malignant human colorectal tumours showed that expression (complementary RNA synthesis) of ras^H and ras^K was elevated at both stages in one study[58], but only at later stages in another[59]. Evidently no general conclusion can be reached on this question at present.

SIGNIFICANCE OF THE CONCEPTS OF INITIATION, PROMOTION AND PROGRESSION FOR CARCINOGENESIS IN MAN

In the previous section evidence was presented ranging from the chemistry of carcinogens to the molecular changes they induce in oncogenes, to support the view that initiation of cancer involves base-substitution mutations. The question then arises whether these mechanisms can provide a plausible quantitative basis for the incidence of cancer.

Early theorists drew attention to the marked age-dependence of this incidence. For example, Nordling[60] considered that the commonly observed relationship between cancer incidence (I) and age (t), $I_t = kt^n$ (often referred to as the 'log-log' relationship, $\log I_t = \log k + n \log t$) with exponents n of around 5 for some common cancers, showed that ($n + 1$) successive discrete steps were necessary in the pathway from normal to malignant cells. Burch[61] later pointed out that if these steps were somatic mutations, the observed incidence would require relatively high rates of mutation, of the order of 10^{-3} per gene per cell per year. Nevertheless, he opted for the view that this was not unreasonable and that such values had in fact been found experimentally, notably for mutation at the H-2 locus in mice. On these grounds he developed a theory of cancer as an 'auto-aggressive' disease resulting from multiple mutations occurring at relatively high rates in growth-controlling stem cells of the lymphoid system. Families of curves could be derived in which age specific death rates *versus* time peaked at various ages according to the type of disease considered (these could include infectious diseases and autoimmune diseases as well as the various forms of cancer), and each curve could fit the observed values with reasonable assumptions regarding the number of cells and proportion of the population at risk.

An alternative option envisages only two discrete steps, and thus resembles the basic theory discussed by Foulds[1] and evidenced by experiments such as those of Mottram[5]; normal cells are converted into intermediate benign cells by an initiating mutation, and a second mutation converts these to malignant cells. The latent period characteristic of the process of carcinogenesis would be interpreted according to this view as reflecting a requirement for clonal growth of initiated cells to such numbers as to permit an appreciable rate of appearance of the second mutation. The acknowledged pioneer of this approach was Platt[62], in a short letter to *The Lancet* in 1955. Subsequently, Armitage and Doll[63] devised a detailed theory that could account for the age-dependence of mortality from several common types of cancer based on the two-stage, as opposed to the previous multi-stage, concept of carcinogenesis.

More recently, Moolgavkar and Knudson[64] have extended this type of model to take account of the concept of tumour promotion. Whereas the earlier theories assumed that initiating mutations of themselves conferred a proliferative growth advantage on the mutant cells, the newer theory introduced a factor expressing the relative 'birth and death rates' of initiated cells, expressed as $\exp(\alpha_2 - \beta_2)$. Together with the product of values of the rates of the first and second mutations $\mu_1 \mu_2$ and certain assumptions regarding the number of cells at risk and their dependence on age, satisfactory agreement with observed data was obtained.

To illustrate the types of curves for age-dependence of cancer incidence, one can mention certain diseases for which these curves peak in childhood (here the number of dividing stem cells at risk declines after a certain age, with no proliferative advantage to initiated cells). Then there is the special case of breast cancer, where incidence rises until around the menopausal age, then flattens, illustrating the decrease in the proliferative factor $(\alpha_2 - \beta_2)$ as oestrogenic stimulus to growth declines in older women. Finally we see the common pattern of the 'log-log' form, characterized by increasing slope 'n' as the value $(\alpha_2 - \beta_2)$ increases. With a typical target tissue, values of the various parameters might be of the order of 10^7 stem cells susceptible to initiating mutations at rates of about 10^{-7} per cell per year; increase in the factor $(\alpha_2 - \beta_2)$ from a value of 0.03 to 0.1 can cause a large (of the order of 20-fold) increase in cancer incidence among older age-groups. The proposed role for promoters, in mouse skin for example, is to increase this factor.

The salient difference between the two approaches is therefore that the hypothesis of two mutational stages presupposes much lower rates of mutation, which are in line with those commonly observed. For example, the most extensively documented mutations in man are those in haemoglobin genes[65]. The majority of mutations are of the base-pair substitution type, and the rate is of the order of 2.5×10^{-9} per base pair per generation (this rate is calculated to result in 17.5 mutations per haploid genome, which Vogel and Motulsky[65] comment is 'frighteningly high'). The rate for mouse or Chinese hamster cells *in vitro* as assessed by mutation to ouabain resistance[66] (as previously noted, probably a good model for tumour-initiating mutation) is about 5×10^{-8} per cell per generation (presumably at a not very large number of sites). Allowing for, say, 50–100 divisions per year of stem cells at risk, the derived rates for cancer initiation at about 10^{-7} per cell per year seem therefore to be reasonable. A further assumption of the theories, that somatic mutation rates are not very age-dependent, is supported by the findings[67] that an increase of only three-fold occurred *in vitro* for human lymphocytes taken from donors aged between 20 and 80 years.

The rates for the second mutational process associated with the step to malignancy may be higher than those for initiation, since tumour progression is associated with increased genetic instability[68]. Evidence to this effect has been obtained by Yamashina and Heppner[69] who compared the rates of mutation (to 6-thioguanine resistance) induced by the alkylating carcinogen, ethyl methanesulphonate, in mouse mammary tumour subpopulation cell lines. The frequency of ethylation-induced mutations was positively correlated with metastatic potential.

The concept that cancer is initiated through somatic mutation due to chemical modification of single base-pair sites in DNA implies that the first stage should be a 'single-hit' process, i.e. that the dose-response relationship should be of the form:

$-\log$ (survival of non-initiated animals) $= k$ (dose of carcinogen)

which may conveniently be abbreviated to $-\log S = k\,d$. Support for this relationship has been obtained from experiments on mouse-skin carcinogenesis using either benzo(a)pyrene[70] or MNU[71] in single applications to induce papillomas, provided that initiation is followed by adequate promotion using croton oil or its active principle, phorbol ester.

However, in most experimental systems intervention through the use of exogenous agents cannot be employed to ensure that promotion does not become rate-limiting and 'complete carcinogenesis' is the end-point. It is not surprising therefore that 'multi-hit' kinetics are generally found, of the form $-\log S = k\,d^n\,t^m$, where $n > 1$, and there is a marked dependence on the time (t) between commencement of treatment and appearance of tumour.

This may at first sight appear to imply that low doses of carcinogens would be very ineffective. Whereas the 'single-hit' kinetics imply that tumour incidence will be proportional to dose at low doses, 'multi-hit' kinetic behaviour predicts tumour incidence proportional to the nth power of dose. However, the existence of a spontaneous background incidence of tumours cannot be ignored, and it seems most reasonable to attribute this background to the operation of the same molecular mechanisms as are involved when exogenous carcinogens are applied, i.e. to assume that it can be represented as the effect of a hypothetical background dose of carcinogen, d_0.

Replacement of the effective dose by $(d_0 + d)$, i.e. $d_0\,(1 + d/d_0)$, then modifies the term for dose-dependence to $k d_0{}^n (1 + d/d_0)^n$; the term in dose will thus be proportional to the first power of dose at low doses where $(d/d_0) \to 0$, and to the nth power as $d > d_0$.

In order to gain experimental support for this concept, a much larger number of animals must be used than are generally available for carcinogenesis studies. Peto et al.[72] have recently reported extensive data from a remarkable study on the effects of continuous feeding of dialkylnitrosamines on rats. As examples of their findings, the use of over four thousand animals with a range of sixteen doses of dimethyl- and diethylnitrosamine led to dose-response relationships for incidence of liver tumours in female rats of:

for dimethylnitrosamine, $-\log_{10} S = 51.45\,(d + 0.1)^6.\,t^7$

and for diethylnitrosamine, $-\log_{10} S = 32.09\,(d + 0.04)^4.\,t^7$

(with dose-rate d in units of mg/kg/day for t years of treatment). The data were sufficient to establish that the increase in incidence of tumours over the spontaneous background was indeed proportional to dose at low doses. The greater effectiveness of diethylnitrosamine is in line with the known lower repair proficiency of rat liver for removal from DNA of promutagenic ethylated bases (particularly of O^4-ethylthymine)[73] compared to products derived from the methyl analogue.

It is known that ingestion of dimethylnitrosamine can induce promutagenic O^6-methylguanine in human liver, from analyses (using a fluorometric technique) of DNA from a victim of poisoning by this carcinogen[74]. This base has also been identified in oesophageal DNA from individuals who underwent surgery for oesophageal cancer in an area of China where ingestion of nitrosamines in food is exceptionally high[75].

Some idea of the order of magnitude of promutagenic alkylation of DNA required for tumorigenesis in mice is provided from the example of induction of thymoma by single intraperitoneal injection of MNU or analogous alkylating carcinogens[76]. In a sensitive strain (RFM) at the mean tumorigenic dose (i.e. for $-\log S = 1$, at $1/e$, (37%) survival of non-tumour-bearing mice) about 60000 O^6-alkylations in a genome of 2.4×10^9 guanine bases were found in DNA of the target organs thymus or bone marrow. This represents a chance of one in 40000 of 'hitting' an individual GC base pair. Since more resistant strains of mice can require up to at least three times higher doses to attain this yield of tumours[77], whereas the extent of alkylation of DNA per unit dose is not strain-dependent[51], the importance of factors other than DNA alkylation as determinants of tumorigenesis is evident. This becomes even more obvious when results from papilloma induction in mouse skin are considered; strain C57BL fails to respond to papilloma induction by MNU applied to skin because it is not susceptible to the promoting action of phorbol ester; nevertheless this treatment causes induction of thymoma. Both types of tumour are readily induced in mice of the RFM strain (G. Harris and P.D. Lawley, unpublished data).

Thus model studies with rodents show that a wide quantitative spectrum of tumour incidence can follow from a given amount of promutagenic damage to DNA, dependent both on subsequent exogenous promotion and, in absence of this, on what may be broadly termed endogenous promotion.

Widening the concept of promotion encompasses a considerable variety of promoters, ranging (for induction of papillomas in mouse skin) from abrasion-induced epidermal hyperplasia without any overt chemical promoter[78], through cytotoxic thiol-reacting alkylating agents that are non-mutagenic[79], to compounds of complex structure with specific receptors[80] such as the well-known phorbol ester and its analogues.

In man, it has been suggested that bile acids[81] may promote colonic cancer through inflammatory action[82] and that acrolein, as a metabolite of cyclophosphamide, may serve as a promoter for bladder tumours induced by this anticancer drug[83]. The positive correlation between consumption of fat and cancer of the endometrium may be mediated through excessive production of oestrogens[84], which may thus be included within the extended definition of promotion.

Epidemiological studies[85] show an inverse relationship between risk of cancer and consumption of foods containing vitamin A or its precursors (such as ß-carotene). In experimental studies, certain derivatives of vitamin A (retinoids such as retinyl acetate) can cause regression of skin papillomas in mice[86] and appear in certain cases to act as 'anti-promoters', but it should be noted that this action is not always found; in fact enhancement of tumour yields occurs in some experimental systems[87,88]. (See also Chapter 6).

A number of studies *in vitro* have suggested the possibility that a significant mechanism of action of promoters[89,90] lies in their ability to inhibit metabolic co-operation between cells. This was detected as increased expression of mutations induced in cells of the V79 Chinese hamster lung cell line. Anti-promoting retinoids had the opposite effect[91].

Complete carcinogenesis, formally equivalent to initiation plus promotion, can be achieved *in vitro* in the form of transformation of rodent cells – either primary embryo cells, or cell lines which do not give tumours when injected into syngeneic animals. Since its discovery by Berwald and Sachs[92], this technique has been extensively studied, in part as a rapid screening test for carcinogens[93].

The use of primary cultures, particularly from Syrian hamsters, showed that a prerequisite for transformation to malignancy is 'immortalization' of cells to give established lines that can be grown indefinitely in conventional media[94]. Immortalizing agents are not identical with either initiators or promoters, but appear to be characterized by their ability to induce chromosomal instability. They include not only classical base-pair mutation-inducing carcinogens, such as MNU and benzo(*a*)pyrene, but also less specifically acting genotoxic agents such as X-rays and methyl methane-sulphonate.

Of particular interest are the studies by Barrett and co-workers[95], showing that the synthetic oestrogen, diethylstilbestrol, a non-mutagen which is established as a carcinogen for humans[96] causing vaginal adenocarcinoma in young women exposed *in utero*, is also effective as an inducer of cell immortalization. Comparative studies of analogues showed this latter action to be independent of oestrogenic activity, to correlate with peroxidase-mediated oxidation, and to involve induction of aneuploidy.

Foulds[97] included *in vitro* transformation, along with carcinogenesis by implantation of plastic films, as 'neoplasia of obscure pathogenesis'. Current opinion places considerable emphasis on the significance of *in vitro* transformation, as indicating the importance of chromosomal rearrangements occurring at possibly the earliest stage in carcinogenesis. Sager[98] has stressed the 'dramatic' ability of human, as opposed to rodent, diploid fibroblasts to maintain the stability of their chromosomes in culture, and the remarkable resistance of these human cells to transformation by procedures that are effective in their counterparts of rodent origin. This may explain how, in the words of Peto *et al.*[72], humans can exert 'controls on the processes of carcinogenesis that are millions of times stricter than those required by small, short-lived rodents.'

Another postulated controlling mechanism without which 'cancer would be more frequent and occur at younger ages' is immunological surveillance, a concept developed by Burnet[99], following a suggestion by Thomas[100]. In its original form surveillance was envisaged as being mediated by thymus-dependent cell-mediated immunity. The hypothesis became experimentally testable[101] with the advent of athymic *nu/nu* strains of mice, which proved to be no more susceptible to chemical carcinogens than were the parent immunocompetent strains, although they were markedly more susceptible to tumour viruses, particularly polyoma.

Patients immunodepressed for organ transplantation showed an increased risk for development of malignancies[102,103], but the diseases were not those typically encountered in the population at large. Rather they were types specifically associated with aetiological involvement of DNA tumour viruses, such as Epstein-Barr virus (non-Hodgkin's lymphoma) and papilloma virus (skin tumours).

As reviewed recently by Klein and Klein[104], the activation of cellular oncogenes by non-viral mechanisms such as point mutations, DNA rearrangements, gene amplification and chromosomal translocations is probably the basis for most tumours of spontaneous origins. Thus the transforming oncogene products will be at most only slightly modified, like the mutated *ras* gene products previously noted, and 'it is difficult to see how they could provide a rejection target for the immune system'[104].

It should not be assumed, however, that immune surveillance plays no role in carcinogenesis. Relatively recent work, notably by Feldman and co-workers[105], has indicated that expression of class I antigens of the major histocompatibility complex (MHC) in mice can profoundly influence the metastatic growth potential of tumours. As an example, decreased metastatic capacity in immunocompetent (but not in immunologically depleted) mice could be induced in a murine sarcoma by transfection of H-2K histocompatibility genes. Mutations, or chromosomal rearrangements, associated with tumour progression may therefore involve MHC genes, and some evidence is available for equivalent phenomena in human melanomas and breast tumours (reviewed[106]).

SUMMARY AND CONCLUSIONS

The concept that tumorigenesis is initiated by somatic mutations now appears to be well established, and from studies with chemical carcinogens the predominant mechanism that has emerged is substitution of a single base-pair in DNA at (perhaps unexpectedly) specific sites. The incidence of human cancer could well be accounted for on the basis of known 'spontaneous' mutation rates, which in turn can be plausibly ascribed to chemical changes in DNA analogous to those induced by experimental carcinogens.

The subsequent stages of carcinogenesis are less well defined. The concept of promotion as permitting growth of initiated cells, sometimes to give benign intermediate tumours, has received experimental support from the 'mouse skin system'. Extension of the concept to universal applicability remains a reasonable assumption.

The acquisition of malignancy is thought to involve further mutagenic change. Studies of these later stages (of progression) of tumours are now beginning to be undertaken using molecular biological techniques analogous to those that have enabled the identification of oncogenes, and will presumably clarify which genes are involved at which stage. At present the most attractive hypothesis is that initiating mutagens and promoters affect certain proteins essential for control of cell division[107] (e.g. initiators cause mutations in the *ras* gene giving altered p21 proteins, and the promoter phorbol ester may bind to protein kinase C) whereas the mutations involved in progression to malignancy alter expression of self-recognition surface antigens of the MHC.

With regard to cancer prevention, the somatic mutation concept has led to the development of excellent methods for screening environmental mutagens of industrial origin as potential initiating carcinogens, but these seem unlikely to account for more than a small proportion (perhaps as low as 1%) of avoidable causes, apart from tobacco smoke[108].

At first sight this seems to contradict the evidence (admittedly from a very limited number of instances) that the oncogene-activating mutations (Table 1.1) are those expected to result from chemically induced damage to DNA, and the question as to how much of the necessary mutagenesis is exogenous as opposed to endogenous appears to remain unresolved. German[109] considered that the lack of cancer of internal tissues in xeroderma pigmentosum (XP) patients (having an inherited deficiency in cellular repair of chemically, as well as sunlight-induced, DNA damage) might indicate that exogenous mutagens did 'not regularly reach body tissues in significant amounts'. Kraemer *et al.*[110] subsequently reported that XP patients do show a much higher rate of early onset of cancers of the oral cavity than the population at large, but suggested that this might be attributed to ingestion of mutagens known to be present in common foods.

The possibility that changed diet could reduce cancer risk through reduced intake of exogenous initiating mutagens cannot therefore be ruled out. However, the major emphasis in the current climate of opinion is that diet predominantly influences the subsequent stage of carcinogenesis, which is included in the broader definition of the term promotion. Change of diet to decrease consumption of fat and increase consumption of vegetables would probably (presumably by decreasing promoting factors) present the best hope for reduction in cancer incidence, but would require drastic re-structuring of agriculture.

The best example of a successful screening procedure is the cytological detection of early-stage cancer of the uterine cervix. As noted by Spriggs[111], 'this has been more thoroughly studied than any other human cancer ... the squamous type could theoretically be prevented ... we still do not know its cause, but that is not necessary for prevention and control'.

Nevertheless the trend towards further defining cancer as a molecular disease, with growth in expenditure on oncogene research, embodies the belief that more detailed knowledge of the causes of cancer at the molecular level will be necessary for future progress in diagnosis as well as prevention and treatment. Possible applications of the new discoveries have recently been reviewed[112].

In the field of carcinogenesis, a shift of emphasis now seems likely towards more precise identification of individuals at risk from carcinogens. With this in mind, studies of genetic polymorphism among oncogenes have already begun[113]. It will also become of interest to find out whether research into oncogenes can specify causative agents of cancer in individual cases, for example by comparing DNA from human tumours with DNA from tumours induced experimentally in animals or from cells transformed *in vitro* by various agents. Already there is evidence for some degree of specificity in the chromosomal changes associated with leukaemias known to have been induced by mutagens[114], whether by industrial exposure or through cancer therapy.

References

1. Foulds, L. (1969, 1975). *Neoplastic Development*. Vols. 1 and 2. (London: Academic Press)
2. Kennaway, E. L. and Hieger, I. (1930). Carcinogenic substances and their fluorescent spectra. *Br. Med. J.*, i, 1044
3. Rous, P. and Kidd, J. G. (1941). Conditional neoplasms and sub-threshold neoplastic states. A study of the tar tumours of rabbits. *J. Exp. Med.*, 73, 365
4. Berenblum, I. (1941). Co-carcinogenic action of croton resin. *Cancer Res.*, 1, 44
5. Mottram, J. C. (1945). Change from benign to malignant in chemically induced warts in mice. *Br. J. Exp. Pathol.*, 26, 1
6. Friedewald, W. F. and Rous, P. (1944). Initiating and promoting elements in tumour production. Analysis of the effects of tar, benzpyrene and methylcholanthrene on rabbit skin. *J. Exp. Med.*, 80, 101
7. Kaplan, H. S. (1972). Mouse leukaemia: interaction of multiple components in a complex oncogenic system. In Emmelot, P. and Bentvelzen, P. (eds.) *RNA Viruses and Host Genome in Oncogenesis*. pp. 143-154. (Amsterdam: North Holland)
8. Lilly, F. and Duran-Reynals, M. L. (1984). Genetics of susceptibility to murine lymphoma. In Bishop, M. J., Rowley, J. D. and Greaves, M. (eds.) *Genes and Cancer*. pp. 51-57. (New York: Alan R. Liss)
9. Huebner, R. J. and Todaro, G. J. (1969). Oncogenes of RNA tumour viruses as determinants of cancer. *Proc. Natl. Acad. Sci. USA*, 64, 1087
10. Cooper, G. M. (1982). Cellular transforming genes. *Science*, 218, 801
11. Land, H., Parada, L. F. and Weinberg, R. A. (1983). Cellular oncogenes and multistage carcinogenesis. *Science*, 222, 771
12. Reddy, E. P., Reynolds, R. K., Santos, E. and Barbacid, M. (1982). A point mutation is responsible for the acquisition of transforming properties by the T24 human bladder carcinoma oncogene. *Nature*, 300, 149
13. Bashford, E. F. and Murray, J. A. (1906). On the occurrence of heterotypical mitoses in cancer. *Proc. R. Soc.*, *Ser. B*, 77, 61
14. Auerbach, C., Robson, J. M. and Carr, J. G. (1947). Chemical production of mutations. *Science*, 105, 243.
15. Heston, W. E. (1950) Carcinogenic action of the mustards. *J. Natl. Cancer Inst.*, 11, 415
16. Lawley, P. D. (1985). Carcinogenesis by alkylating agents. In Searle, C. E., (ed.) *Chemical Carcinogens*. 2nd Edn. *ACS Monograph No. 182*. Vol. 1., pp. 326-484. (Washington: American Chemical Society)
17. Wada, S., Miyanishi, M., Nishimato, Y., Kambe, S. and Miller, R. W. (1968). Mustard gas as a cause of respiratory neoplasia in man. *Lancet*, i, 1611
18. Brookes, P. and Lawley, P. D. (1960). Reaction of mustard gas with nucleic acids *in vitro* and *in vivo*. *Biochem. J.*, 77, 478
19. Lawley, P. D. and Brookes, P. (1961). Acidic dissociation of 7, 9-dialkylguanines and its possible relation to mutagenic properties of alkylating agents. *Nature*, 192, 1081
20. Watson, J. D. and Crick, F. H. C. (1953). Genetical implications of the structure of DNA. *Nature*, 171, 1964
21. Loveless, A. (1969). Possible relevance of O^6-alkylation of deoxyguanosine to mutagenicity of nitrosamines and nitrosamides. *Nature*, 223, 206

22. Loveless, A. and Hampton, C. L. (1969). Inactivation and mutation of coliphage T2 by N-methyl- and N-ethyl-N-nitrosourea. *Mutat. Res.*, **7**, 1

23. Lawley, P. D., Orr, J. D., Shah, S. A., Farmer, P. B. and Jarman, M. (1973). Reaction products from N-methyl-N-nitrosourea and DNA containing thymidine residues: synthesis and identification of a new methylation product O^4-methylthymidine. *Biochem. J.*, **135**, 193

24. Boyland, E. (1952). Different types of carcinogens and their mode of action: a review. *Cancer Res.*, **12**, 77

25. Brookes, P. and Lawley, P. D. (1964). Evidence for binding of polynuclear aromatic hydrocarbons to nucleic acids of mouse skin: relation between carcinogenic power of hydrocarbons and their binding to DNA. *Nature*, **202**, 781

26. Sims, P., Grover, P. L., Swaisland, A., Pal, K. and Hewer, A. (1974). Metabolic activation of benzo(a)pyrene proceeds by a diol-epoxide. *Nature*, **252**, 326

27. Dipple, A., Moschel, R. C. and Bigger, C. A. H. (1985). Polynuclear aromatic hydrocarbons. In Searle, C. E. (ed.) *Chemical Carcinogens*. 2nd ed. *ACS Monograph No. 182*, Vol. I, pp. 42-163. (Washington: American Chemical Society)

28. Coulondre, C. and Miller, J. H. (1977). Genetic studies of the *lac* repressor. IV. Mutagenic specificity in the *lacI* gene of *Escherichia coli*. *J. Mol. Biol.*, **117**, 577

29. Eisenstadt, E., Warren, A. J., Porter, J., Atkins, D. and Miller, J. H. (1982). Carcinogenic epoxides of benzo(a)pyrene and cyclopenta(c,d)pyrene induce base substitutions. *Proc. Natl. Acad. Sci. USA*, **79**, 1945

30. King, H. W. S. and Brookes, P. (1984). On the nature of the mutations induced by the diolepoxide of benzo(a)pyrene in mammalian cells. *Carcinogenesis*, **5**, 965

31. Marshall, C. J., Vousden, K. H. and Phillips, D. H. (1984). Activation of c-Ha-ras-1 proto-oncogene by *in vitro* modification with a chemical carcinogen, benzo(a)pyrene diol-epoxide. *Nature*, **310**, 568

32. Santos, E., Martin-Zanca, D., Reddy, E. P., Pierotti, M. A., Della Porta, G. and Barbacid, M. (1984). Malignant activation of a K-ras oncogene in lung carcinoma but not in normal tissue of the same patient. *Science*, **223**, 661

33. Capon, D. J., Seeburg, P. H., McGrath, J. P., Hayflick, J. S., Edman, W., Levinson, A. D. and Goeddel, P. V. (1983). Activation of Ki-ras 2 gene in human colon and lung carcinogens by two different point mutations. *Nature*, **304**, 507

34. Yuasa, Y., Eva, A., Kraus, M. H., Strivastava, S. K., Needleman, S. W., Pierce, J. H., Rhim, J. S., Gol, R., Reddy, E. P., Tronick, S. R. and Aaronson, S. A. (1984). Ras-related oncogenes of human tumours. In Vande Woude, G. F., Levine, A. J., Topp, W. C. and Watson, J. D. (eds.) *Cancer Cells. 2. Oncogenes and Viral Genes*. pp. 433-439. (New York: Cold Spring Harbor Laboratory)

35. Taparowsky, E., Shimizu, K., Goldfarb, M. and Wigler, M. (1983). Structure and activation of human N-ras gene, *Cell*, **34**, 581

36. Bos, J. L., Toksoz, D., Marshall, C. J., Verlaan-de Vries, M., Veenernan, G. H., van der Eb, A., van Boom, J. H., Janssen, J. W. G. and Steenvoorden, A. C. M. (1985). Amino-acid substitution at codon-13 of the N-ras oncogene in human acute myeloid leukaemia. *Nature*, **315**, 726

37. Sukumar, S., Santos, E., Martin-Zanca, D., Arthur, A. V., Long, L. K. and Barbacid, M. (1984). Transforming *ras* genes in human neoplasia and in chemically induced animal tumour systems. In Bishop, J. M., Rowley, J. D. and Greaves, M. (eds.) *Genes and Cancer*. pp. 353-371. (New York: Alan R. Liss)

38. Zarbl, H., Sukumar, S., Arthur, A. V., Martin-Zanca, D. and Barbacid, M. (1985). Direct mutagenesis of Ha-ras-1 oncogenes by N-methyl-N-nitrosourea during initiation of mammary carcinogenesis in rats. *Nature*, **315**, 382

39. Guerrero, I., Villasante, A., Corces, V. and Pellicer, A. (1984). Activation of a c-K-ras oncogene by somatic mutation in mouse lymphomas induced by γ-radiation. *Science*, **225**, 1159

40. Vousden, K. H., Bos, J. L., Marshall, C. J. and Phillips, D. H. (1986). Mutations activating human c-Ha-ras-1 proto-oncogene (Hras1) induced by chemical carcinogens and depurination. *Proc. Natl. Acad. Sci. USA*, **83**, 1222

41. Wigler, M., Fasano, O., Taparowsky, E., Powers, S., Kataoka, T., Birenbaurn, D., Shimizu, K. and Goldford, M. (1984). Structure and activation of *ras* genes. In Vande Woude, G. F., Levine, A. J., Topp, W. C. and Watson, J. D. (eds.) *Cancer Cells. 2. Oncogenes and Viral Genes*. pp. 419-423. (New York: Cold Spring Harbor Laboratory)

42. Guerrero, I., Villasante, A., D'Eustachio, P. and Pellicer, A. (1984). Isolation, characterization and chromosome assignment of mouse N-*ras* gene from carcinogen-induced thymic lymphoma. *Science*, **225**, 1041

43. Friedrich, U. and Coffino, P. (1977). Mutagenesis in S49 mouse lymphoma cells: induction of resistance to ouabain, 6-thioguanine and dibutyryl cyclic AMP. *Proc. Natl. Acad. Sci. USA*, **74**, 679

44. Arlett, C. F., Turnbull, D., Harcourt, S. A., Lehmann, A. R. and Colella, C. M. (1975). Comparison of 8-azaguanine and ouabain-resistance systems for selection of induced mutant Chinese hamster cells. *Mutat. Res.*, **33**, 261

45. Thacker, J., Stretch, A. and Stephens, M. A. (1977). Induction of thioguanine-resistant mutants of Chinese hamster cells by gamma-rays. *Mutat. Res.*, **42**, 313

46. Yagi, T., Yarosh, D. B. and Day, R. S., III (1984). Comparison of repair of O^6-methylguanine produced by MNNG in mouse and human cells. *Carcinogenesis*, **5**, 593

47. Lawley, P. D. and Orr, D. J. (1970). Specific excision of methylation products from DNA of *Escherichia coli* treated with MNNG. *Chem.-Biol. Interact.*, **2**, 154

48. Jeggo, P. (1979). Isolation and characterization of *E. coli* K-12 mutants unable to induce the adaptive response to simple alkylating agents. *J. Bacteriol.*, **139**, 783

49. Olsson, M. and Lindahl, T. (1980). Repair of alkylated DNA in *E. coli*: methyl group transfer from O^6-methylguanine to a protein cysteine residue. *J. Biol. Chem.*, **255**, 10569

50. Craddock, V. M. and Henderson, A. R. (1984). Repair and replication of DNA in rat and mouse tissues in relation to cancer induction by *N*-nitroso-*N*-alkylureas. *Chem.-Biol. Interact.*, **52**, 223

51. Harris, G., Lawley, P. D. and Olsen, I. (1981). Mode of action of methylating carcinogens: comparative studies of murine and human cells. *Carcinogenesis*, **2**, 403

52. Medcalf, A. S. C. and Lawley, P. D. (1981). Time course of O^6-methylguanine removal from DNA of MNU-treated human fibroblasts. *Nature*, **289**, 796

53. Lawley, P. D., Harris, G., Phillips, E., Irving, W., Colaço, C. B., Lydyard, P. M. and Roitt, I. M. (1986). Repair of chemical carcinogen-induced damage in DNA of human lymphocytes and lymphoid cell lines – studies of the kinetics of removal of O^6-methylguanine and 3-methyladenine. *Chem.-Biol. Interact*, **57**, 107

54. Medcalf, A. S. C. and Wade, M. H. (1983). Comparison of mutagenicity of *N*-methyl-*N*-nitrosourea and *N*-ethyl-*N*-nitrosourea in human diploid fibroblasts. *Carcinogenesis*, **4**, 115

55. Balmain, A., Ramsden, M., Bowden, G. T. and Smith, J. (1984). Activation of mouse cellular Harvey-*ras* gene in chemically induced benign skin papillomas. *Nature*, **307**, 658

56. Bernstein, S. C. and Weinberg, R. A. (1985). Expression of the metastatic phenotype in cells transfected with human metastatic tumour DNA. *Proc. Natl. Acad. Sci. USA*, **82**, 1726

57. Vousden, K. H. and Marshall, C. J. (1984). Three different activated *ras* genes in mouse tumours; evidence for oncogene activation during progression of a mouse lymphoma. *EMBO J.*, **3**, 913

58. Spandidos, D. A. and Kerr, I. B. (1984). Elevated expression of the human *ras* oncogene family in premalignant and malignant tumours of the colerectum. *Br. J. Cancer*, **49**, 681

59. Thor, A., Hand, P. H., Wunderlich, D., Curoso, A., Muraro, R. and Schlom, J. (1984). Monoclonal antibodies define differential *ras* gene expression in malignant and benign colonic disease. *Nature*, **311**, 562

60. Nordling, C. O. (1953). A new theory on the cancer-inducing mechanism. *Br. J. Cancer*, **7**, 68

61. Burch, P. R. J. (1976). *Biology of Cancer, A New Approach*. (Lancaster: MTP)

62. Platt, R. (1955). Clonal ageing and cancer. *Lancet*, **i**, 867

63. Armitage, P. and Doll, R. (1957). A two-stage theory of carcinogenesis in relation to the age-distribution of human cancer. *Br. J. Cancer*, **11**, 161

64. Moolgavkar, S. H. and Knudson, A. G., Jr. (1981). Mutation and cancer: a model for human carcinogenesis. *J. Natl. Cancer Inst.*, **66**, 1037

65. Vogel, F. and Motulsky, A. G. (1982). *Human Genetics, Problems and Approaches*. Chapter 5. (Berlin: Springer Verlag)

66. Baker, R. M., Brunette, D. M., Mankovitz, R., Thompson, L. H., Whitmore, G. F., Siminovitch, L. and Till, J. E. (1974). Ouabain-resistant mutants of mouse and hamster cells in culture. *Cell*, **1**, 9

67. Evans, H. J. (1984). Genetic damage and cancer. In Bishop, M. J., Rowley, J. D. and Greaves, M. (eds.) *Genes and Cancer*, pp. 3-18. (New York: Alan R. Liss)

68. Nowell, P. C. (1976). Clonal evolution of tumour cell subpopulations. *Science*, **194**, 23

69. Yamashina, K. and Heppner, G. H. (1985). Correlation of frequency of induced mutation and metastatic potential in tumor cell lines from a single mouse mammary tumor. *Cancer Res.*, **45**, 4015

70. Albert, R. E. and Burns, F. J. (1977). Carcinogenic atmospheric pollutants and the nature of low level risks. In Hiatt, H. H., Watson, J. D. and Winsten, J. A. (eds.) *Origins of Human Cancer*. pp. 289-292. (New York: Cold Spring Harbor Laboratory)

71. Waynforth, H. B. and Magee, P. N. (1975). Effect of various doses and schedules of administration of MNU, with and without croton oil promotion, on skin papilloma production in Balb/c mice. *Gann Monogr. Cancer Res.*, **17**, 439

72. Peto, R., Gray, R., Brantom, P. and Grasso, P. (1984). Nitrosamine carcinogenesis in 5120 rodents: chronic administration of sixteen different concentrations of NDEA, NDMA and NPYR and NPIP in the water of 4440 inbred rats, with parallel studies on NDEA alone of the effect of age of starting (3, 6 or 20 weeks) and of species (rats, mice or hamsters). In O'Neill, I. K., Von Borstel, R. C., Miller, C. T., Long, J. and Bartsch, H. (eds.) *N-nitroso compounds: occurrence, biological effects and relevance to human cancer. IARC Scientific Publication No. 57*, (Lyon: International Agency for Research on Cancer)

73. Richardson, F. C., Dyroff, M. C., Boucheron, J. A. and Swenberg, J. A. (1985). Differential repair of O^4-alkyl-thymidine following exposure to methylating and ethylating hepatocarcinogens. *Carcinogenesis*, **6**, 625

74. Herron, D. C. and Shank, R. C. (1980). Methylated purines in human liver DNA after probable dimethylnitrosamine poisoning. *Cancer Res.*, **40**, 3116

75. Umbenhauer, D., Wild, C. P., Montesano, R., Saffhill, R., Boyle, J. M., Huh, N., Kirstein, U., Thomale, J., Rajewsky, M. F. and Lu, S. H. (1985). O^6-Methyldeoxyguanosine in oesophageal DNA among individuals at high risk of oesophageal cancer. *Int. J. Cancer*, **36**, 661

76. Frei, J. V., Swenson, D. H., Warren, W. and Lawley, P. D. (1978). Alkylation of DNA *in vivo* in various organs of C57BL mice by EMS, ENU and MNU: some applications of high pressure liquid chromatography. *Biochem. J.*, **174**, 1031

77. Frei, J. V. (1980). MNU-induction of thymomas in AKR mice requires one or two "hits" only. *Carcinogenesis*, **1**, 721

78. Argyris, T. (1980). Tumor promotion by abrasion-induced epidermal hyperplasia in skin of mice. *J. Invest. Dermatol.*, **75**, 360

79. Gwynn, R. H. and Salaman, M. H. (1953). Studies on co-carcinogens. SH-reactors tested for co-carcinogenic action on mouse skin. *Br. J. Cancer*, **7**, 482

80. Hunter, T. (1984). The epidermal growth factor receptor gene and its product. *Nature*, **311**, 414

81. Hill, M. J., Drasar, B. S., Aries, V., Crowder, J. S., Hawksworth, G. and Williams, R. E. O. (1971). Bacteria and aetiology of cancer of large bowel. *Lancet*, i, 95

82. Committee on Diet, Nutrition and Cancer. Assembly of Life Sciences, National Research Council (1982). *Diet, Nutrition and Cancer*. Chapter 5. (Washington: National Academy Press)

83. Cox, P. J. (1979). Cyclophosphamide cystitis – identification of acrolein as the causative agent. *Biochem. Pharmacol.*, **28**, 2045

84. Armstrong, B. K. (1977). Role of diet in human carcinogenesis with special reference to endometrial cancer. In Hiatt, H. H., Watson, J. D. and Winsten, J. A. (eds.) *Origin of Human Cancer*, pp. 557-565. (New York: Cold Spring Harbor Laboratory)

85. Committee on Diet, Nutrition and Cancer. Assembly of Life Sciences, National Research Council (1982). *Diet, Nutrition and Cancer*. Chapter 9. (Washington: National Academy Press)

86. Bollag, W. (1971). Therapy of chemically induced skin tumors of mice with vitamin A palmitate and vitamin A acid. *Experientia*, **27**, 90

87. Hill, D. L. and Grubbs, C. J. (1982). Retinoids as chemopreventive and anticancer agents in intact animals. *Anticancer Res.*, **2**, 111

88. Lower, G. U., Jr. and Kanarek, M. S. (1981). Retinoids, urinary bladder carcinogenesis, and chemoprevention: a review and synthesis. *Mutat. Cancer*, **3**, 109

89. Yotti, L. P., Chang, C. C. and Trosko, J. E. (1979). Elimination of metabolic co-operation in Chinese hamster cells by a tumour promoter. *Science*, **206**, 1089

90. Newbold, R. F. (1982). Metabolic cooperation in tumour promotion and carcinogenesis. In Pitts, J. D. and Finbow, M. E. (eds.) *Functional Integration of Cells in Animal Tissues: British Society for Cell Biology Symposium.* No. 5, pp. 301-307. (Cambridge: Cambridge University Press)

91. Chang, C. -C., Trosko, J. E. and Warren, S. T. (1978). *In vitro* assay for tumor promoters and anti-promoters. *J. Environ. Pathol. Toxicol.*, **2**, 43

92. Berwald, Y. and Sachs, L. (1963). *In vitro cell* transformation with chemical carcinogens. *Nature*, **200**, 1182

93. Mishra, N., Dunkel, V. and Mehlman, M. (eds.) (1980). *Mammalian Cell Transformation by Chemical Carcinogens.* (Princeton Junction, NJ: Senate Press)

94. Newbold, R. F. and Overell, R. W. (1983). Fibroblast immortality is a prerequisite for transformation by EJ c-Ha-*ras* oncogene. *Nature*, **304**, 648

95. Tsutsui, T., Maizumi, H., McLachlan, J. A. and Barrett, J. C. (1983). Aneuploidy induction and cell transformation by diethylstilbestrol: a possible chromosomal mechanism in carcinogenesis. *Cancer Res.*, **43**, 3814

96. Herbst, A. L. and Bern, H. A. (1981). Developmental effect of diethylstilbestrol in progeny. (New York: Thieme-Stratton, Inc.)

97. Foulds, L. (1975). *Neoplastic Development.* Vol. 2, Chapter 7. (London: Academic Press)

98. Sager, R. (1984). Resistance of human cells to oncogenic transformation. In Vande Woude, G. F., Levine, A. J., Topp, W. C. and Watson, J. P. (eds.) *Cancer Cells. 2. Oncogenes and Viral Genes.* pp. 487-500. (New York: Cold Spring Harbor Laboratory)

99. Burnet (Sir) M. F. (1970). *Immunological Surveillance.* (Oxford: Pergamon Press)

100. Thomas, L. (1959). Discussion. In Lawrence, H.S. (ed.) *Cellular and Humoral Aspects of Hypersensitive States.* p. 159. (London: Cassell)

101. Stutman, O. (1975). Immunodepression and malignancy. *Adv. Cancer Res.*, **22**, 261

102. Hoover, R. (1977). Effects of drugs - immunosuppression. In Hiatt, H. H., Watson, J. D. and Winsten, J. A. (eds.) *Origins of Human Cancer. Book A. Incidence of Cancer in Humans.* pp. 369-379. (New York: Cold Spring Harbor Laboratory)

103. Penn, I. (1978). Tumours arising in organ transplant recipients. *Adv. Cancer Res.*, **28**, 32

104. Klein, G. and Klein, E. (1985). Evolution of tumours and the impact of molecular oncology. *Nature*, **315**, 190

105. Wallich, R., Bulbuc, N., Hammerling, G. J., Katzav, S., Segal, S. and Feldman, M. (1985). Abrogation of metastatic properties of tumour cells by *de novo* expression of H-2K antigens following H-2 gene transfection. *Nature*, **315**, 301

106. Hart, J. R. (1985). Molecular basis of tumour spread. *Nature*, **315**, 274

107. Hunter, T. (1984). Proteins of oncogenes. *Sci. Am.*, **251**, 60

108. Doll, R. and Peto, R. (1981). Causes of cancer: Quantitative estimates of avoidable risks of cancer in the United States today. *J. Natl. Cancer Inst.*, **66**, 1192

109. German, J. (1979). Cancers in chromosome breakage syndromes. In Okada, S., Imamura, M., Terashima, T. and Yamaguchi, H. (eds.) *Radiation Research. Proceedings 6th International Congress Radiation Research.* pp. 496-505. (Tokyo: University of Tokyo Press)

110. Kraemer, K. H., Lee, M. M. and Scotto, J. (1982). Early onset of skin and oral cavity neoplasms in xeroderma pigmentosum. *Lancet*, **i**, 56

111. Spriggs, A. I. (1984). Precancerous states of the cervix uteri. In Carter, R. L. (ed.) *Precancerous States.* pp. 317-355. (London: Oxford University Press)

112. Fischinger, P. J. and DeVita, V. T., Jr. (1984). Governance of Science at the National Cancer Institute: Perceptions and opportunities in oncogene research. *Cancer Res.*, **44**, 4693

113. Krontiris, T. G., DiMartino, N. A., Colb, M. and Parkinson, D. R. (1985). Unique allelic restriction fragments of the human Ha-*ras* locus in leukocyte and tumour DNAs of cancer patients. *Nature*, **313**, 369

114. Rowley, J. D. (1983). Chromosome changes in leukaemic cells as indicators of mutagenic exposure. In Rowley, J. D. and Ultmann, J. E. (eds.) *Chromosomes and Cancer from Molecules to Man.* Chapter 8. (New York: Academic Press)

2
Genetic mechanisms in carcinogenesis

D. SHEER AND E. SOLOMON

INTRODUCTION

Research over the last few years has strengthened enormously the evidence that cancer is a genetic disease. That is, heritable changes in the genetic material of a cell are part of a multistep pathway leading to malignancy. That genetics plays some role in cancer development has been known for a long time from observations of certain families in which malignancies are clearly inherited[1,2]. In addition, the observation that both inherited and non-inherited cases could be found for most malignancies suggested that the predisposing mutation in the familial cases was replaced by a somatic mutation in the sporadic cases[3]. Since then, developments in cytogenetics, cell and molecular biology, and gene mapping, have successfully come together to isolate and define some of these specific genetic changes.

Evidence that genetic events are indeed involved in malignant transformation was critically strengthened by improved cytogenetic techniques and, in particular, by advances in chromosome banding. First, the discovery that in some families a consistent constitutional chromosomal abnormality segregated with malignant disease, gave supporting evidence that mutational events were involved in these tumours[4,5]. Second, the finding of consistent chromosomal rearrangements in the malignant cells of some haematological malignancies provided evidence for somatic chromosomal changes also being important in the aetiology of these cancers[6]. Without some further clue to the gene(s) or DNA sequences affected by these changes, however, little could be done towards their isolation. Major progress over the past decade in human gene mapping and molecular genetic techniques, has provided a means by which these chromosomal changes can be examined in detail. The first and best example of this approach was the combined knowledge of the chromosomal location of the Ig heavy and light chain genes, the cellular oncogene *myc*, and the standard and variant translocations in Burkitt's lymphoma, which resulted in detailed molecular knowledge of the genetic changes occurring in this malignancy[7,8].

It has long been known that certain RNA tumour viruses, such as Rous sarcoma virus, are able to 'transform' cells in culture to a neoplastic phenotype with high efficiency and in a short time. These RNA tumour viruses are also known as 'retroviruses' because their RNA genome is copied 'back' into DNA when they enter a cell, and the DNA copy is integrated into the cellular DNA. The retroviral genes responsible for cellular transformation have been identified and called 'oncogenes' (each named after the virus from which it was identified – for example, *src* from the Rous sarcoma virus: see Chapter 1 for a more detailed explanation).

With the development of cytological and mapping techniques and the isolation of cloned DNA sequences, normal cellular sequences homologous to the acute retroviral transforming genes were discovered and defined[9]. They were called 'cellular oncogenes' or 'proto-oncogenes'. Then came the discovery that DNA with transforming activity, isolated from tumours, contained mutated variants of some of these sequences – which were called 'activated' oncogenes[10]. This provided further molecular evidence for mutational changes in tumour cells.

The mapping of cloned DNA sequences to particular chromosomal locations and the discovery of Restriction Fragment Length Polymorphisms (RFLPs) inherited in a Mendelian fashion[11] has greatly increased the possibilities for genetic analysis of familial cases and for following the fate of individual chromosome homologues at the cellular level. Comparison of DNA from normal and tumour tissue from the same individual thus becomes possible at a much finer level than can be done cytologically. These techniques have led to the unmasking of hemizygosity, or homozygosity, of particular chromosomal regions in certain tumours, as compared with normal tissue, leading to the important suggestion that recessively acting genes participate in tumorigenesis[12]. This is described in more detail below in relation to the childhood tumours, retinoblastoma and Wilms' tumour.

That cancer cells have undergone heritable genetic changes is no longer in doubt, and the material that follows will describe the evidence for some of these changes.

SURVEY OF CHROMOSOME ABERRATIONS

Chromosome aberrations have been believed to be important in tumorigenesis for some time. Most tumours can be shown to have structural or numerical chromosome aberrations. The analysis of large numbers of tumours has shown that these aberrations are non-random, with certain aberrations being consistently associated with particular types of tumours[13,14]. Several consistent chromosome aberrations have recently been subjected to rigorous molecular investigation, resulting in the important demonstration that cellular oncogenes and tissue-specific genes can be directly affected by the aberrations. A number of possible genetic consequences from structural chromosome rearrangements could be imagined. Genes could be separated from their normal control sequences and placed near foreign control sequences. A break could occur within the gene to give rise to a fusion gene product. Deletion resulting in hemizygosity could allow the expression of recessive genes. These will be described below in the section on specific genetic changes in tumours.

The most common structural rearrangement is a translocation where part of one chromosome becomes joined on to another, but deletions (losses of material), insertions (gains) and inversions (of a small segment within a chromosome) are also found. Numerical aberrations consist usually of trisomy, the presence of three copies of a chromosome, or much more rarely, monosomy, the presence of only one copy of a chromosome.

Table 2.1 Consistent chromosomal aberrations in leukaemias and lymphomas

Malignancy	Chromosomal aberration
Leukaemias	
Chronic myeloid leukaemia	t(9;22)(q34;q11)
Acute myeloid leukaemias	
myeloblastic (FAB classification: M1)	t(9;22)(q34;q11)
myeloblastic (M2)	t(8;21)(q22;q22)
promyelocytic (M3)	t(15;17)(q22;q12-21)
myelomonocytic (M4) with abnormal eosinophils	inv(16)(p13q22)
monoblastic (M5a)	t(9;11)(p22;q34)
M1, M2, M4 with increased basophils	t(6;9)(p23;q34)
M1, M2, M4, M5, erythroleukaemia (M6)	del(5)(q22q23)
	del(7)(q33q36)
	trisomy 8
Chronic lymphocytic leukaemia	t(11;14)(q13;q32)
	trisomy 12
Acute lymphocytic leukaemia	t(9;22)(q34;q11)
	t(4;11)(q21;q23)
	t(8;14)(q24;q32)
Lymphomas	
Burkitt's lymphoma	t(8;14)(q24;132)
	t(2;8)(p13;q24)
	t(8;22)(q24;q11)
Small non-cleaved cell lymphoma, large cell immunoblastic lymphoma	t(8;14)(q24;q32)
Follicular small cleaved cell lymphoma	t(14;18)(q32;q21)
Small cell lymphocytic lymphoma	trisomy 12
Small cell lymphocytic transformed to diffuse large cell	t(11;14)(q13;q32)

Leukaemias and lymphomas generally have chromosome numbers in the normal (diploid) range with only a few aberrations (Table 2.1, Figures 2.1 and 2.2). Translocations involving the same pairs of chromosomes recur within particular malignancies to varying extents. For example, the Philadelphia chromosome, which is derived from a translocation between chromosomes 9 and 22 – t(9;22) – and the 15;17 chromosome translocation, are present in the leukaemic cells of virtually every patient with chronic myeloid leukaemia (CML) and acute promyelocytic leukaemia (APL), respectively. In contrast, the t(8;21) is present in the leukaemic cells of only approximately 8% of patients with acute myeloid leukaemia (AML), FAB classification[15] M2. The

25

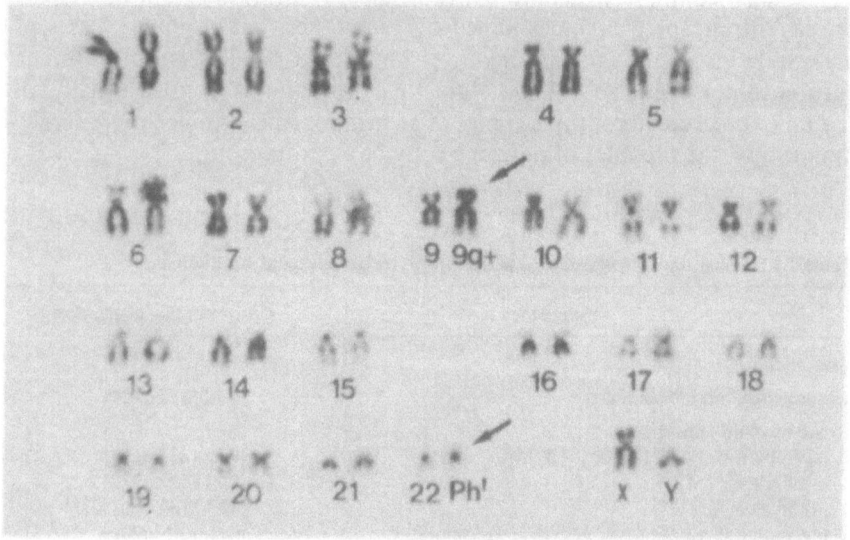

Figure 2.1 G-banded karyotype showing Philadelphia chromosome derived from a t(9;22) (q34;q11) found in most cases of chronic myeloid leukaemia. Note: in chromosome nomenclature, 'p' refers to the short arm, 'q' to the long arm. A t(9;22)(q34;q11) is thus a reciprocal translocation in which the end of the long arm of chromosome 9 is broken off at band q34 and joined onto the long arm of chromosome 22 at band q11, and vice-versa

degree of specificity also varies for the different translocations. For example, the t(15;17) has never been seen in any malignancy besides APL, while the t(8;14) is present in different malignancies of B-cells. This variability could reflect alternative genetic mechanisms for generating some types of tumours. In some cases, the only aberration detected is trisomy, with the most common trisomies being trisomy 8 in AML and trisomy 12 in B-cell chronic lymphocytic leukaemia (CLL).

Table 2.2 Consistent chromosomal aberrations in solid tumours

Malignancy	Chromosomal aberration
Neuroblastoma	del(1)(p31p36)
Small cell lung carcinoma	del(3)(p14p23)
Melanoma	del(6)(q15q23) and t(6q)
Mixed parotid gland tumour	t(3;8)(p25;q21)
Ewing's sarcoma	t(11;22)(q24;q12)
Meningioma	monosomy 22
Wilms' tumour	del(11)(p13)
Retinoblastoma	del(13)(q14)

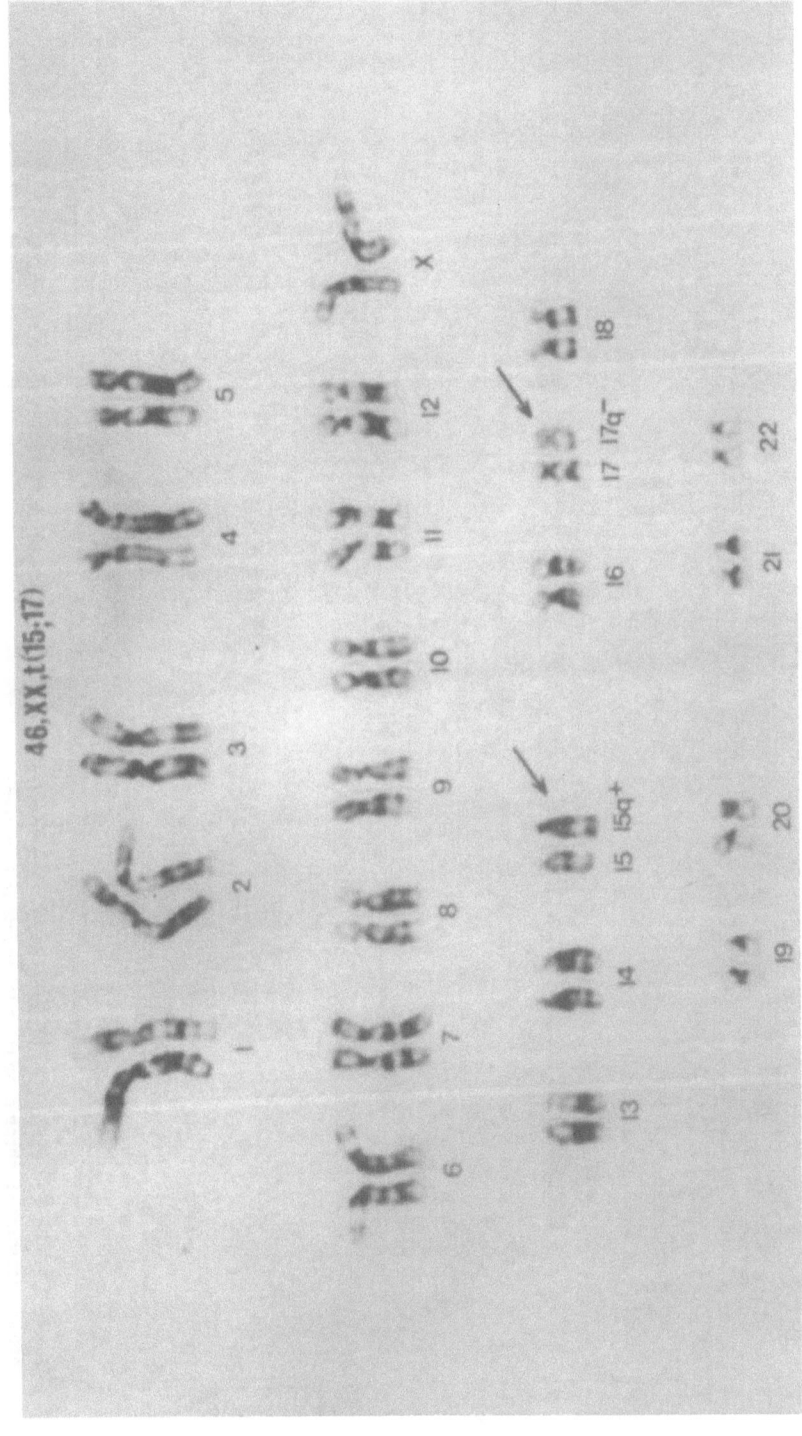

Figure 2.2 G-banded karyotype showing t(15;17)(q22;q12-21) found in most cases of acute promyelocytic leukaemia

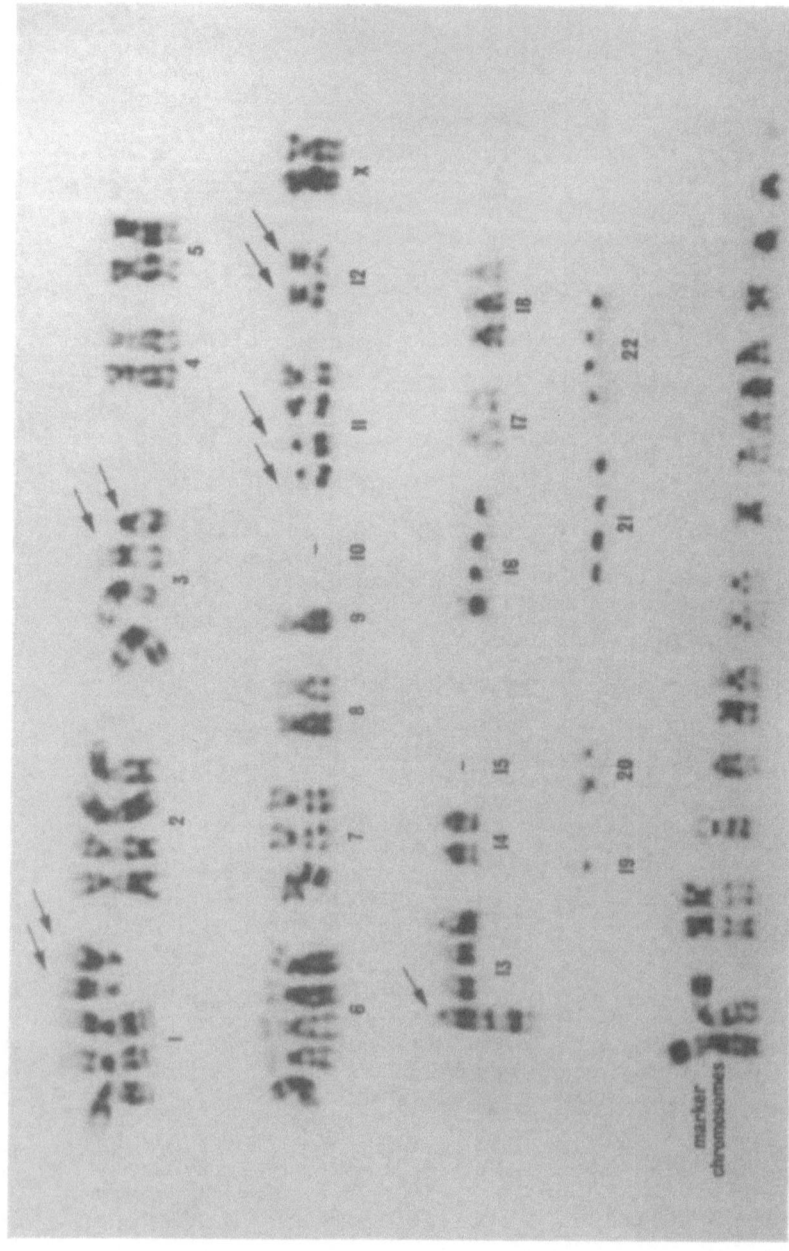

Figure 2.3 G-banded karyotype of cell line SKOV-3 derived from an ovarian serous cystadenocarcinoma. Note large number of marker (rearranged) chromosomes, in lower row and arrowed

Table 2.3 Chromosomal locations of human oncogenes

Oncogene	Chromosomal location	Reference
c-*fgr*	1p36.1–36.2	16
c-*src2*	1p36	17
Blym-1*	1p32	18
L-*myc**	1p32	19
N-*ras**	1p11–12/1p22	20
c-*ski*	1q12-qter	21
N-*myc**	2p23–24	22
c-*rel*	2p	23
c-*raf*1	3p24–25	24
c-*raf*2†	4	24
c-*fms*	5q34	25
c-Ki-*ras*1†	6p23–q12	26
c-*myb*	6q15–24	27
c-*yes2*	6	28
c-*erb*B	7p12–14	29
c-*mos*	8q11	30
c-*myc*	8q24	31
c-*abl*	9q34	32
c-Ha-*ras*1	11p15	33
c-*ets*1	11q23–24	34
int-2*	11q13	35
bcl-1*	11q13.3	36
int-1*	12pter-q14	37
c-Ki-*ras2*	12p12.1	38
c-*fos*	14q21–31	39
akt-1	14q32	39
c-*fes*	15q25–26	40
c-*erb*A1	17q11–21	41
neu*	17q11.2–22	42
c-*yes*1	18q21.3	28
bcl-2*	18q21	43
c-*src*1	20q13	17
c-*ets2*	21	44
c-*sis*	22q12.3–13.1	45
c-Ha-*ras*2†	X	46

Oncogenes marked by (*) are not found in retroviruses.
Oncogenes marked by (†) are pseudogenes.

Solid tumours are far more difficult to karyotype than leukaemias and lymphomas, because they often have few dividing cells and the morphology of the chromosomes is fuzzy and indistinct. They generally have chromosome numbers in the triploid to hypotetraploid range with many aberrations (Figure 2.3). For these reasons, the identification of consistent aberrations in solid tumours has lagged far behind that in leukaemias and lymphomas. A summary of consistent chromosome aberrations in solid tumours is presented in Table 2.2.

SURVEY OF CELLULAR ONCOGENES

Approximately 20 cellular oncogenes have been identified in the human genome by virtue of their homology with retroviral oncogenes[9]. These have been summarized in Table 2.3, together with their chromosomal locations. There is now a large amount of evidence that cellular oncogenes participate in the induction of tumours other than those associated with viruses. This may occur if the oncogene is 'activated' by mutation, or if the unaltered oncogene is abnormally expressed (summarized in Table 2.4).

Table 2.4   Activation of cellular oncogenes

Oncogene	Mechanism	References
N-*ras*	point mutation	47, 48
c–Ha-*ras*	point mutation	49, 50
	amplification	51
c–Ki-*ras*	point mutation	52
	amplification	53, 54
c-*myc*	translocation	7, 8
	amplification	55–58
	viral insertion	59, 60
L-*myc*	amplification	19
N-*myc*	amplification	61
c-*abl*	translocation	62
	amplification	63, 64
c-*erb*B	amplification	65, 66
	rearrangement	66
	viral insertion	67
c-*mos*	rearrangement	68, 69
int-1/2	viral insertion	70, 71
c-*myb*	amplification	72, 73, 112

Activated oncogenes were first recognized in tumours by their ability to transform the pre-neoplastic mouse cell line NIH-3T3 in DNA transfection experiments (see Chapter 1). These oncogenes were shown to belong to the *ras* family, N-*ras*, c-Ha-*ras*1 and c-Ki-*ras*2, and their transforming activity ascribed to point mutations[47-50,52]. Since then several different activated genes that do not appear to be homologous to retroviral oncogenes, such as *Blym*-1[74] and *neu*[75], have also been detected using the transfection assay, but the mechanisms by which they are activated are not yet known. Examples of mechanisms known to lead to abnormal expression of oncogenes, such as chromosomal translocation and gene amplification will be described below in the section on Specific Genetic Alterations in Tumours.

Protein products are known for only a few oncogenes, and much of this information has been deduced from studies of the viral rather than cellular oncogenes. Widely divergent vertebrate species, as well as *Drosophila* and yeast, have been found to have genes homologous to viral oncogenes[76,77]. This degree of evolutionary conservation suggests that cellular oncogenes encode vital functions. An outstanding feature to emerge from studies of viral oncogenes is the high proportion, including *src*, *abl*, *fes*, *yes*, *erb*B and *fms*, which encode tyrosine kinases. Of these, *erb*B encodes the receptor for epidermal growth factor (EGF)[78] while *fms* encodes the receptor for macrophage growth factor, CSF-1[79]. The precise mechanism by which receptors stimulate cell growth is not known, but binding to the appropriate growth factor may initiate a cascade of phosphorylation reactions on the receptor itself and on neighbouring proteins[80] (see also Chapter 3). Of particular interest has been the demonstration that the oncogene v-*erb*B carried by the avian erythroblastosis virus encodes a truncated EGF receptor molecule lacking the external domain which binds EGF[66,78] (see Chapter 9). It has been postulated that this molecule is constitutively activated to trigger cell proliferation, suggesting a possible mechanism whereby a rearrangement within a cellular oncogene encoding a growth factor receptor might precipitate malignant transformation. Further evidence for the direct involvement of certain oncogenes in this mitogenic pathway is provided by the finding that the oncogene c-*sis* encodes the B-chain of platelet derived growth factor[81,82]. The functions of most of the other oncogenes are not known. These include the *ras* family in which there is evidence for GTP- and GDP-binding by the p21 *ras* protein, but inconclusive evidence as to whether it activates adenylate cyclase[83-85].

The patterns of expression of several cellular oncogenes suggest that their products participate in certain differentiation and developmental pathways, i.e. the levels of expression vary in different tissues, at different times. For example, c-*abl* is expressed in mouse tissues to different extents, with particularly high expression in the testes[86]. During mouse embryogenesis, c-*abl* and c-Ki-*ras* are expressed in fluctuating but distinctive patterns, while c-Ha-*ras* is moderately expressed[86]. Expression of c-*myc* and c-Ha-*ras* is elevated during liver regeneration[87,88]. Expression of c-*myb* and c-*myc* is particularly high in haemopoietic tissues[89,90] and decreases dramatically in the promyelocytic leukaemia cell line HL60 when it is induced to differentiate[90]. In all these cases, however, it is still not known whether the oncogenes help direct development or whether they are merely expressed in response to developmental signals.

SPECIFIC GENETIC ALTERATIONS IN TUMOURS

Activation of c-*ras* oncogenes by point mutations (see also Chapter 1)

Activated oncogenes of the *ras* family can be detected in DNA from a variety of human cancers by their ability to transform the pre-neoplastic mouse cell line NIH-3T3 in DNA transfection experiments. Comparison of activated *ras* genes with their normal counterparts reveals point mutations affecting amino acid residues 12, 13 or 61 of the *ras*-coded protein, that confer transforming ability to the protein[48-50,91,92]. It is interesting that amino acid residue 12 is similarly substituted in *ras* genes of Harvey-, BALB- and Kirsten-MSV[93,94]. 10-30% of solid tumours have been found by gene transfection to have activated *ras* genes[9], and in one study, four out of five patients with acute myeloid leukaemia had mutations in the N-*ras* gene affecting amino acid residue 13[48]. The role of the mutated *ras* p21 protein in malignant transformation is not yet understood[95].

Activation of c-*abl* oncogene in CML

Chronic myeloid leukaemia (CML) is an invariably fatal disease characterized by proliferation of myeloid cells and their progenitors. CML was the first malignancy to be associated with a consistent chromosome aberration[96]. The Philadelphia (Ph') chromosome, which is present in over 90% of patients with CML, is derived from a translocation between chromosomes 9 and 22, t(9;22)(q34;q11) which generates the 9q⁺ and 22q⁻ (Ph') chromosomes (Figure 2.1). In the formation of the (Ph') chromosome, the oncogene c-*abl* becomes transferred from chromosome 9 to a region

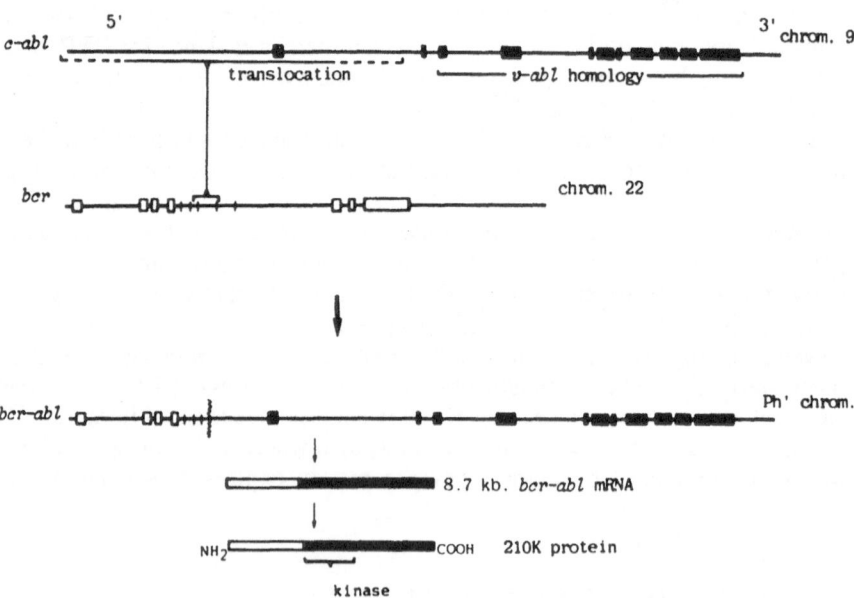

Figure 2.4 Diagrammatic representation of *bcr-abl* fusion arising from the t(9;22) in chronic myeloid leukaemia. Small exons are represented by vertical lines, larger exons by boxes. For c-*abl*, the positions and sizes of the 5' exons are not yet well fixed, nor have the translocation breakpoints been established in most cases, although it is known that they can occur over a wide distance and can be over 50 kb 5' of the c-*abl* gene. For *bcr*, the exons have not yet all been defined, but the breakpoints occur within a much smaller region (bracketed). The precursor RNA produced from the *bcr-abl* fusion gene on the Philadelphia chromosome is believed to be spliced in such a way as to excise sequences of the most 5' *abl* exon (hatched) from the 8.7 kb *bcr-abl* mRNA. (After Adams[125])

of chromosome 22 designated *bcr* (breakpoint cluster region) (Figure 2.4). The translocation breakpoints in different patients can occur on chromosome 9 over a relatively large distance of DNA (50 kb) in the 5′ region of the c-*abl* gene, but on chromosome 22 are restricted to a 5.8 kb region of DNA. CML cells contain an abnormally long mRNA synthesized from a fusion gene in which *bcr* sequences replace part of the 5′ end of the c-*abl* gene[62,97]. Although the breakpoints on chromosome 9 can occur over a large region of DNA in different patients, all CMLs examined so far have the 8 kb transcript. Shtivelman *et al.*[62] suggest that a much larger transcript is synthesized initially from the entire *bcr-abl* gene, but that subsequent splicing generates an 8 kb transcript that is identical in each patient. All CML cells examined so far contain a c-*abl* polypeptide of approximate M_r 210 000 while normal cells have a c-*abl* polypeptide of approximate M_r 145 000[98,99]. The abnormal molecule has the amino terminal of the normal c-*abl* polypeptide (at least 25 residues) replaced by 600–700 residues from the amino terminal of the *bcr* locus.

It is still not known how the *bcr-abl* gene product promotes myeloid tumorigenesis. The product of the normal *bcr* gene is not known. In common with the v-*abl* gene product, but unlike that of its normal homologue c-*abl*, the fusion polypeptide has tyrosine kinase activity[62]. The fusion polypeptide may therefore function as a receptor for a growth factor, since several such receptors have been shown to be tyrosine kinases. Substitution of the amino terminus of the molecule might result in constitutive phosphorylating activity of the molecule thus promoting cell proliferation[62].

Activation of c-*myc* oncogene in Burkitt's lymphoma

The c-*myc* oncogene is activated by consistent chromosome translocations in Burkitt's lymphoma, which is a B-cell malignancy. An (8;14)(q24;q32) chromosome translocation is present in the malignant cells of 90% of patients with Burkitt's lymphoma. One of two variant translocations, t(2;8)(p12;q24) or t(8;22)(q24;q11) is present in approximately 10% of patients with this disease. All three translocations are also present in B-cell acute lymphoblastic leukaemia. Chromosomes 14, 2 and 22 carry the immunoglobulin heavy chain gene (IgH), and the immunoglobulin kappa (Igκ) and lambda (Igλ) light chain genes, respectively, at the sites of the breakpoints on each of these chromosomes. In the typical t(8;14), the oncogene c-*myc* which is normally located at band q24 of chromosome 8, translocates into the IgH locus on chromosome 14[100]. In the variant translocations, c-*myc* remains on chromosome 8 while sequences from the Igκ and Igλ loci translocate into the vicinity of the c-*myc* gene[101,102]. Analogous translocations between c-*myc* and the IgH or Igκ are present in rat and mouse plasmacytomas, which are also derived from B-cells[103]. All three translocations in Burkitt's lymphoma, and those in rat and mouse plasmacytomas, result in enhanced transcription of the c-*myc* gene by replacing the normal control sequences upstream of the c-*myc* gene with Ig sequences[7-9].

Immunoglobulin genes in B-cell malignancies

The IgH genes are also directly involved in recurring translocations in other B-cell malignancies. Some small cell lymphocytic lymphomas and diffuse large cell lymphomas have a t(11;14)(q13;q32), while follicular lymphomas have a t(14;18)(q32;q21). Sequences designated bcl-1 and bcl-2 (B-cell lymphoma/leukaemia) have been shown to become translocated from their normal locations on chromosomes 11 and 18, respectively, into the immediate vicinity of the IgH locus on chromosome 14[36,43,104,105]. There is some evidence that in some cases the translocation between chromosomes 14 and 18 occurs as a result of a mistake during the immunoglobulin VDJ-joining at the pre B-stage of differentiation, so that there is an interchromosomal rather than an intrachromosomal joining[106]. Neither bcl-1 nor bcl-2 is homologous to any known retroviral oncogene, but it is possible that these genes are activated as a result of their juxtaposition with IgH genes.

T-cell receptor genes in T-cell malignancies

The direct involvement of Ig genes in B-cell malignancies illustrates what may be a more common phenomenon, i.e. subversion of tissue-specific genes in tumorigenesis. A second example of this has recently been demonstrated in T-cell malignancies, many of which have chromosome rearrangements involving the 14q11-13 region, where the gene coding the α-chain of the T-cell receptor has been mapped[107]. Translocation breakpoints in leukaemic cells of two patients with T-cell acute lymphoblastic leukaemia showing a t(11;14)(p13;q13) were found to occur between the variable and constant (C) region genes of the α-chain of the T-cell receptor, resulting in the C-region genes being transferred to chromosome 11[108]. It has been postulated that juxtaposition of genes from the α-chain of the T-cell receptor with sequences, as yet unidentified, from chromosome 11 leads to activation of these sequences as occurs for c-myc in B-cell malignancies.

Activation of oncogenes by amplification

Inappropriate gene expression, i.e. the expression of otherwise normal genes in the wrong cells or at the wrong time, is believed to be an important contributing factor in malignant transformation. The example of enhanced expression of c-myc in Burkitt's lymphomas as a result of chromosome translocation has been described above. Enhanced gene expression in tumours can also be achieved by increasing the copy number of a gene, known as gene amplification. Gene amplification has been recognized for some time as one way in which cells gain resistance against selective drugs[109]. Cytogenetic studies of drug-resistant cell lines demonstrated that amplified genes were found in homogeneously staining regions (HSRs) of chromosomes, or in double minutes (DMs). The term HSR comes from the unusually uniform staining of these chromosome regions, while DMs are small paired chromosome structures which lack centromeres and therefore do not segregate symmetrically at mitosis. Cells generally contain either HSRs or DMs but not both, and there is some evidence that they are alternative manifestations of gene amplification. There are many examples of amplified cellular oncogenes in tumours, often in association with the presence of HSRs or DMs. Some of these have been listed in Table 2.5. A particularly important finding has emerged from studies of amplified *myc* genes in certain tumours. Amplification of N-*myc* in neuroblastomas[111], and either c-*myc* or N-*myc* in human lung carcinomas[113] is associated with more aggressive forms of these malignancies. This suggests that enhanced expression of these genes helps drive the tumours towards a more malignant phenotype.

Table 2.5 Amplification of cellular oncogenes

Oncogene	Malignancy	References
c-Ha-*ras*	lung carcinoma	51
c-Ki-*ras*	SW480 (colon carcinoma cell line)	53
	YI (mouse adrenocortical tumour cell line)	54
c-*myc*	HL60 (promyelocytic cell line)	55-57
	COLO320 (malignant neuro-endocrine cell line)	58
	lung carcinoma cell lines	110
L-*myc*	small cell lung carcinomas	19
N-*myc*	neuroblastomas	61,111
	lung carcinomas	113
c *abl*	K562 (CML cell line)	63, 64
c-*erb*B	glial tumours	65
	A431 (epidermoid carcinoma cell line)	66
c *myb*	ML-1, -2, -3 (AML cell lines)	72
	COLO 201, 205 (colon carcinoma cell lines)	73, 112

Recessive genes in Wilms' tumour and retinoblastoma

While findings on the role of certain activated cellular oncogenes in malignancy suggest that these genes behave in a dominant fashion, studies of a rather different nature reveal that other genes may act recessively in tumorigenesis. These very important studies do not deal with isolated genes *per se*, but rather with chromosomal regions implicated through cytogenetic studies in the genesis of particular tumours. This work also provides very interesting data on the genetic mechanisms through which such recessive genes may be revealed or expressed.

The technical basis of all these studies is the use of cloned DNA fragments that detect restriction fragment length polymorphisms (RFLPs). Restriction enzymes cut DNA at particular nucleotide sequences, generating so-called restriction fragments. These can be visualized on agarose gels with radiolabelled cloned probes which hybridize to the region of DNA containing the particular cutting site. The length of these fragments is obviously determined by the distance between cutting sites. Should such a cutting site be mutated or deleted such that the enzyme does not cut, a longer fragment will be generated. Similarly, mutations or insertions which generate new sites will result in new, shorter fragments. It appears that normal variation within the genome results in stably inherited differences in these sites, or RFLPs. These segregate in a Mendelian fashion and individuals may be homozygous for the presence or absence of a site (++, --), or heterozygous (+ -). As with any polymorphic marker, inheritance of the alleles may be followed through families and used in linkage studies. Many probes detecting RFLPs have now been assigned to individual chromosomes. These probes provide an enormous source of polymorphic markers and allow detailed examination of the fate of chromosome homologues which are heterozygous for these markers.

Retinoblastoma (rb) is a childhood tumour which exists in both dominantly inherited and sporadic forms. The familial cases generally exhibit bilateral disease and the sporadic cases, unilateral. This pattern of expression initially led Knudson to propose a 'two hit' model for the disease, i.e. inherited cases carry a constitutional, or germ-line, mutation in all cells of the body, and a second mutation, presumably in the retinal cells, is necessary to cause the disease[3]. In sporadic cases, both mutations must occur as somatic events. Several lines of evidence suggested that the gene or genes involved in this mutation reside on chromosome 13, in or near band q14. First, among the hereditary cases, a small percentage carry a constitutional deletion in chromosome 13, which includes band 13q14[5,114]. Second, in non-deletion families with retinoblastoma, tight linkage to the enzyme esterase D has been demonstrated, and this enzyme mapped to 13q14[115]. Third, a patient with no family history of the disease had esterase D levels 50% of normal in the peripheral blood, suggesting a submicroscopic deletion in this region of chromosome 13[116]. This patient's tumour had no detectable esterase D activity, i.e. there was total loss of genetic information at 13q14 in the tumour, which led the author to propose a recessive rb gene, both copies of which must be mutated or lost for tumour development to occur. Fourth, several individuals heterozygous for esterase D expressed only one esterase D allele in their tumours[117]. Finally, careful karyotypic analyses of rb tumours, both hereditary and non-hereditary, revealed non-random loss of chromosome 13, and deletions including 13q14[118].

From the use of DNA probes, there is now conclusive evidence that the gene involved in the aetiology of rb resides in this region of chromosome 13, and that gross chromosomal changes can lead to the expression of recessive mutations in this gene. Using probes which cover loci along the length of chromosome 13 and which detect RFLPs, the genotypes of rb tumours have been compared with the genotypes of normal tissue from the same individuals[12]. In approximately 50% of cases, the tumour exhibits loss of the heterozygosity seen in the normal tissue. That is, the tumour has become hemizygous or homozygous for markers on chromosome 13. Examination of either the karyotype of the tumour or densitometric measurements of DNA blots reveal that this can come about by several mechanisms, including non-disjunction leading to monosomy for chromosome 13, non-disjunction followed by reduplication leading to two identical chromosomes 13, or mitotic non-disjunction so that the markers in the region of 13q14 are homozygous, but crossover has occurred so that the markers on the rest of chromosome 13 are heterozygous. As Knudson suggested, the model proposed as a result of this evidence is that one chromosome 13 carries a mutation at the rb locus, either constitutionally or acquired through somatic mutation. A second mutational event then occurs so that the corresponding normal allele is lost, thereby allowing expression of a recessively acting gene. The two conclusions of major importance from these studies are first, of course, that genes which are involved in the development of cancer may act recessively, and second, that the mutational events leading to their expression involve not only submicroscopic events such as point mutations, frame shifts, etc., but in at least 50% of cases gross chromosomal changes.

More recently, similar studies have been performed on osteosarcomas[119]. This bone cancer occurs with higher than expected frequency as a second tumour in patients with rb, whether or not they have received radiotherapy, which raised the suspicion that the same genetic locus might be involved in its aetiology. DNA from normal and osteosarcoma tissue from non-rb patients was examined with chromosome 13 probes. In approximately half the cases in which the DNA from normal tissue showed heterozygosity at the chromosome 13 marker locus, loss of one allele was found in the tumour. This fascinating finding suggests that the gene or genes at 13q14 are more general than for just rb tumours, giving impetus to the general effort to clone and define these genes.

Another childhood tumour, Wilms' tumour, has been examined with the same rationale[120-123]. This malignancy, again with both sporadic and dominantly inherited cases, is known occasionally to occur in patients with constitutional deletions in the short arm of chromosome 11 at band 11p13. Using probes on the short arm of chromosome 11 which detect RFLPs to compare DNA from normal and tumour tissue from the same patient, once again, hemi- or homozygosity was revealed in the tumour, suggesting a recessively acting gene at this locus as well. Even more interesting is the finding that when these studies of 11p were extended to other embryonic tumours such as those seen in the Beckwith-Wiedemann syndrome, i.e. rhabdomyosarcoma and hepatoblastoma, the same result was seen, i.e. hemi- or homozygosity at 11p in the tumour but not at control loci on other chromosomes or in other tumours[124]. As with the 'rb' locus, considerable effort is now being directed at the cloning of this region of 11p.

CONCLUSIONS

The types of genetic alterations which appear to lead to tumour formation include a wide range - from point mutations, to amplification of segments of DNA, to whole chromosome loss. These are all rather universal genetic mechanisms leading to mutations, or alteration of function, and that they are involved in carcinogenesis is not surprising. Of greater importance, now, is the identification of the particular gene(s) affected by these mutations and an understanding of how their malfunction contributes to tumorigenesis. While in a few cases enormous progress has been made at the molecular level in defining the genetic alterations, there still remains a large gap between this molecular definition and functional understanding, even where the specific genes involved are known. For example, in chronic myeloid leukaemia and Burkitt's lymphomas it is known that c-*abl* and c-*myc* respectively are altered but the exact effect of the alterations is not known. Similarly the point mutations and amplifications so clearly defined in the *ras* gene family still do not reveal the nature of the abnormal functioning of these genes. What is awaited is a more precise biological understanding of how some of the mutations detected in tumours lead to carcinogenesis.

In the current development of this field it is of interest that analysis of solid tumours, on the one hand, and leukaemias and lymphomas, on the other, have contributed such very different kinds of approaches and information. Because consistent cytogenetic alterations in most solid tumours are far less obvious than in haematological malignancies, and because more 'functional' or 'biological' assays have been available, almost all of the work on solid tumours has involved the detection of transforming activity in the DNA of these tumours. The limitation here has been that the transforming activity as detected in recipient NIH 3T3 cells has been restricted mainly to the c-*ras* family. A much wider range of recipient cells and assays is needed. The exceptions in terms of solid tumours are the cases of retinoblastoma and Wilms' tumour where consistent chromosome deletions led to the observation of recessively acting genes. This very important discovery, however, stands at the other end of the spectrum of understanding insofar as no information whatsoever is yet afforded as to the nature of the genes involved.

The haematological malignancies have contributed other types of information. In most of these cases transformation of NIH 3T3 cells has been unsuccessful, so that altered biological activity has not been defined. By virtue of gene mapping it has been possible to 'guess' at the genes involved in some of the breakpoints and thereby to clone these regions. One of the long outstanding questions regarding these translocations has been answered: although they may involve the same pairs of genes in cytologically identical translocations, they are not always at the same nucleotides. Still outstanding in molecular terms in the aetiology of these diseases are those cases with identical clinical features where no rearrangements are seen. Do other mechanisms operate to generate the same genetic end-product, or mutation, or are other genes in a common pathway involved? Why in some disorders such as acute promyelocytic leukaemia is the same chromosome translocation seen in every case, so that there is apparently no other mechanism of generating this disease? There remain large numbers of leukaemias and lymphomas with consistent chromosome translocations, but where no clue is available as to which genes are involved. Here, techniques are needed for isolating and cloning these regions. Assays of transforming activity also need to be developed for these malignancies.

We have discussed how heritable changes leading to tumour formation both in germ-line and somatic cells are becoming clearly defined in classical genetic terms. In some cases the genes involved are known. Further developments must surely focus on the normal and abnormal functioning of these genes.

References

1. Dukes, C. (1930). The hereditary factor in polyposis intestini, or multiple adenomata. *Cancer Rev.*, **4**, 242-251
2. Harnden, D., Morten, J. and Featherstone, T. (1984). Dominant susceptibility to cancer in man. *Adv. Cancer Res.*, **41**, 185-255
3. Knudson, A. G. (1971). Mutation and cancer: a statistical study of retinoblastoma. *Proc. Natl. Acad. Sci. USA*, **68**, 820-823
4. Yunis, J. J. and Ramsey, N. (1978). Retinoblastoma and subband deletion of chromosome 13. *Am. J. Dis. Child.*, **132**, 161-163
5. Cohen, A. J., Li, F.P., Berg, S., Marchetto, D. J., Tsai, S., Jacobs, S. C. and Brown, R. (1979). Hereditary renal-cell carcinoma associated with a chromosomal translocation. *N. Engl. J. Med.*, **301**, 592-595
6. Rowley, J. D. and Testa, J. R. (1982). Chromosome abnormalities in malignant haematologic diseases. *Adv. Cancer Res.*, **36**, 103-148
7. Leder, P., Battey, J., Lenoir, G., Moulding, C., Murphy, W., Potter, H., Stewart, T. and Taub, R. (1983). Translocations among antibody genes in human cancer. *Science*, **222**, 765-771
8. Robertson, M. (1983). Paradox and paradigm: the message and meaning of *myc*. *Nature*, **306**, 733-736
9. Marshall, C. (1985). Human oncogenes. In Weiss, R., Teich, N., Varmus, H. and Coffin, J. (eds.) *RNA Tumour Viruses*. 2nd Edn., pp. 487-558. (New York: Cold Spring Harbor Laboratory)
10. Pulciani, S., Santos, E., Lauver, A. V., Long, L. K., Aaronson, S. A. and Barbacid, M. (1982). Oncogenes in solid human tumours. *Nature*, **300**, 539-542
11. Botstein, D., White, R. L., Skolnick, M. and Davis, R. (1980). Construction of a genetic linkage map in man using restriction fragment length polymorphisms. *Am. J. Hum. Genet.*, **32**, 314-331
12. Cavanee, W. K., Dryja, T. P., Phillips, R. A., Benedict, W. F., Godbout, R., Gallie, B. L., Murphee, A. L., Strong, L. C. and White, R. L. (1983). Expression of recessive alleles by chromosomal mechanisms in retinoblastoma. *Nature*, **305**, 779-784
13. Yunis, J. J. (1983). The chromosomal basis of human neoplasia. *Science*, **221**, 227-236
14. Rowley, J. D. (ed.) (1984). Consistent chromosomal aberrations and oncogenes in human tumours. *Cancer Survey*. Vol 3
15. Bennett, J. M., Catovsky, D., Daniel, M. T., Flandrin, G., Galton, D. A. G., Gralnick, H. R. and Sultan, C. (1976). Proposals for the classification of the acute leukaemias. *Br. J. Haematol.*, **33**, 451-458
16. Tronick, S. R., Popescu, N. C., Cheah, M. S. C., Swan, D. C., Amsbaugh, S. C., Lengel, C. R., DiPaolo, J. A. and Robbins, K. A. (1985). Isolation and chromosomal localisation of the human *fgr* protooncogene, a distinct member of the tyrosine kinase gene family. *Proc. Natl. Acad. Sci. USA*, **82**, 6595-6599
17. Le Beau, M. M., Westbrook, C. A., Diaz, M. O. and Rowley, J. D. (1984). Evidence for two distinct c-*src* loci on human chromosomes 1 and 20. *Nature*, **312**, 70-71
18. Morton, C. C., Taub, R., Diamond, A., Lane, M. A., Cooper, G. M. and Leder, P. (1984). Mapping of the human *Blym*-1 transforming gene activated in Burkitt lymphomas to chromosome 1. *Science*, **223**, 173-175
19. Nau, M. M., Brooks, B. J., Battey, J., Sausville, E., Gazdar, A. F., Kirsch, I. R., McBride, O. W., Bertness, V., Hollis, G. F. and Minna, J. D. (1985). L-*myc*, a new *myc*-related gene amplified and expressed in human small cell lung cancer. *Nature*, **318**, 69-72

20. Povey, S., Morton, N. E., and Sherman, S. L. (1985). Report of the committee on the genetic constitution of chromosomes 1 and 2. Human Gene Mapping 8. *Cytogenet. Cell Genet.*, **40**, 67-106

21. Balazs, I., Greschik, K. H. and Stavnezer, E. (1984). Assignment of the human homologue of a chicken oncogene to chromosome 1. Human Gene Mapping 7. *Cytogenet. Cell Genet.*, **37**, 410-411

22. Schwab, M., Varmus, H. E., Bishop, J. M., Grzeschik, K. H., Naylor, S. L., Sakaguchi, A. Y., Brodeur, G. and Trent, J. (1984). Chromosome localization in normal human cells and neuroblastomas of a gene related to c-*myc*. *Nature*, **308**, 288-291

23. Brownell, E., O'Brien, S. J., Nash, W. G. and Rice, N. (1985). Genetic characterisation of human c-*rel* sequences. *Mol. Cell. Biol.*, **5**, 2826-2831

24. Bonner, T., O'Brien, S. J., Nash, W. G., Rapp, U. R., Morton, C. C. and Leder, P. (1984). The human homologues of the *raf* (*mil*) oncogene are located on human chromosomes 3 and 4. *Science*, **233**, 71-74

25. Groffen, J., Heisterkamp, N., Spurr, N., Dana, S., Wasmuth, J. J. and Stephenson J. R. (1983). Chromosomal localisation of the human c-*fms* oncogene. *Nucl. Acids Res.*, **11**, 6331-6339

26. Sakaguchi, A. Y., Zabel, B. U., Grzechick, K-H., Law, M. L., Ellis, R. W., Scolnick, E. M. and Naylor, S. L. (1984). Regional localisation of two human cellular kirsten *ras* genes on chromosomes 6 and 12. *Mol. Cell. Biol.*, **4**, 989-993

27. Robson, E. B. and Lamm, L. U. (1984). Report of the committee of the genetic constitution of chromosome 6. Human Gene Mapping 7. *Cytogenet. Cell Genet.*, **37**, 47-70

28. Semba, K., Yamanashi, Y., Nishizawa, M., Sukegawa, J., Yoshida, M., Sasaki, M., Yamamoto, T. and Toyoshima, K. (1984). Location of the c-*yes* gene on the human chromosome and its expression in various tissues. *Science*, **227**, 1038-1040

29. Shimizu, N., Hunts, J., Merlino, G., Wang-Peng, J., Xu, Y-H., Yamamoto, T., Toyoshima, K. and Pastan, I. (1985). Regional mapping of the EGF receptor (EGFR)/c-erbB protooncogene. Human Gene Mapping 8. *Cytogenet. Cell Genet.*, **40**, 743-744

30. Caubet, J-F., Maphieu-Mahul, D., Bernheim, A., Larsen, C-J. and Berger, R. (1985). Human proto-oncogene c-*mos* maps to 8q11. *EMBO J.*, **4**, 2245-2248

31. Dalla-Favera, R., Bregni, M., Erikson, J., Patterson, D., Gallo, R. C. and Croce, C. M. (1982). Human c-*myc onc* gene is located on the region of chromosome 8 that is translocated in Burkitt lymphoma cells. *Proc. Natl. Acad. Sci. USA*, **79**, 7824-7827

32. De Klein, A., van Kessel, A. G., Grosveld, A. G., Bartram, C. R., Hagemeijer, A., Bootsma, D., Spurr, N. K., Heisterkamp, N., Groffen, J. and Stephenson, J. R. (1982). A cellular oncogene is translocated to the Philadelphia chromosome in chronic myelocytic leukaemia. *Nature*, **300**, 765-767

33. Sheer, D., Spurr, N. K. and Solomon, E. (1984). Gene mapping and human malignant diseases. *Cancer Surv.*, **3**, 543-566

34. de Taisne, C., Gegonne, A., Stehelin, D., Bernheim, A. and Berger, R. (1984). Chromosomal localisation of the human proto-oncogene c-*ets*. *Nature*, **310**, 581-583

35. Casey, G., Smith, R., McGillivray, D., Peters, G. and Dickson, C. (1986). Characterisation and chromosome assignment of the human homolog of *INT-2*, a potential proto-oncogene. *Mol. Cell. Biol.*, **6**, 502-510

36. Tsujimoto, Y., Yunis, J., Onorato-Showe, L., Erikson, J., Nowell, P. C. and Croce, C. M. (1984). Molecular cloning of the chromosomal breakpoint of B-cell lymphomas and leukaemias with the t(11;14) chromosome translocation. *Science*, **224**, 1403-1406

37. van't Veer, L. J., van Kessel, A. G., van Heerikhuizen, H., van Ooyen, A. and Nusse, R. (1984). Molecular cloning and chromosomal assignment of the human homolog of *int*-1, a mouse gene implicated in mammary tumorigenesis. *Mol. Cell. Biol.*, **4**, 2532-2534

38. Barker, P. E., Rabin, M., Watson, M., Breg, W. R., Ruddle, F. H. and Verma, I. M. (1984). Human c-*fos* oncogene mapped within chromosomal region 14q21-q31. *Proc. Natl. Acad. Sci. USA*, **81**, 5826-5830

39. Testa, J. R., Huebner, K., Croce, C. M. and Staal, S. (1985). The *AKT1* gene, the human homologue of a retroviral oncogene, is located on chromosome 14 at band q32. Human gene mapping 8. *Cytogenet. Cell Genet.*, **40**, 761

40. Harper, M. E., Franchini, G., Love, J., Simon, M. I., Gallo, R. C. and Wong-Staal, F. (1983). Chromosomal sublocalization of human c-*myb* and c-*fes* cellular *onc* genes. *Nature*, **304**, 169-171

41. Sheer, D., Sheppard, D. M., Le Beau, M., Rowley, J. D., San Roman, C. and Solomon, E. (1985). Localisation of the oncogene c-erbA1 immediately proximal to the acute promyelocytic leukaemia breakpoint on chromosome 17. *Ann. Hum. Genet.*, **49**, 167-171

42. Schechter, A. L., Hung, M. C., Vaidyanathan, L., Weinberg, R. A., Yang-Feng, T. L., Francke, U., Ullrich, A. and Coussens, L. (1985). The *neu* gene: an *erb*B-homologous gene distinct from and unlinked to the gene encoding the EGF receptor. *Science*, **229**, 976-978

43. Tsujimoto, Y., Finger, R., Yunis, J. J., Nowell, P. C. and Croce, C. M. (1985). Cloning of the chromosome breakpoint of neoplastic B cells with the t(14;18) chromosome translocation. *Science*, **226**, 1097-1099

44. Watson, D. K., McWilliams-Smith, M. J., Nunn, M. F., Duesberg, P. H., O'Brien, S. J. and Papas, T. S. (1985). The *ets* sequence from the transforming gene of avian erythroblastosis virus, E36, has unique domains on human chromosomes 11 and 21: both loci are transcriptionally active. *Proc. Natl. Acad. Sci. USA*, **82**, 7294-7298

45. Bartram, C. R., De Klein, A., Hagemeijer, A., Grosveld, G., Heisterkamp, N. and Groffen, J. (1984). Localization of the human c-*sis* oncogene in Ph'-positive and Ph'-negative chronic myelocytic leukaemia by in situ hybridisation. *Blood*, **63**, 223-225

46. O'Brien, S. J., Nash, W. G., Goodwin, J. L., Lowry, D. R. and Chang, E. H. (1983). Dispersion of the ras family of transforming genes to four different chromosomes in man. *Nature*, **302**, 839-842

47. Taparowsky, E., Shimizu, K., Goldfarb, M. and Wigler, M. (1983). Structure and activation of the human N-*ras* gene. *Cell*, **34**, 581-586

48. Bos, J. K., Toksoz, D., Marshall, C. J., Verlaan-de Vries, M., Veeneman, G. H., van der Eb, A. J., van Boom, J. H., Janssen, J. W. G. and Steenvoorden, A. C. M. (1985). Amino-acid substitutions at codon 13 of the N-*ras* oncogene in human acute myeloid leukaemia. *Nature*, **315**, 726-730

49. Reddy, E. P., Reynolds, R. K., Santos, E. and Barbacid, M. (1982). A point mutation is responsible for the acquisition of transforming properties by the T24 human bladder carcinoma oncogene. *Nature*, **300**, 149-152

50. Yuasa, Y., Srivastava, S. K., Dunn, C. Y., Rhim, J. S., Reddy, E. P. and Aaronson, S. A. (1983). Acquisition of transforming properties by alternative point mutations within c-*has/has* human proto-oncogene. *Nature*, **303**, 775-779

51. Pulciani, S., Santos, E., Long, L. K., Sorrentino, V. and Barbacid, M. (1985). *ras* gene amplification and malignant transformation. *Mol. Cell. Biol.*, **5**, 2836-2841

52. Capon, D. J., Seeburg, P. H., McGrath, J. P., Hayflick, J. S., Edman, U., Levinson, A. D. and Goeddel, D. V. (1983). Activation of Ki-*ras2* gene in human colon and lung carcinomas by two different point mutations. *Nature*, **11**, 507-513

53. McCoy, M. S., Toole, J. J., Cunningham, J. M., Chang, E. H. Lowy, D. R. and Weinberg, R. A. (1983). Characterization of a human colon/lung carcinoma oncogene. *Nature*, **302**, 79-81

54. Schwab, M., Alitalo, K., Varmus, H. E., Bishop, J. M. and George, D. (1983). A cellular oncogene (c-Ki-*ras*) is amplified, overexpressed, and located within karyotypic abnormalities in mouse adrenocortical tumour cells. *Nature*, **309**, 497-501

55. Dalla Favera, R., Wong-Staal, F. and Gallo, R. C. (1982). *onc* gene amplification in promyelocytic leukaemia cell line HL-60 and primary leukaemic cells of the same patient. *Nature*, **299**, 61-65

56. Collins, S. and Groudine, M. (1982). Amplification of endogenous *myc*-related DNA sequences in a human myeloid leukaemia cell line. *Nature*, **298**, 679-681

57. Nowell, P., Finan, J., Dalla Favera, R., Gallo, R. C., Ar-Rushdi, A., Romanczuk, H., Selden, J. R., Emanuel, B. S., Rovera, G. and Croce, C. M. (1983). Association of amplified oncogene c-*myc* with an abnormally banded chromosome 8 in a human leukaemia cell line. *Nature*, **306**, 494-496

58. Alitalo, K., Schwab, M., Lin, C. C., Varmus, H. E. and Bishop, J. M. (1983). Homogeneously staining chromosomal regions contain amplified copies of an abundantly expressed cellular oncogene (c-*myc*) in malignant neuroendocrine cells from a human colon carcinoma. *Proc. Natl. Acad. Sci. USA*, **80**, 1707-1711

59. Hayward, W. S., Neel, B. G. and Astrin, S. M. (1981). Activation of a cellular *onc* gene by promoter insertion in ALV-induced lymphoid leukosis. *Nature*, **290**, 475-479

60. Steffen, D. (1984). Proviruses are adjacent to c-*myc* in some murine leukaemia virus-induced lymphomas. *Proc. Natl. Acad. Sci. USA*, **81**, 2097-2101

61. Kohl, N. E., Kanda, N., Schreck, R. R., Bruno, G., Latt, S. A., Gilbert, F. and Alt, F. W. (1983). Transposition and amplification of oncogene-related sequences in human neuroblastomas. *Cell*, **35**, 359-367

62. Shtivelman, E., Lifshitz, B., Gale, R. P. and Canaani, E. (1985). Fused transcript of *abl* and *bcr* genes in chronic myelogenous leukaemia. *Nature*, **315**, 550-554

63. Collins, S. J. and Groudine, M. T. (1983). Rearrangement and amplification of c-*abl* sequences in the human chronic myelogenous leukaemia cell line K-562. *Proc. Natl. Acad. Sci. USA*, **80**, 4813-4817

64. Yamamoto, T., Kamata, N., Kawano, H., Shimizu, S., Kuroki, T., Toyoshima, K., Rikimaru, K., Nomura, N., Ishizaki, R., Pastan, I., Gamou, S. and Shimizu, N. (1986). High incidence of amplification of the epidermal growth factor receptor gene in human squamous carcinoma cell lines. *Cancer Res.*, **46**, 414-416

65. Libermann, T. A., Nusbaum, H. R., Razon, N., Kris, R., Lax, I., Soreq, H., Whittle, N., Waterfield, M. D., Ullrich, A. and Schlessinger, J. (1985). Amplification, enhanced expression and possible rearrangement of EGF receptor gene in primary human brain tumours of glial origin. *Nature*, **313**, 144-149

66. Ullrich, A., Coussens, L., Hayflick, J. S., Dull, T. J., Gray, A., Tam, A. W., Lee J., Yarden, Y., Libermann, T. A., Schlessinger, J., Downward, J., Mayes, E. L. V., Whittle, N., Waterfield, M. D. and Seeburg, P. H. (1984). Human epidermal growth factor receptor cDNA sequence and aberrant expression of the amplified gene in A431 epidermoid carcinoma cells. *Nature*, **309**, 418-425

67. Fung, Y. K. T., Lewis, W. G., Kung, H. J. and Crittenden, L. B. (1983). Activation of the cellular oncogene c-*erb*B by LTR insertion: Molecular basis for induction of erythroblastosis by avian leukosis virus. *Cell*, **33**, 357-368

68. Rechavi, G., Givol, D. and Canaani, E. (1982). Activation of a cellular oncogene by DNA rearrangement: possible involvement of an IS-like element. *Nature*, **300**, 607-611

69. Canaani, E., Dreazen, O., Klar, A., Rechavi, G., Ram, D., Cohen, J. B. and Givol, D. (1983). Activation of the c-*mos* oncogene in a mouse plasmaytoma by insertion of an endogenous intracisternal A-particle genome. *Proc. Natl. Acad. Sci. USA.*, **80**, 7118-7122

70. Nusse, R., van Ooyen, A., Cox, D., Fung, Y. K. T. and Varmus, H. (1984). Mode of proviral activation of a putative mammary oncogene (*int-1*) on mouse chromosome 15. *Nature*, **307**, 131-136

71. Dickson, C., Smith, R., Brookes, S. and Peters, G. (1984). Tumorigenesis by mouse mammary tumour virus: Proviral activation of a cellular gene in the common integration region int-2. *Cell*, **37**, 529-536

72. Pelicci, P-G., Lanfrancone, L., Brathwaite, M. D., Wolman, S. R. and Dalla-Favera, R. (1984). Amplification of the c-*myb* oncogene in a case of human acute myelogenous leukemia. *Science*, **224**, 1117-1121

73. Alitalo, K., Winqvist, R., Lin, C. C., de la Chapelle, A., Schwab, M. and Bishop, J. M. (1984). Aberrant expression of an amplified c-*myb* oncogene in two cell lines from a colon carcinoma. *Proc. Natl. Acad. Sci. USA*, **81**, 4534-4538

74. Diamond, A., Cooper, G. M., Ritz, J. and Lane, M. A. (1983). Identification and molecular cloning of the human *Blym* transforming gene activated in Burkitt's lymphomas. *Nature*, **305**, 112-115

75. Schechter, A. L., Stern, D. F., Vaidyanathan, L., Decker, S. J., Drebin, J. A., Greene, M. I. and Weinberg, R. A. (1984). The *neu* oncogene: an *erb*-B-related gene encoding a 185,000-M tumour antigen. *Nature*, **312**, 513-516

76. Hoffman-Falk, H., Einat, P., Shilo, B-Z. and Hoffman, F. M. (1983). *Drosophila melanogaster* DNA clones homologous to vertebrate oncogenes: Evidence for a common ancester to *src* and *abl* cellular genes. *Cell*, **32**, 393-401

77. DeFeo-Jones, D., Scolnick, E. M., Koller, R. and Dhar, R. (1983). *ras*-related gene sequences identified and isolated from *Saccharomyces cerevisiae*. *Nature*, **306**, 707-709

78. Downward, J., Yarden, Y., Mayes, E., Scrace, G., Totty, N., Stockwell, P., Ullrich, A., Schlessinger, J. and Waterfield, M. D. (1984). Close similarity of epidermal growth factor receptor and v-*erb*-B oncogene protein sequences. *Nature*, **307**, 521-527

79. Sherr, C. J., Rettenmier, C. W., Sacca, R., Roussel, M. F., Look, A. T. and Stanley E. R. (1985). The c-*fms* proto-oncogene product is related to the receptor for the mononuclear phagocyte growth factor, CSF-1. *Cell*, **41**, 665-676

80. Pike, L. J., Bowen Pope, D. F., Rosse, D. R. and Krebs, E. G. (1983). Characterisation of platelet-derived growth factor-stimulated phosphorylation in cell membranes. *J. Biol. Chem.*, **258**, 9383-9390
81. Waterfield, M. D., Scrace, G. T., Whittle, N., Stroobant, P., Johnsson, A., Wasteson, A., Westermark, B., Heldin, C-H., Huang, J. S. and Deuel, T. F. (1983). Plated derived growth factor is structurally related to the putative transforming protein p28^{sis} of simian sarcoma virus. *Nature*, **304**, 35-39
82. Sporn, M. B. and Roberts, A. B. (1985). Autocrine growth factors and cancer. *Nature*, **313**, 745-747
83. Papageorge, A., Lowy, D. and Scolnick, E. M. (1982). Comparative biochemical properties of p21 *ras* molecules coded for by viral and cellular *ras* genes. *J. Virol.*, **44**, 509-519
84. Kataoka, T., Powers, S., Cameron, S., Fasano, O., Goldfarb, M., Broach, J. and Wigler, M. (1985). Functional homology of mammalian and yeast *ras* genes. *Cell*, **40**, 19-26
85. Beckner, S. K., Hattori, S. and Shih, T. Y. (1985). The *ras* oncogene product p21 is not a regulatory component of adenylate cyclase. *Nature*, **317**, 71-72
86. Muller, R., Slamon, D. J., Tremblay, J. M., Cline, M. J., Verma, I. M. (1982). Differential expression of cellular oncogenes during pre- and postnatal development of the mouse. *Nature*, **299**, 640-643
87. Goyette, M., Petropoulos, C. J., Shank, P. R. and Fausto, N. (1983). Expression of a cellular oncogene during liver regeneration. *Science*, **219**, 510-511
88. Goyette, M., Petropoulos, C. J., Shank, P. R. and Fausto, N. (1984). Regulated transcription of c-Ki-*ras* and c-*myc* during compensatory growth of rat liver. *Mol. Cell. Biol.*, **4**, 1493-1498
89. Westin, E. H., Gallo, R. C., Arya, S. K., Eva, A., Souza, L. M., Baluda, M. A., Aaronson, S. A. and Wong-Staal, F. (1982). Differential expression of the AMV gene in human hematopoietic cells. *Proc. Natl. Acad. Sci. USA*, **79**, 2194-2198
90. Westin, E. H., Wong-Staal, F., Gelmann, E. P., Dalla Favera, R., Papas, T. S., Lautenberger, J. A., Eva, A., Reddy, E. P., Tronick, S. R., Aaronson, S. A. and Gallo, R. A. (1982). Expression of cellular homologues of retroviral *onc* genes in human hemato-poietic cells. *Proc. Natl. Acad. Sci. USA*, **79**, 2490-2494
91. Tabin, C. J., Bradley, S. M., Bargmann, C. I., Weinberg, R. A., Papageorge, A. G., Scolnick, E. M., Dhar, R., Lowy, D. R. and Chang, E. H. (1982). Mechanism of activation of a human oncogene. *Nature*, **300**, 143-149
92. Taparowsky, E., Suard, Y., Fasano, O., Shimizu, K., Goldfarb, M. and Wigler, M. (1982). Activation of the T24 bladder carcinoma transforming gene is linked to a single amino acid change. *Nature*, **300**, 762-765
93. Dhar, R., Ellis, R. W., Shih, T. Y., Oroszlan, S., Shapiro, B., Maizel, J., Lowy, D. and Scolnick, E. M. (1982). Nucleotide sequence of the p21 transforming protein of Harvey murine sarcoma virus. *Science*, **217**, 934-937
94. Tsuchida, N., Ryder, T. and Ohtsubo, E. (1982). Nucleotide sequence of oncogene encoding the p21 transforming protein of Kirsten murine sarcoma virus. *Science*, **217**, 937-939
95. Der, C. J., Finkel, T. and Cooper, G. M. (1986). Biological and biochemical properties of human *ras*^{H} genes mutated at codon 61. *Cell*, **44**, 167-176
96. Nowell, P. C. and Hungerford, D. A. (1960). A minute chromosome in human granulocytic leukemia. *Science*, **132**, 1497
97. Heisterkamp, N., Stam, K., Groffen, J., de Klein, A. and Grosveld, G. (1985). Structural organisation of the *bcr* gene and its role in the Ph' translocation. *Nature*, **315**, 758-761
98. Konopka, J. B., Wanatabe, S. M. and Witte, O. N. (1984). An alteration of the human c-*abl* protein in K562 leukemia cells unmasks associated tyrosine kinase activity. *Cell*, **37**, 1035-1042
99. Konopka, J. B., Wanatabe, S. M., Singer, J. W., Collins, S. J. and Witte, O. N. (1985). Cell lines and clinical isolates derived from Ph'-positive chronic myelogenous leukemia patients express c-*abl* proteins with a common structural alteration. *Proc. Natl. Acad. Sci. USA*, **82**, 1810-1814
100. Taub, R., Kirsch, I., Morton, C., Lenoir, G., Swan, D., Tronick, S., Aaronson, S. and Leder, P. (1982). Translocation of the c-*myc* gene into the immunoglobulin heavy chain locus in human Burkitt's lymphoma and murine plasmacytoma cells. *Proc. Natl. Acad. Sci. USA*, **79**, 7837-7841

101. Erikson, J., Nishikura, K., Ar-Rushdi, A., Finan, J., Emanuel, B., Lenoir, G., Nowell, P. C. and Croce, C. M. (1983). Translocation of an immunoglobulin k locus to a region 3' of an unrearranged c-*myc* oncogene enhances c-*myc* transcription. *Proc. Natl. Acad. Sci. USA*, **80**, 7581-7585

102. Croce, C. M., Thierfelder, W., Erikson, J., Nishikura, K., Finan, J., Lenoir, G. M., and Nowell, P. C. (1983). Transcriptional activation of an unrearranged and untranslocated c-*myc* oncogene by translocation of a Cλ locus in Burkitt lymphoma cells. *Proc. Natl. Acad. Sci. USA*, **80**, 6922-6926

103. Klein, G. (1983). Specific chromosomal translocations and the genesis of B-cell-derived tumors in mice and men. *Cell*, **32**, 311-315

104. Erikson, J., Finan, J., Tsujimoto, Y., Nowell, P. C. and Croce, C. M. (1984). The chromosome 14 breakpoint in neoplastic B-cells with the t(11;14) translocation involves the immunoglobulin heavy chain locus. *Proc. Natl. Acad. Sci. USA*, **81**, 4144-4148

105. Cleary, M. L. and Sklar, J. (1985). Nucleotide sequence of a t(14;18) chromosomal breakpoint in follicular lymphoma and demonstration of a breakpoint-cluster region near a transcriptionally active locus on chromosome 18. *Proc. Natl. Acad. Sci. USA*, **82**, 7439-7443

106. Tsujimoto, Y., Gorham, J., Cossman, J., Jaffe, E. and Croce, C. M. (1985). The t(14;18) chromosome translocations involved in B-cell neoplasms result from mistakes in VDJ joining. *Science*, **229**, 1390-1393

107. Collins, M. K. L., Goodfellow, P. N., Spurr, N. K., Solomon, E., Tanigawa, G., Tonegawa, S. and Owen, M. J. (1985). The human T-cell receptor α-chain gene maps to chromosome 14. *Nature*, **314**, 273-274

108. Lewis, W. H., Michalopoulos, E. E., Williams, D. L., Minden, M. D. and Mak, T. W. (1985). Breakpoints in the human T-cell antigen receptor α-chain locus in two T-cell leukaemia patients with chromosomal translocations. *Nature*, **317**, 544-546

109. Shimke, R. T. (1984). Gene amplification in cultured animal cells. *Cell*, **37**, 705-713

110. Little, C. D., Nau, M. M., Carney, D. N., Gazdar, A. F. and Minna, J. D. (1983). Amplification and expression of the c-*myc* oncogene in human lung cancer cell lines. *Nature*, **306**, 194-196

111. Brodeur, G. M., Seeger, R. C., Schwab, M., Varmus, H. E. and Bishop, J. M. (1984). Amplification of N-*myc* in untreated human neuroblastomas correlates with advanced disease stage. *Science*, **224**, 1121-1124

112. Winqvist, R., Knuutila, S., Leprince, D., Stehelin, D. and Alitalo, K. (1985). Mapping of amplified c-*myb* oncogene, sister chromatid exchanges, and karyotypic analysis of the COLO 205 colon carcinoma cell line. *Cancer Genet.Cytogenet.*, **18**, 251-264

113. Nau, M. M., Carney, D. N., Battey, J., Johnson, B., Little, C., Gazdar, A. and Minna, J. D. (1984). Amplification, expression and rearrangement of c-*myc* and N-*myc* oncogenes in human lung cancer. *Curr. Top. Microbiol. Immunol.*, **113**, 172-177

114. Sparkes, R. S., Sparkes, M. C., Wilson, W. G., Towner, J. W., Benedict, W. F., Murphree, A. L. and Yunis, J. J. (1980). Regional assignment of genes for human esterase D and retinoblastoma to chromosome band 13q14. *Science*, **208**, 1042-1044

115. Sparkes, R. S., Murphree, A. L., Lingua, R. W., Sparkes, M. C., Field, L. L., Funderburk, S. J. and Benedict, W. F. (1983). Gene for hereditary retinoblastoma assigned to human chromosome 13 by linkage to esterase D. *Science*, **219**, 971-973

116. Benedict, W. F., Murphree, A. L., Banerjee, A., Spina, C. A., Sparkes, M. C. and Sparkes, R. S. (1983). Patient with 13 chromosome deletion: evidence that the retinoblastoma gene is a recessive cancer gene. *Science*, **219**, 973-975

117. Godbout, R., Dryja, T. P., Squire, J., Gallie, B. L. and Phillips, R. A. (1983). Somatic inactivation of genes on chromosome 13 is a common event in retinoblastoma. *Nature*, **304**, 451-453

118. Benedict, W. F., Banerjee, A., Mark, C. and Murphree, A. L. (1983). Nonrandom chromosomal changes in untreated retinoblastomas. *Cancer Genet. Cytogenet.*, **10**, 311-333

119. Hansen, M. F., Koufos, A., Gallie, B. L., Phillips, R. A., Fodstad, O., Brogger, A., Gedde-Dahl, T. and Cavenee, W. K. (1985). Osteosarcoma and retinoblastoma: A shared chromosomal mechanism revealing recessive predisposition. *Proc. Natl. Acad. Sci. USA*, **82**, 6216-6220

120. Koufos, A., Hansen, M. F., Lampkin, B. C., Workman, M. L., Copeland, N. G., Jenkins,

N. A. and Cavenee, W. K. (1984). Loss of alleles at loci on human chromosome 11 during genesis of Wilms' tumour. *Nature*, **309**, 170-172

121. Orkin, S. H., Goldman, D. S. and Sallan, S. E. (1984). Development of homozygosity for chromosome 11p markers in Wilms' tumour. *Nature*, **309**, 172-174

122. Reeve, A. E., Housiaux, P. J., Gardner, R. J. M., Chewings, W. E., Grindley, R. M. and Millow, L. J. (1984). Loss of a Harvey *ras* allele in sporadic Wilms' tumour. *Nature*, **309**, 174-176

123. Fearon, E. R., Vogelstein, B. and Feinberg, A. P. (1984). Somatic deletion and duplication of genes on chromosome 11 in Wilms' tumour. *Nature*, **309**, 176-178

124. Koufos, A., Hansen, M. F., Copeland, N. G., Jenkins, N. A., Lampkin, B. C. and Cavenee, W. B. (1985). Loss of heterozygosity in three embryonal tumours suggests a common pathogenetic mechanism. *Nature*, **316**, 330-334

125. Adams, J. M. (1985). Oncogene activation by fusion of chromosomes in leukemia. *Nature*, **315**, 542-543

3
Growth control in normal cells and in relation to carcinogenesis

D. J. VENTER AND W. J. GULLICK

INTRODUCTION

In this chapter, we will describe some of the molecular mechanisms involved in the control of normal cell growth. In addition we will discuss abnormalities in these mechanisms which are found in neoplastic cells, and which may be active in carcinogenesis.

PROCESSES OCCURRING IN NORMAL GROWTH AND DEVELOPMENT

Growth can be defined as an increase in the size of an organism or organ due to a net proliferation of its constituent cells. Proliferation (an increase in the number of viable cells) is ultimately dependent on the rate of cell division coupled with the rate of cell death. In this chapter we will focus on the mechanisms controlling cell division. In multicellular organisms this proliferation is always accompanied by differentiation of the majority of the cells to form various phenotypes, each capable of performing a specific function.

In the developing embryo, organogenesis requires that cells divide, migrate to the appropriate position in the organism and differentiate (see Chapter 5 for a more detailed discussion of cell growth in relation to embryogenesis). In the mature animal, optimal function of an organ may necessitate the replacement of senescent or damaged cells by sufficient numbers of new cells capable of differentiating to perform the desired function. All these events require the interaction of a complex network of control mechanisms, and, *in vivo*, the rate of cell division is controlled by events occurring both inside and outside the cell. Growth control is a delicate interplay between multiple synergistic and antagonistic forces, and any attempt to define, on the basis of experimental work, how these mechanisms interact must at present be an oversimplification.

REQUIREMENTS FOR CONTROL OF THESE PROCESSES

In order for normal growth and development to occur the following are necessary conditions.

Normal intermediary metabolism

Cells must take up and metabolise nutrients at a sufficient rate to store excess energy and to manufacture macromolecules for use in synthesis of cellular components. These functions are under enzymatic control, with the activities of the enzymes themselves regulated by various mechanisms.

Appropriate gene expression

The production of proteins coded for by the genome is necessary to perform the myriad cellular functions. Gene expression must occur in the correct sequence, depending on the stage of the cell cycle and the degree of differentiation[1,2] and at the appropriate rate to furnish optimal amounts of the protein in question[3].

Interactions between cells

In a multicellular organism, intercellular communication serves to regulate diverse functions such as the rate of cell proliferation and the release of substances involved in homeostasis. Here are some examples:

(1) Hormones. These are chemicals produced by glandular structures which are transported in the circulation to target cells defined by the expression of appropriate receptors. They frequently have multiple functions, depending on the target cell studied, and often act synergistically with other secreted molecules. Some hormones which regulate cell growth are: insulin, growth hormone, thyroxine, glucocorticoids, androgens, oestrogens, prolactin and glucagon.

(2) Polypeptide Growth Factors (see below in the section on Growth Factors for definition and detailed discussion).

(3) Direct intercellular communication. Gap junctions are protein structures which form a channel between two adjacent cell membranes through which ions and other molecules may pass. Their function is regulated in part by the intracellular Ca^{2+} concentration[4].

(4) Neural communication by synaptic transmission.

Cell migration and motility

The migration of a cell from one area of an embryo or organ to its final anatomical resting place depends on a complex series of interactions between specific cell surface adhesion molecules and molecules present in the extracellular matrix as well as on adjacent cells. For a discussion of how knowledge of these processes may contribute to our understanding of mechanisms involved in metastasis and tumour spread, see Chapters 4 and 5, and refs. 5–9.

All cells perform mechanical work such as movement during organogenesis, cleavage during mitosis, and endocytosis. These functions are carried out by an intracellular network of filaments called the cytoskeleton, composed primarily of actin filaments, microtubules and intermediate filaments[10,11]. Several proteins appear to have a role in controlling cell shape and adhesion, one example of which is vinculin which is thought to link actin bundles to the cell surface membrane. It appears to be phosphorylated by both tyrosine kinases and protein kinase C (see later), which may have an effect on its function[12,13], although the evidence for this remains to be firmly substantiated.

GROWTH REGULATORY CONTROL MECHANISMS

In this section we will describe some of the mechanisms responsible for controlling normal cell growth and development. Briefly stated, growth factors act by modifying the activity of enzymes and other proteins with resultant effect on gene expression and, ultimately, cell division.

Growth factors

The observation that the majority of cultured cell types required serum for their continued proliferation led to the hypothesis that the serum contained growth factors[14]. Many of these have now been purified and defined biochemically. The majority are polypeptides, and it is the function of these which will be described here. However, it should be borne in mind that many cell types require additional non-polypeptide molecules for normal growth and differentiation (such as steroid hormones for normal proliferation of mammary epithelium). Some well-defined polypeptide growth factors and the cell types affected by them are listed in Table 3.1.

Origins of growth factors

The growth factors which act to control normal cell proliferation and differentiation may act by three different mechanisms. They may be hormones such as insulin synthesised in a discrete organ and having their effect on distant cells – a process known as endocrine control. Alternatively, a

Table 3.1 Polypeptide growth factors

Growth factor	Target cell type	Reference
Epidermal growth factor (EGF)	Epithelial and fibroblastic cells	15
Transforming growth factors (TGF) α and β	Mesenchymal and epithelial cells	24–27
Vaccinia virus growth factor	Unknown	32
Platelet-derived growth factor (PDGF)	Mesenchymal cells, glia	16–19
Insulin and insulin-like growth factors (IGF-I and II)	Mesenchymal cells	20, 21
Nerve growth factor (NGF)	Sympathetic and sensory neurons	22, 23
Bombesin	Fibroblasts	29, 30
Angiogenin	Endothelial cells	31*
Substance P Substance K	Mesenchymal cells	33
Granulocyte-macrophage colony stimulating factors	Bone marrow cells of granulocyte and monocyte-macrophage lineage	34
Interleukin-2 (IL-2) (formerly T-cell growth factor)	T-lymphocytes	28

*Review

growth factor may be released from a cell in the immediate vicinity of the target cells and diffuse to reach its site of action. This is known as paracrine control and is seen, for example, in the action of PDGF which promotes division of smooth muscle cells at the site of arterial injury[35]. Finally, growth factors may be synthesized by a cell and act on that same cell – a process called 'autocrine' stimulation. Autocrine stimulation has been reported to operate normally as a transient phenomenon during embryological development and also during repair of tissue injury[36].

Mechanisms of action of polypeptide growth factors

Growth factors such as platelet-derived growth factor (PDGF), epidermal growth factor (EGF) and insulin bind to well-defined specific glycoprotein receptors embedded in the cell membrane. It is hypothesized that binding may affect the conformation of the receptor in such a way that a signal is transmitted to the interior of the cell. In the case of many growth factor receptors, one of the common results of ligand binding is the activation of a tyrosine kinase, with resulting phosphorylation of proteins (including enzymes) and presumably, alteration in their activity[21]. Binding of PDGF to its receptor, for instance, initiates a series of events including the generation of second messengers and alteration of ionic fluxes with resultant effects on proteins and, ultimately, the cell cycle[17,37]. One of the major pathways thought to be responsible for conveying messages from ligand-receptor complexes to the interior of the cell employs the membrane phospholipid phosphatidylinositol 4,5-bisphosphate (PIP2). Following binding of the ligand such as PDGF to its receptor, PIP2 is hydrolysed by the enzyme PIP2 phosphodiesterase (PDE) to yield inositol triphosphate (IP3) and diacylglycerol (DG). The IP3 is thought to act as a second messenger leading to mobilisation of intracellular Ca^{2+} stores. Also functioning as a second messenger the DG is capable of activating protein kinase C, an enzyme thought to be active in a number of important cellular growth-controlling processes (for review of this mechanism and its putative role in growth factor-induced metabolic changes and tumour promotion see refs. 37–40).

The binding of EGF to its receptor also gives rise to a combination of tyrosine kinase activation and increased ionic fluxes, as well as numerous other effects[41] (see later for full discussion of EGF receptor structure and function).

In addition the binding affinity of the growth factors for their receptors and their ability to generate intracellular signals are both capable of being modulated by additional protein kinases, providing yet another level of growth control.

Protein phosphorylation

Reversible phosphorylation is one of the major mechanisms for the regulation of protein function in eukaryotes[42-44]. The addition of phosphate to serine, threonine or tyrosine residues on enzymes and other proteins can result in conformational changes. These may affect sites necessary for enzyme activity, which result in an increase or decrease in their rates of catalysis, depending on the enzyme and the amino acids phosphorylated. This process of covalent modification is reversible, the phosphate group being cleaved off by phosphatases.

Protein phosphorylation may occur following binding of a growth factor to its target cell, such as the increase in tyrosine-kinase activity seen after binding of EGF, PDGF and insulin to their specific receptors[21,41]. The protein phosphorylation which occurs following binding of a growth factor to its specific receptor may represent the mechanism by which these growth factors control cell division and differentiation. It is thought that the tyrosine kinase activity has the effect of activating enzymes critical for control of gene expression and the mitotic process.

It should be noted that insulin and several other polypeptide growth factors such as bombesin and substance P are capable of functioning either as hormones or as growth factors, dependent on as yet undefined intracellular events which occur following binding to the specific receptor[21]. Thus insulin functions as a hormone promoting the synthesis of glycogen when binding to adult skeletal muscle cells and hepatocytes[44]. When binding to rat hepatoma cells in culture, however, it functions as a mitogen[45,46] in conjunction with EGF.

Regulation of gene expression

The production of a specific protein required by the cell is the end result of a sequence of molecular events, each of which is subject directly or indirectly to regulation. Control can occur at the level of chromatin structure and DNA methylation which affects access of transcription enzymes to the gene; at the level of initiation of RNA transcription; post-transcriptional modification; or translation itself (see refs. 8, 3, 47–50).

One facet of transcriptional control involves the attachment of specific proteins to enhancer sequences which affect binding of RNA polymerase[3] to the promoter region[51]. The affinity of these binding proteins may be modified by phosphorylation (see preceding section and ref. 52) thereby influencing transcription. Two groups of proteins which might fulfil this role and thus have an effect on contolling normal cell division and embryological development are those encoded by the homeo box[2,53] and the protein products of the c-*myc*, c-*fos*, *myb*, and possibly the *p53* and N-*myc* oncogenes[54].

THE EPIDERMAL GROWTH FACTOR RECEPTOR

In this section we will describe the structure and function of one molecule, the EGF receptor, in some detail in an attempt to illustrate the general principles of growth factor receptor function.

Distribution

The epidermal growth factor receptor (EGFR) is a glycoprotein found on the cell membranes of a wide variety of cell types derived from ectodermal, mesodermal and endodermal layers, including fibroblasts, glia, keratinocytes, placental membranes and endothelial cells[55]. Its presence has been established both in cultured cells (by means of ^{125}I-EGF binding, cell proliferation and immunoprecipitation assays), and *in situ* in normal and neoplastic tissue using immunocytochemical methods on tissue sections.

Biological effects

Studies in intact animals, organ cultures and cell culture systems have shown that the binding of EGF to specific EGF receptors results in a wide variety of effects[15]. Some early responses which occur within minutes of binding are:

increased ion transport;
activation of glycolysis;
increased nutrient uptake;
membrane ruffling and micropinocytosis;
stimulation of tyrosine kinase activity; and
increased phosphatidyl inositol turnover.

The last of these effects has so far been seen only in A431 squamous carcinoma cells.

Late responses seen hours after binding are:

stimulation of RNA synthesis;
stimulation of protein synthesis;
stimulation of DNA synthesis; and
enhanced cell proliferation.

In cell culture systems, these effects may be observed both in non-transformed cells (e.g., human fibroblasts, glia, mammary epithelium and keratinocytes) and in transformed cell types, e.g. HeLa cells. It should be noted that not all of these effects have been observed in any one cell type. It is not known what mechanisms are responsible for determining the varied effects seen in different tissues.

Structure

An account of technical aspects of the purification and sequencing of the EGFR is given in reference 41. The primary amino acid sequence suggests, on the basis of hydrophobicity plots, that the molecule can be divided into three main regions (Figure 3.1).

(1) An amino-terminal portion, 621 amino acids long, which lies external to the cell membrane. This portion forms the EGF binding domain and is glycosylated. It contains 51 cysteine residues, many or all of which may

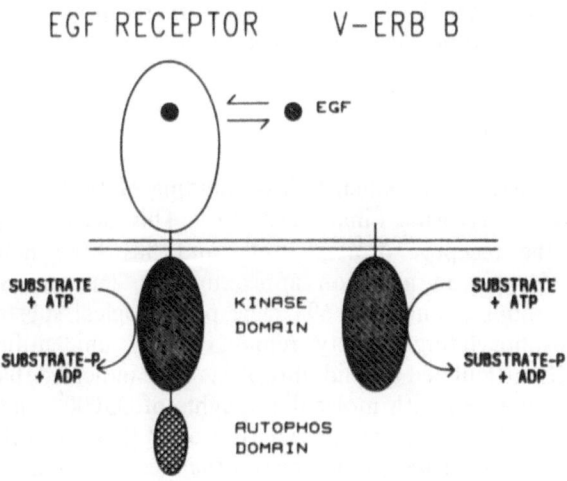

Figure 3.1 Diagrammatic representation of the transmembrane arrangement of the epidermal growth factor receptor compared to the v-*erb* B protein

form disulphide bonds, giving rise to a highly cross-linked globular structure.

(2) A hydrophobic transmembrane region 23 amino acids long arranged in an α-helix.

(3) An intracytoplasmic C-terminal domain 542 amino acids long which can be divided (on the basis of protease mapping) into a kinase domain and an autophosphorylation site domain[56].

Biochemical events following EGF binding

EGF binding is followed by a series of biochemical processes capable of producing the biological effects noted above. Several of these will be described below, although it is by no means clear exactly how they are linked with complex events such as cell division.

Transmembrane signalling

Attachment of EGF to the external (ligand-binding) portion of the receptor is followed by transduction of the signal to the internal (cytoplasmic) portion. It would appear unlikely that the predicted single α-helical transmembrane domain would be capable of transmitting either a conformational or ionic signal, and thus it is possible that transduction requires interaction between receptors. Following binding of the ligand, EGF-receptor complexes are known to cluster in coated pits prior to being internalised and degraded in lysosomes[57,58]. It is possible that this clustering results in the bringing together of several receptor cytoplasmic domains, causing receptor interactions which result in the observed biochemical effects.

Tyrosine kinase activity

One of the earliest events which follows binding of EGF to its receptor is increased protein tyrosine kinase activity[59]. This activity appears to be intrinsic to the receptor protein itself, and has been mapped to the cytoplasmic domain in a region approximately 250 amino acids long, beginning at about amino acid 694. The physiological substrates for this tyrosine phosphorylating activity remain largely unidentified, although studies on EGF-stimulated diploid fibroblasts have indicated that a variety of proteins including two with molecular weights of $35\,000$[60] and $43\,000$[61] are phosphorylated. Obviously, the characterisation of these and other substrates is desirable in order further to understand the mechanism of action of EGF on the cell[62].

The binding of PDGF, insulin and IGF-1 to their specific receptors also induces tyrosine kinase activity. In addition proteins encoded by members of the *src* family of oncogenes (*src, erb*-B, *yes, fps, fms, abl, fgr*) show similar protein tyrosine kinase activities. Thus it is likely that the phosphorylation of proteins on tyrosine residues plays a key role in the regulation of cell growth[62]. For a review of protein-tyrosine kinases see ref. 63.

Autophosphorylation activity

The intrinsic tyrosine kinase activity not only phosphorylates exogenous substrates but also phosphorylates three tyrosine residues on the C-terminal portion of the EGF receptor itself, at amino acids 1173, 1148 and 1068[64]. The possible significance of this autophosphorylation will be discussed in the next section.

Modulation of EGF receptor function

There is a wide degree of variation in the biological responses following the binding of EGF to its receptor in different cell types. It is known that several factors act on the receptor itself to modulate its response (for general review see ref. 65).

Phosphorylation of the receptor by cellular enzymes

As described above the activity of enzymes can be modulated by phosphorylation. Recent results have shown that the ubiquitous Ca^{2+} and phospholipid-dependent enzyme, protein kinase C, can phosphorylate the EGF receptor on threonine residue 654, which lies close to the cell membrane on the cytoplasmic portion of the receptor. Phosphorylation of purified EGFR at this site *in vitro* causes a three-fold decrease in both the EGF binding affinity and the receptor kinase activity[62,64]. In support of this, treatment of cells with the tumour promoting phorbol ester phorbol myristyl acetate (PMA) reduces the binding of EGF. PMA is known to activate protein kinase C directly, mimicking the effect of diacylglycerol. Such modulation of growth factor binding affinity may be one of the mechanisms by which tumour promoters act[66]. The binding of PDGF to its receptor stimulates the production of diacylglycerol thereby activating protein kinase C which amongst other targets phosphorylates the EGF receptor. The affinity of the EGF receptor for EGF is thus decreased. This 'crosstalk' between growth factor receptors has been termed transmodulation[67].

Autophosphorylation

The EGF receptor protein is itself one of the major substrates for its own kinase activity. Three distinct tyrosine residues in the carboxy terminal region of the protein are phosphorylated[56]. It is not known precisely what physiological function, if any, phosphorylation at these sites may perform.

Thus far studies on the effect of autophosphorylation on EGF receptor tyrosine kinase activity have revealed conflicting results[64,65].

Receptor internalisation

Following binding of EGF, the EGF-receptor complexes form clusters in coated pits and are internalised. The internalised complexes subsequently fuse with lysosomes, and are degraded[55]. Receptor internalisation *per se* does not appear to mediate the mitogenic response to EGF stimulation nor does it appear to affect the intrinsic tyrosine kinase activity of the receptor. It does however serve as a method of down regulating the number of cell surface EGF receptors, thus modifying the subsequent response of the cells to EGF[57].

The EGF receptor gene

The EGF receptor gene is situated on chromosome 7 (p14–p12), is approximately 110 kb in length, and contains at least 26 exons. Two RNA transcripts of 10 and 5.6 kb are produced in normal cells, the difference thought to occur in the length of the 3′ untranslated sequences. For a more detailed discussion of the gene and mechanisms which may control its expression see ref. 68.

ABNORMALITIES OF GROWTH CONTROL

The above description of mechanisms involved in the control of normal growth suggests that abnormalities occurring at any one of several control points may contribute toward the neoplastic phenotype (Figure 3.2). Experiments based on this supposition have shown aberrations in growth control at each of the following levels: growth factor; receptor; post-receptor signal transduction; and gene expression. Much of the recent progress in this area has been enhanced by the finding that the products of many oncogenes resemble specific molecules involved in the normal processes of growth control (see Chapter 2 and refs. 12, 69–73).

Abnormal secretion of growth factors: autocrine stimulation

The role of autocrine stimulation in controlling normal growth has been discussed above. Evidence has accumulated that this process can occur in an abnormal manner, leading to the cells involved becoming independent of external growth control and thus contributing to the establishment of the neoplastic phenotype[24,35,54]. The observation that the B chain of PDGF is structurally similar to the transforming protein p28sis of simian sarcoma virus[17], which is known to be expressed at high levels in these transformed cells, led to the suggestion that the mechanism for transformation might

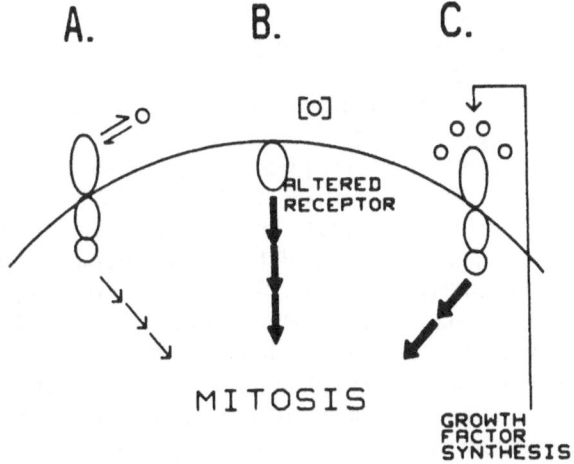

Figure 3.2 Models for: (A) normal growth factor interaction with its receptor leading to controlled cell division; (B) altered receptor leading to uncontrolled signal generation; and (C) autocrine stimulation of cell growth by the overproduction of a growth factor

reside in the secretion of a protein which has growth factor activity and which acts to alter cell growth abnormally in an autocrine manner[35,36,74-77].

In addition to cells transformed by simian sarcoma virus, platelet-derived growth factor-like peptides have also been found to be produced by a number of other transformed cell types, such as human osteosarcoma cells[74], the human breast cancer cell line T47D[75] and SV40-transformed BHK cells[17].

Cells transformed by viruses containing certain cytoplasmic oncogenes (e.g. *src*, *ras* and *mos*) release growth factors into their culture medium. These growth factors have subsequently been purified, and have been called transforming growth factors. They are coded for by the host cell genome and their synthesis is induced by the transforming oncogene via an unknown mechanism. Their precise role in cellular transformation is still under investigation, and it is not known what part they play in normal growth control[25,26]. The above examples suggest, however, that the abnormal production of growth factors acting on the same cell which produces them may be causally related to the neoplastic transformation of these cells. Additional examples where such abnormal autocrine control may be operative are the production of bombesin-like peptides in human small-cell lung cancer[78] and the production of B-cell growth factor by human lymphocytes transformed by Epstein-Barr virus[79].

Abnormal growth factor receptor function and signal transduction

Growth factor receptors generate a signal on binding of their ligand which is then conveyed to the cytoplasm, a process known as signal transduction. It is possible that abnormalities involving the signal transduction process could result in altered growth control. This could be due to a net increase or decrease in the activity of the receptor proteins themselves, brought about either by an alteration in the tyrosine kinase coding domain, or by the presence of greater or lesser numbers of receptor molecules.

The v-*erb*-B oncogene is the active transforming gene present in the avian erythroblastosis virus AEV-H[80]. The predicted protein sequence of the v-*erb*-B oncogene closely matches the sequence of part of the EGF receptor protein[81], corresponding to residues 551–1154. Thus, most of the extracellular EGF binding domain is missing, as is a small length of C-terminus which contains the major autophosphorylation site (tyrosine 1178). It thus appears that this viral oncogene protein is a truncated form of the EGF receptor. Protein tyrosine kinase activity has been demonstrated *in vitro* in this molecule, and therefore one could hypothesise that in this instance cell transformation may be brought about by continuously elevated levels of tyrosine kinase activity which do not require the presence of bound EGF. The C-terminal truncation and resultant deletion of the major auto-phosphorylation site may also result in abnormally high tyrosine kinase activity or alteration in the specificity of substrate phosphorylation. This hypothesis remains to be proved conclusively *in vitro*, however.

The *neu* oncogene which has recently been isolated from an ethyl nitrosourea-induced rat neuro/glioblastoma, has since been found to have a normal cellular counterpart in rats and man which codes for a 185 kd protein similar in structure to the EGF receptor[82]. It is not presently known how the transforming *neu*-encoded protein differs in structure from its normal cellular counterpart and experiments are in progress to determine whether it shows abnormal tyrosine kinase activity. A third transforming oncogene product which may function by an analogous mechanism is the v-*fms* protein, an altered version of the normal cellular c-*fms* product, which appears to code for the murine macrophage colony stimulating factor (CSF-1) receptor[83].

As stated above, an increase in the total signal following binding of a growth factor to its receptor could also occur due to the presence of increased numbers of that receptor. Elevated levels of EGF receptor have been found in several types of malignant tumour, including squamous carcinomas arising in the skin[84], lung[85,86] and cervix[87]; gliomas[88,89]; and transitional cell carcinomas of the bladder[90]. A similar finding has been reported in cell lines derived from ovarian and breast carcinomas[91] and the vulval squamous carcinoma cell line A431[92]. DNA from the A431 cells and from a number of human glioma biopsies shows amplification (i.e. increased copy number) and rearrangement of the EGF receptor gene[89,93]. The amplification may account for an increase in gene expression with the result that more EGF receptors are expressed on the cell surface, while the rearrangement may give rise to the production of the truncated EGF receptor proteins.

Abnormal signalling could also occur due to changes in the molecules generating the so-called second messengers. The G proteins are a family of guanine nucleotide-binding proteins which are functionally associated with many receptors including those for β-adrenergic agonists, gonadotropins and possibly some growth factors. These G proteins regulate the activity of adenylate cyclase, and thus the production of cyclic AMP (reviewed[94]). The proteins coded for by the normal cellular *ras* genes (Ha-, Ki-, and N-*ras*) show structural homology with the G proteins and may have a similar function in signal transduction. Comparison between the normal Ha-*ras* protein and the transforming T24 human bladder carcinoma Ha-*ras* oncogene product shows a single amino acid substitution, that of valine for glycine at residue 12. At a functional level, this amino acid substitution results in impaired GTPase activity in the oncogenic protein[95] but it is not clear whether this alteration in activity is critical for transformation[96]. The Ki-*ras*, N-*ras* and Ha-*ras* transforming proteins found in primary tumours can also show other point mutations resulting in amino acid changes at residues 13 and 61. The fact that these oncogenes are detectable by transfection assays in a wide variety of tumours suggests that their abnormal function may play an important part in the process of malignant transformation[95].

Abnormal expression of nuclear oncogenes

The protein product of the c-*myc* oncogene is located in the nucleus and may bind to DNA, thereby playing a role in control of RNA transcription and gene expression[97-100]. The N-*myc* oncogene shows homology to c-*myc*, and it is thought that the putative protein product of this gene may serve a similar function[101,102]. Increased levels of transcription of c-*myc* are found in Burkitt's lymphoma, and of N-*myc* in some neuroblastomas, suggesting that this overexpression may play a role in cell transformation. In the case of c-*myc*, 75% of cases of Burkitt's lymphoma (a neoplasm derived from B-lymphocytes) show a translocation of the c-*myc* locus from its normal site on band q24 of chromosome 8 to the immunoglobulin heavy chain locus on chromosome 14. As the tumour cell is derived from a B-lymphocyte the immunoglobulin heavy chain is expressed at a high level and it is thought that the enhancer sequence of the immunoglobulin gene has the effect of increasing transcription of the translocated c-*myc* gene[54,103-105].

The increased levels of N-*myc* RNA found in several human neuroblastomas are associated with amplification of the gene, which may be present in as many as 300 copies in the genome. It is interesting that there is a strong correlation between the degree of amplification and severity of disease, with the highest level of amplification being found in the more widely disseminated tumours[106,107]. This finding may be of use in determining prognosis and possibly in the choice of treatment regimen.

DIRECTION FOR FUTURE RESEARCH

Perhaps the most pressing need is to define the physiological substrates for the protein kinase activity displayed by many growth factor receptors following ligand binding. This will aid in building up a picture of the sequence of events occurring between binding of growth factor and initiation of cell division. Establishing how the proteins of different oncogenes interact to control normal and abnormal cell growth and relating these functions to the steps involved in cell maturation will be an equally absorbing task.

Acknowledgements

We would like to thank Audrey Becket for secretarial assistance. D.V. is grateful to the Sir Jules Thorn Charitable Trust for financial assistance and would like to thank Professor P.L. Lantos and Dr M.D. Waterfield for their continued support. We are grateful to Drs P. Parker and M. Berger for reading the manuscript prior to publication. W.G. acknowledges the support of the Imperial Cancer Research Fund.

References

1. Curran, T., Miller, A. D., Zokas, L. and Verma, I. M. (1984). Viral and cellular *fos* proteins: A comparative analysis. *Cell*, **36**, 259-268
2. Manley, J. L. and Levine, M. S. (1985). The homeo box and mammalian development. *Cell*, **43**, 1-2
3. Nomura, M. (1984). The control of ribosome synthesis. *Sci. Am.*, **250**, 72-83
4. Loewenstein, W. R. (1979). Junctional intercellular communication and the control of growth. *Biochim. Biophys. Acta*, **560**, 1-65
5. D'Ardenne, A. J. and McGee, J. O'D. (1984). Fibronectin in disease. *J. Pathol.*, **142**, 235-251
6. Edelman, G. M. (1984). Cell-adhesion molecules: A molecular basis for animal form. *Sci. Am.*, **250**, 80-91
7. Stern, C. D. (1984). Mini-review: Hyaluronidases in early embryonic development. *Cell Biol. Int. Rep.*, **8**, 703-717
8. Poste, G. and Fidler, I. J. (1980). The pathogenesis of cancer metastasis. *Nature*, **283**, 139-146
9. Iozzo, R. V. (1984). Proteoglycans and neoplastic-mesenchymal cell interactions. *Hum. Pathol.*, **15**, 2-10
10. Clarke, M. and Spudich, J. A. (1977). Nonmuscle contractile proteins: The role of actin and myosin in cell motility and shape determination. *Annu. Rev. Biochem.*, **46**, 797-822
11. Lazarides, E. and Revel, J. P. (1979). The molecular basis of cell movement. *Sci. Am.*, **240**, 88-100
12. Hunter, T. (1984). The proteins of oncogenes. *Sci. Am.*, **251**, 60-69
13. Werth, D. K., Niedel, J. E. and Pastan, I. (1983). Vinculin, a cytoskeletal substrate of protein kinase C. *J. Biol. Chem.*, **258**, 11 423-11 426
14. Rozengurt, E. (1983). Growth factors, cell proliferation and cancer: An overview. *Mol. Biol. Med.*, **1**, 169-181
15. Carpenter, G. and Cohen, S. (1979). Epidermal growth factor. *Annu. Rev. Biochem.*, **48**, 193-216
16. Heldin, C-H., Westermark, B. and Wasteson, A. (1981). Specific receptors for platelet-derived growth factor on cells derived from connective tissue and glia. *Proc. Natl. Acad. Sci. USA*, **78**, 3664-3668
17. Waterfield, M. D., Scrace, G. T., Whittle, N., Stroobant, P., Johnsson, A., Wasteson, A., Westermark, B., Heldin, C-H., Huang, J. S. and Deuel, T. F. (1983). Platelet-derived growth factor is structurally related to the putative transforming protein p28sis of simian sarcoma virus. *Nature*, **304**, 35-39
18. Antoniades, H. N., Scher, C. D., and Stiles, C. D. (1979). Purification of human platelet-derived growth factor. *Proc. Natl. Acad. Sci. USA*, **76**, 1809-1813
19. Stroobant, P. and Waterfield, M. D. (1984). Purification and properties of porcine platelet-derived growth factor. *EMBO J.*, **3**, 2963-2967

20. Froesch, E. R., Zapf, J., Rinderknecht, E., Morell, B., Schoenie, E. and Humbel, R. E. (1979). Insulin-like growth factor (IGF-NSILA). Structure, function and physiology. In Sato, G. H. and Ross, R. (eds.) *Hormones and Cell Culture*. Cold Spring Harbor Conferences on Cell Proliferation. Book A, pp. 61-77. (New York: Cold Spring Harbor)
21. Ullrich, A., Bell, J. R., Chen, E. Y., Herrera, R., Petruzzelli, L. M., Dull, T. J., Gray, A., Coussens, L., Liao, Y-C., Tsubokawa, M., Mason, A., Seeburg, P. H., Grunfeld, C., Rosen, O. M. and Ramachandran, J. (1985). Human insulin receptor and its relationship to the tyrosine kinase family of oncogenes. *Nature*, **313**, 756-761
22. Calissano, P., Cattaneo, A., Biocca, S., Aloe, L., Mercanti, D. and Levi-Montalcini, R. (1984). The nerve growth factor. *Exp. Cell Res.*, **154**, 1-9
23. Lillien, L. E. and Claude, P. (1985). Nerve growth factor is a mitogen for cultured chromaffin cells. *Nature*, **317**, 632-634
24. Todaro, G. J. and De Larco, J. E. (1978). Growth factors produced by sarcoma-virus-transformed cells. *Cancer Res.*, **38**, 4147-4154
25. Lawrence, D. A. (1985). Transforming growth factors - An overview. *Biol. Cell*, **53**, 93-98
26. Massague, J. (1985). Transforming growth factors. Isolation, characterisation, and interaction with cellular receptors. *Prog. Med. Virol.*, **32**, 142-158
27. Derynck, R., Jarrett, J. A., Chen, E. Y., Eaton, D.H., Bell, J. R., Assoian, R. K., Roberts, A. B., Sporn, M. B. and Goeddel, D. V. (1985). Human transforming growth factor-β complementary DNA sequence and expression in normal and transformed cells. *Nature*, **316**, 701-705
28. Taniguchi, T., Matsui, H., Fujita, T., Takaoka, C., Kashima, N., Yoshimoto, R., and Hamiro, J. (1983). Structure and expression of a cloned cDNA for human interleukin-2. *Nature*, **302**, 305-310
29. Rozengurt, E. and Sinnett-Smith, J. (1983). Bombesin stimulation of DNA synthesis and cell division in cultures of Swiss 3T3 cells. *Proc. Natl. Acad. Sci. USA*, **80**, 2936-2940
30. Zachary, I. and Rozengurt, E. (1985). High-affinity receptors for peptides of the bombesin family in Swiss 3T3 cells. *Proc. Natl. Acad. Sci. USA*, **82**, 7616-7620
31. Liotta, L. (1985). Isolation of a protein that stimulates blood vessel growth. *Nature*, **318**, 14
32. Stroobant, P., Rice, A. P., Gullick, W. J., Cheng, D. J., Kerr, I. M. and Waterfield, M. D. (1985). Purification and characterisation of Vaccinia virus growth factor. *Cell*, **42**, 383-393
33. Nilsson, J., von Euler, A. M., and Dalsgaard, C. J. (1985). Stimulation of connective tissue cell growth by substance P and substance K. *Nature*, **315**, 61-63
34. Metcalf, D. (1985). The granulocyte-macrophage colony-stimulating factors. *Science*, **229**, 16-22
35. Heldin, C-H. and Westermark, B. (1984). Growth factors: mechanism of action and relation to oncogenes. *Cell*, **37**, 9-20
36. Sporn, M. B. and Roberts, A. B. (1985). Autocrine growth factors and cancer. *Nature*, **313**, 745-747
37. Berridge, M. J. (1985). The molecular basis of communication within the cell. *Sci. Am.*, **253**, 124-134
38. Nishizuka, Y. (1984). The role of protein kinase C in cell surface signal transduction and tumour promotion. *Nature*, **308**, 693-698
39. Berridge, M. J. and Irvine, R. F. (1984). Inositol triphosphate, a novel second messenger in cellular signal transduction. *Nature*, **312**, 315-321
40. Coughlin, S. R., Lee, W. M. F., Williams, P. M., Giels, G. M. and Williams, L. T. (1985). *c-myc* gene expression is stimulated by agents that activate protein kinase C and does not account for the mitogenic effect of PDGF. *Cell*, **43**, 243-251
41. Downward, J. and Waterfield, M. D. (1985). The structure and function of the epidermal growth factor receptor: Its relationship to the protein product of the v-*erb*-B oncogene. In Andersson, L. C., Gahmberg, C. G. and Ekblom, P. (eds.) *Gene Expression During Normal and Malignant Differentiation*. pp. 237-243. (London: Academic Press Inc.)
42. Cohen, P. (1980). *Molecular Aspects of Cell Regulation*. Vol. 1 and Vol. 3. (Amsterdam, New York: Elsevier Biomedical Press)
43. Cohen, P. (1982). The role of protein phosphorylation in neural and hormonal control of cellular activity. *Nature*, **296**, 613-620
44. Cohen, P. (1985). The role of protein phosphorylation in the hormonal control of enzyme activity. *Eur. J. Biochem.*, **151**, 439-448

45. Podskalny, J. N., Takeda, S., Silverman, R. E., Tran, D., Carpentier, J-L., Orci, L. and Gorden, P. (1985). Insulin receptors and bioresponses in a human cell line (HEPG-2). *Eur. J. Biochem.*, **150**, 401-407

46. Van Wyk, J. J., Graves, D. C., Casella, S. J. and Jacobs, S. (1985). Evidence from monoclonal antibody studies that insulin stimulates deoxyribonucleic acid synthesis through the Type I somatomedin receptor. *J. Clin. Endocrinol. Metab.*, **61**, 639-643

47. Hochhauser, S. J., Stein, G. S., Stein, J. L. (1981). Regulation of gene expression in normal and neoplastic cells - a review. *Pathobiol. Annu.*, **11**, 1-29

48. Jacob, F. and Monod, J. (1961). Genetic regulatory mechanisms in the synthesis of proteins. *J. Mol. Biol.*, **3**, 318-356

49. Miller, J. H. and Reznikoff, W. S. (eds.) (1978). *The Operon.* (New York: Cold Spring Harbor Laboratory)

50. Serfling, E., Jasin, M. and Schaffner, W. (1985). Enhancers and eukaryotic gene transcription. *Trends Genet.*, **1**, 224-230

51. Yaniv, M. (1984). Regulation of eukaryotic gene expression by transactivating proteins and cis acting DNA elements. *Biol. Cell.*, **50**, 203-216

52. Nagamine, Y. and Reich, E. (1985). Gene expression and cAMP. *Proc. Natl. Acad. Sci. USA*, **82**, 4606-4610

53. Gehring, W. J. (1985). The molecular basis of development. *Sci. Am.*, **253**, 136-146

54. Weinberg, R. A. (1985). The action of oncogenes in the cytoplasm and nucleus. *Science*, **230**, 770-776

55. Adamson, E. D. and Rees, A. R. (1981). Epidermal growth factor receptors. *Mol. Cell Biochem.*, **34**, 129-152

56. Gullick, W. J., Downward, J. and Waterfield, M. D. (1985). Antibodies to the autophosphorylation sites of the epidermal growth factor receptor protein-tyrosine kinase as probes of structure and function. *EMBO J.*, **4**, 2869-2877

57. Gregoriou, M. and Rees, A. R. (1984). Properties of monoclonal antibody to epidermal growth factor receptor with implications for the mechanism of action of EGF. *EMBO J.*, **3**, 929-937

58. Cohen, S. and Fava, R. A. (1985). Internalization of functional epidermal growth factor receptor-kinase complexes in A-431 cells. *J. Biol. Chem.*, **260**, 12351-12358

59. Cohen, S., Carpenter, G. and King, L. (1980). Epidermal growth factor-receptor-protein kinase interactions. *J. Biol. Chem.*, **255**, 4834-4842

60. Giugni, T. D., James, L. C. and Haigler, H. T. (1985). Epidermal growth factor stimulates tyrosine phosphorylation of specific proteins in permeabilized human fibroblasts. *J. Biol. Chem.*, **260**, 15081-15090

61. Cooper, J. A., Bowen-Pope, D. F., Raines, E., Ross, R. and Hunter, T. (1982). Similar effects of platelet-derived growth factor and epidermal growth factor on the phosphorylation of tyrosine in cellular proteins. *Cell*, **31**, 263-273

62. Foulkes, J. G. and Rich-Rosner, M. R. (1985). Tyrosine-specific protein kinase as mediators of growth control. In Cohen, P. and Houslay, M. D. (eds.) *Molecular Aspects of Cellular Regulation*. Vol. 4, pp. 217-252. (Amsterdam, New York, London: Elsevier)

63. Hunter, T. and Cooper, J. A. (1985). Protein-tyrosine kinases. *Annu. Rev. Biochem.*, **54**, 897-930

64. Downward, J., Waterfield, M. D. and Parker, P. (1985). Autophosphorylation and protein kinase C phosphorylation of the epidermal growth factor receptor. *J. Biol. Chem.*, **260**, 14538-14546

65. Bertics, P. J., Weber, W., Cochet, C. and Gill, G. N. (1985). Regulation of the epidermal growth factor receptor by phosphorylation. *J. Cell Biochem.*, **29**, 195-208

66. Fearn, J. C. and King, A. C. (1985). EGF receptor affinity is regulated by intracellular calcium and protein kinase C. *Cell*, **40**, 991-1000

67. Collins, M. K. L., Sinnett-Smith, J. W. and Rozengurt, E. (1983). Platelet-derived growth factor treatment decreases the affinity of the epidermal growth factor receptor of Swiss 3T3 cells. *J. Biol. Chem.*, **258**, 11689-11693

68. Haley, J., Kinchington, D., Whittle, N., Ullrich, A. and Waterfield, M. D. (1986). The epidermal growth factor receptor gene. In Guroff, G. (ed.) *Growth and Maturation Factors*. Vol. 4. (New York: John Wiley and Sons) (In press)

69. Bishop, J. M. (1983). Cellular oncogenes and retroviruses. *Annu. Rev. Biochem.*, **52**, 301-354

70. Bishop, J. M. (1985). Viral oncogenes. *Cell*, **42**, 23-38
71. Slamon, D. J., de Kernion, J. B., Verma, I. M. and Cline, M. J. (1984). Expression of cellular oncogenes in human malignancies. *Science*, **224**, 256-262
72. Marshall, C. J. (1985). Human oncogenes. In Weiss, R., Teich, N., Varmus, H. and Coffin, J. (eds.) *RNA Tumor Viruses*. Vol. 2, pp. 487--558. (New York: Cold Spring Harbor Laboratory)
73. Weinberg, R. A. (1983). A molecular basis for cancer. *Sci. Am.*, **249**, 102-116
74. Heldin, C. H., Johnsson, A., Wennergren, S., Wernstedt, C., Betsholtz, C. and Westermark, B. (1986). A human osteosarcoma cell line secretes a growth factor structurally related to a homodimer of PDGF A-chains. *Nature*, **319**, 511-514
75. Rozengurt, E., Sinnett-Smith, J. and Taylor-Papadimitriou, J. (1985). Production of PDGF-like growth factor by breast cancer cell lines. *Int. J. Cancer*, **36**, 247-252
76. Duel, T., Huang, J. S., Huang, S. S., Stroobant, P. and Waterfield, M. D. (1983). Expression of a platelet-derived growth factor-like protein in simian sarcoma virus transformed cells. *Science*, **221**, 1348-1350
77. Heldin, C. H., Wasteson, A. and Westermark, B. (1985). Platelet-derived growth factor. *Mol. Cell. Endocrinol.*, **39**, 169-187
78. Cuttitta, F., Carney, D. N., Mulshine, J., Moody, T. W., Fedorko, J., Fischler, A. and Minna, J. D. (1985). Bombesin-like peptides can function as autocrine growth factors in human small-cell lung cancer. *Nature*, **316**, 823-826
79. Gordon, J., Ley, S. C. Melamed, M. D., English, L. S. and Hughes-Jones, N. C. (1984). Immortilized B lymphocytes produce B-cell growth factor. *Nature*, **310**, 145-147
80. Frykberg, L., Palmieri, S., Beug, H., Graf, T., Hayman, M. J. and Vennstrom, B. (1983). Transforming capacities of avian erythroblastosis virus mutants deleted in the *erb* A or *erb* B oncogenes. *Cell*, **32**, 227-238
81. Downward, J., Yarden, Y., Mayes, E., Scrace, G., Totty, N., Stockwell, P., Ullrich, A., Schlessinger, J. and Waterfield, M.D. (1984). Close similarity of epidermal growth factor receptor and v-*erb*-B oncogene protein sequences. *Nature*, **307**, 521-527
82. Bargmann, C., Hung, M-C., and Weinberg, R. A. (1986). The *neu* oncogene encodes an epidermal growth factor receptor-related protein. *Nature*, **319**, 226-230
83. Sherr, C. J., Rettenmier, C. W., Sacca, R., Roussel, M. F., Look, A. T. and Stanley, E. R. (1985). The c-*fms* proto-oncogene product is related to the receptor for the mononuclear phagocyte growth factor, CSF-1. *Cell*, **41**, 665-676
84. Bauknecht, T., Gross, G. and Hagedorn, M. (1985). Epidermal growth factor receptors in different skin tumors. *Dermatologica*, **171**, 16-20
85. Hendler, F. J. and Ozanne, B. W. (1984). Human squamous cell lung cancers express increased epidermal growth factor receptors. *J. Clin. Invest.*, **74**, 647-651
86. Ozanne, B., Shum, A., Richards, C. S., Cassells, D., Grossman, D., Trent, J., Gusterson, B. and Hendler, F. (1985). Evidence for an increase of EGF receptors in epidermoid malignancies. *Cancer Cells*, **3**, 41-49
87. Gullick, W. J., Marsden, J. J., Whittle, N., Ward, B., Bobrow, L. and Waterfield, M.D. (1986). Expression of epidermal growth factor receptors on human cervical, ovarian, and vulval carcinomas. *Cancer Res.*, **46**, 285-292
88. Libermann, T. A., Razon, N., Bartal, A. D., Yarden, Y., Schlessinger, J. and Soreq, H. (1984). Expression of epidermal growth factor receptors in human brain tumors. *Cancer Res.*, **44**, 753-760
89. Libermann, T. A., Nusbaum, H. R., Razon, N., Kris, R., Lax, I., Soreq, H., Whittle, N., Waterfield, M., Ullrich, A. and Schlessinger, J. (1985). Amplification, enhanced expression and possible rearrangement of EGF receptor gene in primary human brain tumors of glial origin. *Nature*, **313**, 144-147
90. Neal, D. E., Marsh, C., Bennett, M. K., Abel, P. D., Hall, R. R., Sainsbury, J. R. C. and Harris, A. L. (1985). Epidermal growth factor receptors in human bladder cancer: comparison of invasive and superficial tumors. *Lancet*, i, 366-368
91. Xu, Y-H., Richert, N., Ito, S., Merlino, G. T. and Pastan, I. (1984). Characterization of epidermal growth factor receptor gene expression in malignant and normal cell lines. *Proc. Natl. Acad. Sci. USA*, **81**, 7308, 7312
92. Stoscheck, C. M. and Carpenter, G. (1983). Biology of the A431 cell: A useful organism for hormone research. *J. Cell. Biochem.*, **23**, 191-202
93. Lin, C. R., Chen, W. S., Kruiger, W., Stolarsky, L. S., Weber, W., Evans, R. M., Verma, I.

M., Gill, G. N. and Rosenfeld, M. G. (1984). Expression cloning of human EGF receptor complementary DNA; gene amplification and three related messenger RNA products in A431 cells. *Science*, **224**, 843-848

94. Gilman, A. G. (1984). G proteins and dual control of adenylate cyclase. *Cell*, **36**, 577-579
95. McGrath, J. P., Capon, D. J., Goeddel, D. V. and Levinson, A. D. (1984). Comparative biochemical properties of normal and activated human *ras* p21 protein. *Nature*, **310**, 644-649
96. Reddy, E. P., Reynolds, R. K., Santos, E. and Barbacid, M. (1982). A point mutation is responsible for the acquisition of transforming properties by the T24 human bladder carcinoma oncogene. *Nature*, **300**, 149-152
97. Persson, H. and Leder, P. (1984). Nuclear location and DNA binding properties of a protein expressed by human c-*myc* oncogene. *Science*, **225**, 718-721
98. Ralston, R. and Bishop, J. M. (1983). The protein products of the *myc* and *myb* oncogenes and adenovirus Ela are structurally related. *Nature*, **306**, 803-806
99. Pfeifer-Ohlsson, S., Rydnert, J., Goustin, A. S., Larsson, E., Betsholtz, C. and Ohlsson, R. (1985). Cell-type-specific pattern of *myc* protooncogene expression in developing human embryos. *Proc. Natl. Acad. Sci. USA*, **82**, 5050-5054
100. Thompson, C. B., Challoner, P. B., Neiman, P. E. and Groudine, M. (1985). Levels of c-*myc* oncogene mRNA are invariant throughout the cell cycle. *Nature*, **314**, 363-366
101. Kohl, N. E., Legouy, E., DePinho, R. A., Nisen, P. D., Smith, R. K., Gee, C. E. and Alt, F. W. (1986). Human N-*myc* is closely related in organization and nucleotide sequence to c-*myc*. *Nature*, **319**, 73-77
102. Schwab, M., Varmus, H. E. and Bishop, J. M. (1985). Human N-*myc* contributes to neoplastic transformation of mammalian cells in cell culture. *Nature*, **316**, 160-162
103. Croce, C. M., Tsujimoto, Y., Erikson, J. and Nowell, P. (1984). Chromosomal translocations and B cell neoplasia. *Lab. Invest.*, **51**, 258-267
104. Klein, G. and Klein, E. (1985). Evolution of tumors and the impact of molecular oncology. *Nature*, **315**, 190-195
105. Land, H., Parada, L. F. and Weinberg, R. A. (1983). Cellular oncogenes and multi-step carcinogenesis. *Science*, **222**, 771-778
106. Schwab, M., Ellison, J., Busch, M., Rosenau, W., Varmus, H. E. and Bishop, J. M. (1984). Enhanced expression of the human gene N-*myc* consequent to amplification of DNA may contribute to malignant progression of neuroblastoma. *Proc. Natl. Acad. Sci. USA*, **81**, 4940-4944
107. Seeger, R. C., Brodeur, G. M., Sather, H., Dalton, A., Siegel, S. E., Wong, K. Y. and Hammond, D. (1985). Association of multiple copies of the N-*myc* oncogene with rapid progression of neuroblastomas. *N. Engl. J. Med.*, **313**, 1111-1116

4
The cellular basis of carcinogenesis

D.C. BENNETT

INTRODUCTION

Cellular oncology covers an ill-delineated set of topics, some of which overlap with the clinical level of analysis, like 'invasiveness', others with the molecular level, like 'autocrine growth stimulation', and yet others which are more essentially biological, like questions of cell lineage. Our knowledge of the cellular basis of carcinogenesis includes subjects from each of these areas. To review this large field it will be helpful to divide it on the basis firstly of the initiation of cancers - in other words the cells from which cancers arise - and secondly of cancer growth. Both these topics are far from completely understood, and are the subjects of a variety of research. Some major aspects, especially of cancer growth are treated in other chapters. Here I shall survey the types of evidence available and some current ideas, concluding with possible applications and future prospects for research. This short review will not be comprehensive, but where possible the issues will be argued from selected concrete examples rather than in the abstract.

Carcinogenesis will be taken to mean the production of a malignant (invasive) tumour from normal tissue. Haemopoietic neoplasms will be included for convenience in the term 'tumour'. Benign tumours cannot be altogether excluded from the discussion, partly because of the possibility that malignant tumours develop from benign ones and partly because it is impossible in practice to draw a clear line between the two. Instead tumours show a spectrum of different degrees of malignancy[1-4].

CELLS FROM WHICH CANCERS ARISE

Clonal origin of cancers

A central aspect of the origin of cancers is the question of the number of normal cells from which a cancer arises. It is widely believed that the answer is one - that cancers are monoclonal. The evidence behind this belief will now be examined.

Firstly there is a statistical argument: for a cancer to contain two or more clones, all component steps of carcinogenesis[1,2] (Chapters 1 and 2) must occur separately in two or more normal cells. The incidence of this should be no higher than the incidence of two separate cancers in one patient which is normally very low. This is a strong argument unless there is a positive interaction between neighbouring clones at an early stage, as some have suggested[5-7]; see also Chapter 9.

The remaining arguments are empirical, and are well reviewed by Fialkow[8,9]. These are based on evidence for the monoclonal *composition* of tumours, which is not the same as monoclonal *origin* because several abnormal clones present at an early stage might later be superseded by a single one[10,5-7]. There is evidence that this can occur in experimental carcinogenesis[5-7] (Chapter 9). A powerful indicator of monoclonal composition is the synthesis of a single species of immunoglobulin by the neoplastic cells in multiple myeloma, chronic lymphocytic leukaemia and other lymphoproliferative disorders[8]. For other human tumours the chief method of analysis has involved women heterozygous for two alleles of the X-linked gene for glucose-6-phosphate dehydrogenase (G6PD). These women are mosaics of many patches of about 1000–10 000 cells[8], each descended from a single cell at the time of X-chromosome inactivation, and thus containing only one of the two isoenzymes[7-9]. Their tumours almost invariably contain only one isoenzyme. From the number of tumours studied it can be concluded that most tumours are monoclonal in composition. However, the possibility of polyclonal origin from cells which were originally in close proximity cannot be excluded by such data, for such cells will almost always share the same isoenzyme.

There are manifest exceptions: G6PD studies show specific types of benign tumour to be multiclonal[8,9,11]. Not surprisingly these include some virally-caused tumours such as venereal warts[8]. The rest involve an hereditary predisposition, where the individual tends to have numerous tumours, such as multiple neurofibromatosis and polyposis coli[11]. It is interesting that malignant neurofibrosarcoma, when developed within such a neurofibroma, appears monoclonal in composition, as does hereditary thyroid carcinoma, which is thought to arise in one of multiple hyperplastic thyroid cell clones[12]. In considering whether to view these cancers as monoclonal in origin, a useful criterion would be whether the several component clones in each benign lesion grew independently; if they grew interdependently then the cancer would be considered polyclonal in origin. I am not aware of evidence on this, but it may also be relevant to non-hereditary human cancers. These too commonly arise from discrete 'premalignant' lesions, which may represent the expression of some early step(s) of carcinogenesis[2,13] (Chapter 1); and benign lesions are often numerous in a cancer-bearing organ[2,13,14].

In summary, all human non-viral cancers appear to be monoclonal in composition, but it is not certain whether an early stage of carcinogenesis sometimes involves an interaction between more than one abnormal clone.

Stem cells: concepts

To our next question, as to what types of cells are targets for carcinogenesis, a

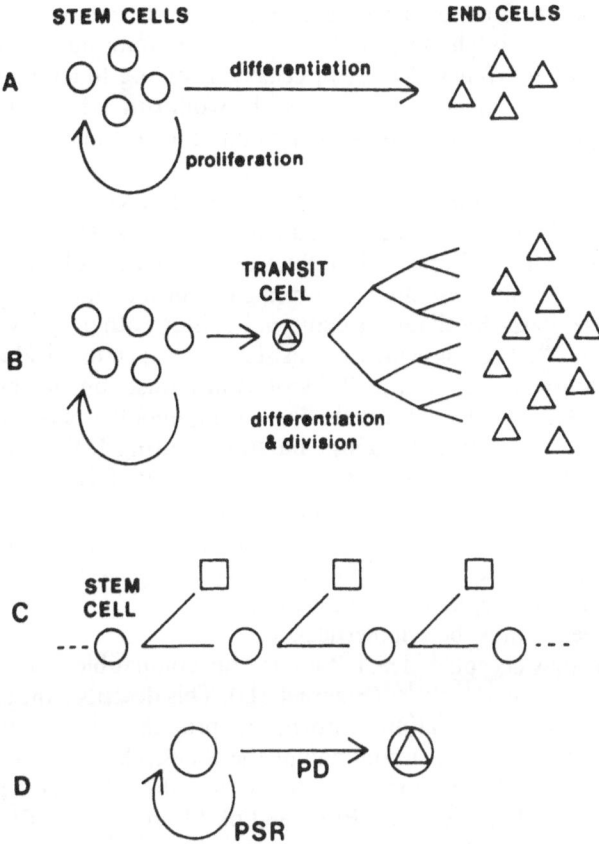

Figure 4.1 Stem cell concepts. In (D), PSR means probability of self-renewal and PD means probability of differentiation. See text for further explanation

popular reply would be that cancers arise from and contain stem cells. I shall argue that at present there is little evidence for this as a generality; but to examine the evidence critically, one needs a clear definition of a stem cell. Unfortunately, there are several conflicting views as to what stem cells are[6,15].

Few authors would disagree with the broad but vague idea that normal stem cells are proliferative reserve cells which produce and maintain a non-proliferative, specialized cell population ('end cells') by both differentiation and production of more stem cells ('self-renewal')[15-22] (Figure 4.1A). It is well established that mature vertebrate tissues with rapid cellular turnover, such as most blood cells, epidermis and digestive tract epithelia, are maintained in this way but with each differentiating ('transit') cell proliferating to produce a number of end cells[15-19] (Figure 4.1B). Viewed in this way, stem cells of this kind and in these tissues are physically different from end cells, largely lacking their distinctive shapes, sizes and products. Some tissues like liver and kidney, in which cellular turnover is normally slow and is apparently achieved by division of mature functional cells, are thought not to contain any stem cells as thus defined, although this has not been proven. Some authors describe all cells capable of self-renewal as stem cells[17], including functional liver cells and, presumably, amoebae. I agree with Woodruff[6] that such a broad definition renders the term almost redundant, and this meaning will not be used here.

One specific definition is that a stem cell is a cell which undergoes asymmetrical division – always producing one new stem cell and one differentiating cell[20-22] (Figure 4.1C). Such cells have been observed in insects and nematodes[20], but there are no proven cases in mammals. Asymmetrical division occurs in the 8-cell mouse embryo, but here both progeny differ from the parent cell[23,20]. There is evidence consistent with asymmetrical retention of radiolabelled DNA after some cell divisions in mouse tongue and intestinal epithelium[21]. This would support the interesting hypothesis of Cairns[22] that stem cells may be protected against mutations during DNA replication by (asymmetrical) segregation of the newly-synthesised DNA strands into a transit cell at each division. However the evidence is inconclusive[21]. Moreover, asymmetrical division can at most maintain a constant number of stem cells, whereas stem cells of blood and epithelia are known to increase their number after depletion by tissue damage[15-19,21]. Thus some stem cell divisions, at least, must be symmetrical.

An increasingly accepted idea, but not readily compatible with the previous one, is that of Till et al.[15-18,24,25] (Figure 4.1D). This describes the initiation of self-renewal and differentiation as stochastic (probabilistic) events, generally occurring in interphase. To accommodate the changeable rates of production of stem cells and end cells in response to varying physiological requirements, the probabilities of self-renewal (PSR) and of differentiation (PD) are often considered to be changeable in response to homeostatic signals. Stochastic models fit the kinetics of differentiation for a number of cell types[16,17,24,25], although they cannot be considered as proven without some information on the molecular basis of the putative control events. A related idea of potential importance in the context of carcinogenesis is the 'stem cell continuum' model[19,15]. This suggests that in stem cell progeny which have initiated differentiation, possibly by movement away from a localized 'stem cell niche', the potential for self-renewal is lost, not abruptly but gradually, over several divisions. In terms of the stochastic model, the PSR would fall gradually and the PD would also rise gradually[19]: thus commitment to differentiate would also not be abrupt. This accounts for observations that the number of 'potential' stem cells (capable of regeneration after damage) in certain tissues is greater than the number of stem cells normally functional in turnover[19,15]. It is also consistent with evidence for gradual commitment in cultured cells[25].

There are also some operational definitions of stem cells, that is, assays. Radiobiological assays for 'functional' and 'potential' stem cells in vivo are reviewed by Wright and Alison[15]. There are also assays applicable in vitro (Figure 4.2). In what is sometimes called the 'tumour stem cell' assay[27,28], a tissue is disaggregated to single cells which are cultured for some weeks in soft agar by one of two main methods[27,29] (Figure 4.2A). Usually a very small proportion of tumour cells, and no cells from normal tissues, form

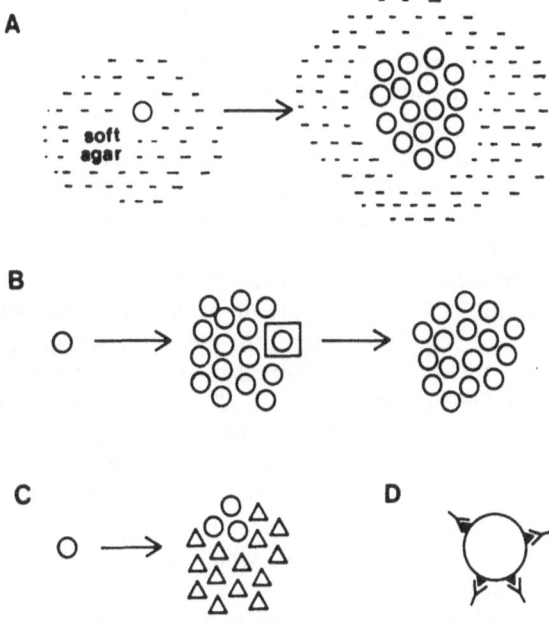

Figure 4.2 Operational definitions of stem cells
(A) For 'tumour clonogenic cells': colony formation in soft agar under specific conditions.
(B) Production of secondary colonies after recloning, a test applied under various conditions of culture, not necessarily in soft agar, or *in vivo*[16]. In (A) and (B) the symbols indicate 'cells of unspecified type(s)'. (C) Clonal analysis. The cells may be grown in culture under various conditions[12,13,16] or *in vivo*[16]. The stem cell is defined as producing a clone containing cells both like itself and more mature. Criteria for identifying the different cells depend on the particular lineage studied. (D) Specific cellular markers (see text)

macroscopic colonies (of at least about 20 cells). These cells were originally postulated to be tumour stem cells[27]. The term 'clonogenic' cells is now prevalent however[26,29,30], and is preferable because, among other reasons, some transit cells can apparently produce much more than 20 progeny[17]. The idea is that possibly only a fraction of tumour cells can renew themselves (discussed below); that these are the important cells in maintaining tumour growth, and hence cultures of such cells might be used for the testing of chemotherapeutic regimes before treatment of the patient (see for example refs. 26–30). Some predictive value has already been claimed[26]. However, these findings require substantial confirmation and considerable problems remain, as reviewed by Hill[30]. In particular there is evidence that the few cells which form colonies are not a unique subpopulation. From studies with cell lines, the apparent proportion of clonogenic cells in a given population varies widely with varying culture conditions[30,31]. Some tumours, including breast cancers, yield a negligible number of colonies or none[26]. Reproducibility of the results is often very poor[26]. A good deal more work is therefore required on these points. The exact nature of the cells isolated is, of course, much less important than the question of whether responses to therapy can be predicted.

Normal haemopoietic stem cells are sometimes distinguished from transit cells in culture by the ability of cells from a primary colony to form new colonies after replating, a crude test of 'self-renewal'[32] (Figure 4.2B). It does not seem helpful at present to apply this double test to human tumour primary cultures, despite a few attempts[26]; the problems of low yield and variability are much exacerbated, and again the population obtained is unlikely to be unique.

Stem cells can be defined more specifically, by clonal analysis, as cells of which one can produce a colony containing both similar and differentiating progeny cells (Figure 4.2C). This requires the use of specific morphological or antigenic markers, at least for the differentiated cells. Indeed the stem cells themselves can be defined by the possession of specific markers (Figure 4.2D), where this correlates with stem cell behaviour, say by clonal analysis. These last two tests are valuable, allowing the direct identification and characterization of stem cells and indeed other populations from various tissues[32-36], including cancers. This could lead to a more rational classification of cancers, and more precise prognoses, which are already beginning to be achieved with the leukaemias[34].

In the remainder of this chapter, 'stem cells' will be defined as in Figure 4.1B, and, where applicable, Figures 4.2C and 4.2D.

Stem cells: targets of carcinogenesis?

For some target tissues the degree of morphological differentiation of tumours is roughly inversely correlated to their malignancy[1,3,4], although the two trends are separable[2]. A possible and widely-suggested explanation is that it is stem cells which become malignant and that this entails impaired differentiation[3,28,34,37]. An analysis of the evidence for this idea, rather as with monoclonality, resolves into two parts: do cancers *contain* malignant stem cells, and do they *originate* from normal stem cells?

The former part can be clearly answered for some types of cancer. The answer varies, as a few examples will illustrate. Certain transplantable rodent squamous-cell and embryoid carcinomas continually produce histologically well-differentiated areas after transplantation. If the differentiated areas are transplanted separately, no tumour develops[38]. The conclusion is that the original malignant cells are behaving like stem cells, and producing differentiated progeny which, however, are non-neoplastic. With squamous skin cancers the histological organization suggests that cells equivalent to normal stem cells of the basal layer - or to those of the suprabasal layer, thought to be potential stem cells[2] - are present and are malignant. Teratocarcinomas yield a rather different result, which illustrates a wider problem of terminology. It is believed that teratocarcinomas arise from embryonic primordial germ cells. Now these cells are not stem cells, because normally all of them are thought to mature into late germ cell precursors rather than reproducing themselves indefinitely. Should cells which acquire stem-cell characteristics only when neoplastic be called stem cells? It is a widespread practice and so dispute may well be futile. However in that case it is important to realise that neoplastic 'stem cells' may not have arisen from normal stem cells. I prefer to describe the neoplastic self-renewing cells by a term such as 'generative cells', which does not allow this misleading implication.

There has recently been much progress in the identification of the malignant cell populations present in human leukaemias (for reviews see refs. 8, 18, 33, 34). Chronic myelocytic (or myeloid) leukaemia (CML) provides a most illuminating example. CML is characterized as an overabundance of immature granulocytes in the blood and bone marrow. Numbers of mature blood cells of other lineages are close to normal, but progenitors of granulocytes, erythrocytes and megakaryocytes are all overabundant[39,40]. Moreover all the normal blood cells except some lymphocytes are descended from the same clone as the leukaemic cells; they all contain the same G6PD isoenzyme in heterozygotes and all nucleated cells show the mutant Philadelphia chromosome, when present in the leukaemic cells[39,8,7,34]. These findings imply that pluripotent stem cells are mutant and hyperplastic – cells capable of engendering all the blood cell lineages[8,34,39]. However malignancy is overt only in the granulocyte lineage, where maturation is also deficient[33,34]. Thus one could say that the pluripotent stem cells are not exactly malignant in CML but they do appear to be generative cells of the leukaemia. This behaviour perhaps involves translocation of an oncogene close to a transcriptional promoter active in granulocyte precursors, by analogy with mechanisms in other cancers (Chapter 2).

Permanent cultured cell lines have been derived from a number of human (as well as animal) leukaemias, of which many resemble unipotent myeloid precursors such as pre-erythroid or pregranulocytic cells[32]. This suggests that transit cells have gained or retained self-renewal potential in these leukaemias, as discussed by Greaves[34] and Sachs[41]. It is also possible however that normal, unipotent, myeloid stem cells exist and are targets for carcinogenesis; our understanding of haemopoietic lineages is good but nonetheless incomplete[32,34]. Perhaps there is a 'stem cell continuum' (as discussed above) in bone marrow. If pregranulocytic cells are self-renewing in CML then this disease is characterized by at least two generative cell populations, these and pluripotent cells.

The last example in this section will be breast cancer. Normal female breast epithelium has an unusual proliferative pattern, with rapid division only in pregnancy and full differentiation only in lactation[42,43]. Our understanding of breast cell lineages is still largely speculative, although the rat has perhaps provided a useful model system[36,44-47], and analytical lineage studies on the human breast and its tumours have begun[48-51]. Studies of rat mammary glands and tumours, using cell culture, ultrastructural and immunological markers, suggest that there are bipotent stem cells which can generate both the secretory and myoepithelial cells of the lactating gland[36,44-47]. These stem cells are probably found principally in the growing tips of immature glands[45,46], and appear to be capable of becoming malignant in the rat[36]. In the human breast, bipotent stem cells have not been unequivocally identified, but a luminal epithelial subpopulation has tentatively been identified as a later type of stem cell, possibly unipotent and presecretory, on the basis of a cytoskeletal antigen and cell culture studies[49,51]. These cells were not overabundant but apparently absent in nearly all of 141 breast carcinomas examined[50]. The carcinoma cells instead usually carried an antigen present in more mature presecretory cells. Consistently, a study using other specific markers indicated that myoepithelial cells were rare or absent in most ductal breast carcinomas[48]. A tentative conclusion is that late, presecretory cells may be the commonest malignant cells present in human breast cancer, although alternatively these may be benign and maintained by a small malignant stem cell population[50]. These conclusions are vague, and much more work is needed to account for the many subclasses of breast cancer[1-3].

To conclude this section it will be helpful to summarize the reasons why the cells which are finally malignant may differ in type from the normal cells which originally underwent carcinogenesis - the true target cells. Let us suppose that we have identified a malignant population as equivalent to a particular normal precursor cell type, P. Then there are many possible target cells (Figure 4.3). These may have been P cells. They may have been an earlier precursor cell type E, as seems to be the case with CML. The target may have been a more mature cell type M, provided such cells are long-lived (this might occur in the breast, for example), as carcinogenesis takes many years in

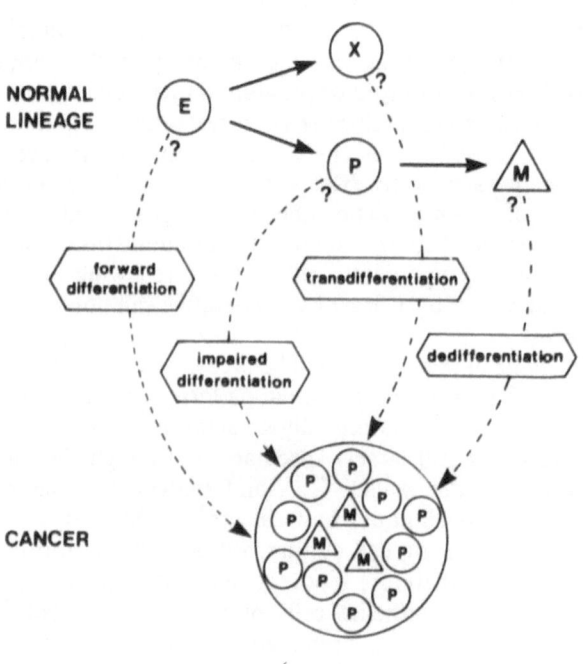

Figure 4.3 Possible target cells of carcinogenesis. See text for explanation

humans (Chapter 1). This would require dedifferentiation of the M cells, a concept which some readers may find hard to accept. However it was supported by Foulds[2], and several recent reports have presented strong evidence for true destabilization and regression of normally stable forms of mammalian cell differentiation (reviewed[52,53]). The phenomenon is well established in other vertebrates and other phyla.

Mammalian cells are also capable of 'transdifferentiation' or switching to a different lineage (reviewed[52,53]), as in the production of muscle cells by a cloned rat neuroblastoma. Many of the known cases have involved cultured tumour cells, leading to the idea that the stability of differentiation might sometimes be disrupted in neoplasia[53,54]. There is also widespread but inconclusive evidence for transdifferentiation in tumours *in vivo*, in the form of metaplasia, altered differentiation in an intact tissue[2,4,54]. For example some breast cancers contain bone and cartilage[2]. However, metaplasia may also result from selective growth of a rare cell type. Farber argues that normal cells, such as liver cells, may enter unusual but entirely physiological states of differentiation in metabolic response to unusual stimuli such as carcinogens, and that some precancerous lesions represent just such altered states rather than mutations[13]. Bissell has similarly suggested that cells in culture can adopt unusual states of differentiation[55]. Thus we cannot exclude the possibility of transdifferentiation (Figure 4.3), or even less readily classifiable changes of cellular state, in carcinogenesis.

To summarize, there seem to be few cases where we can even guess at the true target cell for specific cancers. These are generally cases where only one long-lived cell type is known in the affected tissue, such as mature hepatocytes.

CELLULAR ENVIRONMENT AND CANCER DEVELOPMENT

We now turn from the initiation to the growth of cancers and factors affecting that growth. Intracellular mechanisms and specific growth factors are discussed in Chapters 2 and 3, and systemic host effects in Chapter 9. It remains here to review local environmental influences on tumour development.

Biologists commonly assert that tumour growth differs from that of normal tissues in being autonomous or independent of the host organism. This is perhaps a case where the biologist could have been enlightened by the clinician. Even if we exclude as trivial the fact that the tissue environment supplies nutrients to and elutes waste products from a tumour, there is much and diverse evidence that tumour growth is influenced by this environment.

Effects of stroma

Normal stromal components are often interspersed with a solid tumour. The stroma may include blood vessels, leukocytes and fibroblasts with various types of extracellular matrix[1-3]. Vascularization and the roles of infiltrating leukocytes are included in Chapter 9; see also articles discussing host defences in relation to metastasis[4,56-58]. Before considering the effects of fibrous stroma on tumours, some perspective may be provided by a brief review of the influences of mesenchyme on normal epithelia and other cells.

These interactions have often been studied by separating pieces of epithelium and mesenchyme from various animal organs, physically recombining these in various ways and observing the results after culture or re-implantation. Morphogenesis of embryonic epithelia was often changed by the presence of a foreign mesenchyme[59]. For example mouse mammary epithelium apposed to salivary gland mesenchyme grew with a salivary-like branching pattern[60]. In this case only shape was changed, not biochemical differentiation, for such salivary-like glands could still respond to hormonal stimuli *in vivo* by apparent lactation and synthesis of α-lactalbumin[61]. Conversely pancreatic mesenchyme apparently could induce pancreatic differentiation and secretion by salivary epithelium, as judged by electron microscopy[62]. Persistence of this effect when the tissues were separated by a filter indicated a diffusible mediator, possibly unpolymerized collagen[62]. Many such inductive influences of mesenchyme have since been described, on neural crest and mesenchymal cell types as well as on epithelia[59]. There is evidence that many of these effects are mediated by the extracellular matrix, which includes collagen, fibronectin, hyaluronate and other glycos-aminoglycans (reviewed[59]).

Studies of the influence of mesenchyme and its matrix on tumour cells are much less numerous, but include some striking observations. One is the induction of tubular morphogenesis in an anaplastic mouse mammary adenocarcinoma by embryonic mammary mesenchyme; tumour cell proliferation was also slightly reduced[63]. Cloned rat mammary carcinoma cells were used to show that the morphogenesis of branching tubules did not require stromal cells at all, a gel of tendon collagen being sufficient[64]. Fibronectin was isolated as a 'transformation-sensitive' protein; virally-transformed fibroblasts apparently failed to synthesize it and moreover the purified protein could change the morphology of such transformed cells back to that of normal fibroblasts in culture[65]. Now transformation of cultured cells, especially as described for fibroblasts, is not the same as malignancy, as cell biologists fortunately now realise[66]. Nonetheless, exposure to fibronectin was recently found to decrease the experimental metastatic potential in mice (a true aspect of malignancy) of B16 melanoma cells[67]. Laminin, a component of basement membrane, increased this potential[67]. These and other isolated observations suggest that further investigations of stromal effects on tumour growth and malignancy may be medically useful.

Effects of stroma on a tumour cannot be viewed independently of reciprocal effects of the tumour upon the stroma. The very maintenance of a stroma by tumour tissue is one such effect, and is to some extent a favourable prognostic feature[3,4]. Growth of a fibrous capsule around a tumour is a classical, although not universal, sign of benign nature, and may be a form of defence by the host[1,3]. In this connection an assay has been developed for a 'host mesodermal response', comprising implantation of tumour cells into early chick embryos in short-term culture[4]. In a positive response, chick mesenchymal cells move to surround the implant. The extent of this response does correlate inversely with estimates of malignancy of the implanted cells, when animal tissues or tumours are tested. This and other responses of the chick embryonic tissue are under study as possible prognostic indicators in human cancer[4].

Other environmental influences

The 'seed and soil' idea, that tumour growth depends both on the particular tumour (seed) and its location in the body (soil), was attributed to Fuchs by Paget[68]. Over nearly a century the idea has been well substantiated. Some clear evidence arises from the transplantation of replicate samples of animal tumours to different sites. One surprising result involved the cranio-caudal axis. A transplantable mammary tumour and a sarcoma, implanted subcutaneously in mice at points along this axis, both showed maximum growth rates near the head, decreasing progressively in the caudal and cranial directions[69]. A perhaps more explicable variation was shown by an oestrogen-responsive human mammary tumour cell line. When implanted in immunodeficient mice, these cells formed small, benign tumours in lung and subcutaneous sites, but large, invasive lesions in brain, uterus and other organs which had the common property of being rich in oestrogen[70]. It is significant that not only the proliferation but also the invasiveness of these cells varied with location. As mentioned earlier, malignancy is not a unitary property but a variable quantity[1-4]. It can now be added that this quantity is not specified completely in the genes of the tumour, but can also depend on the environment (discussed further below).

Paget's original observation was that breast cancers metastasized to specific sites, such as liver and bone, more often than expected by chance[68]. Other classes of cancer also show preferred sites of secondary growth[3,4,56,58]. The factors affecting metastatic spread have been reviewed comprehensively and recently[4,56,58], and therefore this important field will not be discussed at length. Briefly to summarize, there are general factors, like the physical routes available for dissemination, which affect metastatic spread and there are also more specific factors. For example different sublines of the same mouse tumours were developed, which selectively metastasized to various different organs, simply by serial transplantation of secondary tumours which did arise in each chosen organ[56,71]. The molecular bases of these specificities are not known, although a number of possibilities are under investigation[58,67].

The environmental factors affecting tumour cell growth include the effects of other tumour cells, and not only simple autocrine effects (see Chapter 3). Tumours and especially human cancers are often highly heterogeneous[1-4,6,10,56,58,72]. Some of the heterogeneity is environmental, as where non-vascularized tumours show central necrosis[1]. Some is genetic[72]; some is epigenetic (clonally heritable without primary genetic coding, like states of differentiation)[4,73]. Epigenetic variation includes the occurrence of cell differentiation in tumours (see above), and may include less well-understood phenomena[58,73]. For example subclones of the B16 melanoma show widely divergent metastatic potentials in mice[72], and the metastatic properties of a given subclone can shift rapidly in culture[73], apparently too rapidly for genetic mutation[58]. However these rapid shifts were not observed in mixtures of the subclones, suggesting some stabilizing interaction between the clones[73,58]. It is possible that these effects were connected with spontaneous cell differentiation: our recent observations reveal that differentiated, pigmented B16 cells exhibit a markedly higher rate of experimental metastasis than do unpigmented cells[74]. Different clones in the same tumour may interact, then (reviewed[75]); there is also evidence for interaction between different tumours in the same host, with mutual effects on growth rates[75].

An extreme type of environmental effect on tumour growth occurs where malignancy is completely abolished by transplantation to a particular site. A famous experiment was the implantation of single cells of a highly malignant mouse teratocarcinoma into early mouse embryos, which were then replaced to develop in female mice. Often the progeny of the malignant cell became normal, differentiating into many types of cell and tissue, sometimes including germ cells from which normal mice could be bred[76-78]. This remarkable result indicated that some teratocarcinoma cells were genetically normal and diploid: their malignancy was not genetically determined. Now cancer cells are not in general genetically normal and diploid (Chapter 2). Nonetheless even presumably aneuploid tumour cells can sometimes be similarly 'normalized' by transplantation, although not to the extent of producing normal germ cells and descendant mice. These include mouse neuroblastoma cells put into neurula-stage embryos[79], myeloid leukaemic cells implanted in placenta[80] and mouse erythroleukaemic spleen cells transferred to irradiated mice[81]. In the latter two cases, differentiated progeny of the tumour cells were detected[80,81]. It has been speculated that such observations reflect a retention of responsiveness to signals which induce differentiation of the corresponding normal cells[78,41].

PERSPECTIVE: APPLICATIONS AND POSSIBLE DEVELOPMENTS

This last section will be concerned with the extent to which the topics discussed above may prove relevant to the prevention or treatment of human cancer, now or through future research.

It is appropriate to begin with the 'clonogenic tumour cells' assay, some of whose proponents envisage a time when its use to select chemotherapeutic agents and to monitor treatment will be as routine as the culture of bacteria to test their susceptibility to antibiotics[26]. This seems a worthy goal but, as already discussed, there is no evidence yet that the assay will be useful for many forms of cancer. Much more work is needed, on such problems as improvement of the culture methods and examining their possible diversification for application to more types of cancer[30].

The further problem of which cells grow in such assays[30] is connected with the next subject: the identity of the generative cells and of the malignant cells in particular cancers. Leukaemia research has demonstrated that progress on this subject depends on a detailed understanding of normal cell lineages.

Although knowledge of even the haemopoietic lineages is incomplete[34,32], the known cell-type-specific markers can be used to classify leukaemias more precisely[34]. This in turn permits the study of whether the sub-classes of leukaemia have different prognoses and responses to therapy. Lineage analysis has also brought about the realization that the generative cells of a cancer may include cells (such as pluripotent stem cells in CML) distinct from the overtly malignant cells (precursors of granulocytes in CML). One wonders which of these would proliferate in current 'tumour clonogenic cells' assays. Clearly all the generative cells of a tumour need to be monitored for the projected uses of these assays.

It will be a long time before we have an equally sophisticated understanding of cell lineage in the major solid cancers and their target organs. This will probably require, as with haemopoiesis, a combination of clonal analysis in culture and establishment of an appreciable collection of specific antigens and other markers. In several cases this will require improved techniques of epithelial cell culture. Lineage studies have begun with breast epithelium, as mentioned above[47,48], but there is still difficulty with the culture of human breast carcinomas[82]. The evidence that human cancers often contain only a small proportion of generative cells is at present circumstantial[26,28]. There is good evidence that some cancer cells differentiate, but the actual proportion of generative cells in human cancers will remain unknown until and unless we develop proven techniques to identify these cells. Once again a better understanding of normal cell lineages should help.

The value of knowing the original, normal target cells for carcinogenesis lies less in treatment than in aetiology and possible prevention. For example the important features of the metabolism of chemical carcinogens in target cells may not be observed if that metabolism is studied in other cells. Rapid progress on this problem cannot be expected at present, however, because of the difficulty of identifying early stages in human carcinogenesis[82].

Lastly, the relevance of understanding the effects of the cellular environment on tumour growth and malignancy lies in the obvious possibility that factors responsible for negative effects, or inhibitors of the action of factors with positive effects, might be isolated and put to therapeutic use. The possible correlation between induced loss of malignancy and differentiation seems particularly interesting. Pierce suggests that embryonic inducers of differentiation are more likely than other inducers to regulate cancer cells, which are perhaps not normally exposed to the former[78]. However there is also interest in differentiation-inducing factors present postnatally[41,83]. Caution will be needed with such approaches since opposite effects can also be produced. Hormonally-induced differentiation of mouse melanoma cells was associated with an *increased* rate of experimental metastasis[74], while induced differentiation of three leukaemic cell lines reduced their susceptibility to lysis by natural killer cells, cells which may contribute to the suppression of metastasis[84]. Again we cannot expect all cancer cells to respond to natural inducers of differentiation[41]. Nonetheless there have been preliminary successes in increasing the survival of tumour-bearing animals by treatment of the animals with normal or pharmacological inducers of differentiation[85,86] (reviewed[83,74]). It has also been argued that important chemotherapeutic agents may act largely through the induction of cell differentiation[83]. This surely merits further research.

In conclusion, studies of the cellular basis of cancer initiation and growth are still at an early stage. Pursuit of these problems can be expected to offer attractive possibilities for the future attack on cancer, not least in respect of more specific diagnosis and treatment, and the use of more physiological and less toxic therapeutic agents.

Acknowledgements

Ian Hart and Nick Wright are thanked for constructive comments. The author's research is supported by the Cancer Research Campaign. Melanie Coulton is also thanked for her patient and efficient typing of the manuscript.

References

1. Anderson, J. R. (ed.) (1985). *Muir's Textbook of Pathology.* 12th Edn. (London: E. Arnold)
2. Foulds, L. (1975). *Neoplastic Development.* (New York: Academic Press)
3. Willis, R. A. (1967). *Pathology of Tumours.* 4th Edn. (London: Butterworth and Company)
4. Sherbet, G. V. (1982). *The Biology of Tumour Malignancy.* (New York: Academic Press)
5. Woodruff, M. F. A., Ansell, J. D., Forbes, G. M., Gordon, J. C., Burton, D. I. and Micklem, H. S. (1982). Clonal interaction in tumours. *Nature,* **299**, 822-826
6. Woodruff, M. F. A. (1983). Cellular heterogeneity in tumours. *Br. J. Cancer,* **7**, 589-594
7. Alexander, P. (1985). Do cancers arise from a single transformed cell or is monoclonality of tumours a late event in carcinogenesis? *Br. J. Cancer,* **51**, 453-457
8. Fialkow, P. J. (1976). Clonal origin of human tumors. *Biochim. Biophys. Acta,* **458**, 281-321
9. Fialkow, P. J. (1979). Clonal origin of human tumors. *Annu. Rev. Med.,* **30**, 135-153
10. Mintz, B. (1978). Genetic mosaicism and in vivo analysis of neoplasia and differentiation. In Saunders, G. F. (ed.) *Cell Differentiation and Neoplasia.* pp. 27-53. (New York: Raven Press)
11. Hsu, S. H., Luk, G. D., Krush, A. J., Hamilton, S. R. and Hoover, H. H. (1983). Multiclonal origin of polyps in Gardner syndrome. *Science,* **221**, 951-953
12. Jackson, C. E., Block, M. A., Greenawald, K. A. and Tashjian, A. H. (1979). The two-mutational-event theory in medullary thyroid cancer. *Am. J. Hum. Genet.,* **31**, 704-710
13. Farber, E. (1984). Pre-cancerous steps in carcinogenesis. Their physiological adaptive nature. *Biochim. Biophys. Acta,* **738**, 171-180
14. Wellings, S. R., Jensen, H. M. and Marcus, R. G. (1975). An atlas of subgross pathology of the human breast with special reference to possible precancerous lesions. *J. Natl. Cancer Inst.,* **55**, 231-273
15. Wright, N. and Alison, M. (1984). *The Biology of Epithelial Cell Populations.* (Oxford: Clarendon Press)
16. Till, J. E., McCulloch, E. A. and Siminovitch, L. (1964). A stochastic model of stem cell proliferation, based on the growth of spleen colony-forming cells. *Proc. Natl. Acad. Sci. USA,* **51**, 29-36
17. Lajtha, L. G. (1979). Stem cell concepts. *Differentiation,* **14**, 23-34
18. Till, J. E. and McCulloch, E. A. (1980). Haemopoietic stem cell differentiation. *Biochim. Biophys. Acta,* **605**, 431-459
19. Potten, C. S., Schofield, R. and Lajtha, L. G. (1979). A comparison of cell replacement in bone marrow, testis and three regions of surface epithelium. *Biochim. Biophys. Acta,* **560**, 281-299

20. Slack, J. M. W. (1983). *From Egg to Embryo*. (London: Cambridge University Press)
21. Potten, C. S., Hime, W. J., Reid, P. and Cairns, J. (1978). The segregation of DNA in epithelial stem cells. *Cell*, **15**, 899–906
22. Cairns, J. (1975). Mutation selection and the natural history of cancer. *Nature*, **255**, 197–200
23. Johnson, M. H., McConnell, J. and Van Blerkom, J. (1984). Programmed development in the mouse embryo. *J. Embryol. Exp. Morphol.*, **83** (Supplement), 197–231
24. Levenson, R. and Housman, D. (1981). Commitment: how do cells make the decision to differentiate? *Cell*, **25**, 5–6
25. Bennett, D. C. (1983). Differentiation in mouse melanoma cells: Initial reversibility and an on-off stochastic model. *Cell*, **34**, 445–453
26. Salmon, S. E. and Trent, J. M. (eds.) (1984). *Human Tumor Cloning*. (Orlando: Grune and Stratton, Inc.)
27. Hamburger, A. W. and Salmon, S. E. (1977). Primary bioassay of human tumour stem cells. *Science*, **197**, 461–463
28. Buick, R. N. and Pollack, M. N. (1984). Perspectives on clonogenic tumor cells, stem cells, and oncogenes. *Cancer Res.*, **44**, 4909–4918
29. Courtenay, V. D. and Mills, J. (1978). An *in vitro* colony assay for human tumours grown in immune-suppressed mice and treated *in vivo* with cytotoxic agents. *Br. J. Cancer*, **37**, 261–268
30. Hill, B. T. (1984). Summary Perspectives. In Salmon, S. E. and Trent, J. M. (eds.) *Human Tumor Cloning*. pp. 629–645. (Orlando: Grune and Stratton, Inc.)
31. Brooks, R. F., Richmond, F. N., Riddle, P. N. and Richmond, K. M. V. (1984). Apparent heterogeneity in the response of quiescent Swiss 3T3 cells to serum growth factors: implications for the transition probability model and parallels with "cellular senescence" and "competence". *J. Cell Physiol.*, **121**, 341–350
32. McCulloch, E. A. (ed.) (1984). *Clinics in Haematology. Vol. 13:2 Cell culture techniques*. (Eastbourne: W. B. Saunders Co.)
33. Janossy, G., Greaves, M. F., Capellaro, D., Roberts, M. and Goldstone, A. H. (1977). Membrane marker analysis of "lymphoid" and myeloid blast crisis in Ph¹ positive (chronic myeloid) leukaemia. *Haematol. Blood Transfus.*, **20**, 97–107
34. Greaves, M. F., Delia, D., Newman, R. and Vodinelich, L. (1982). Analysis of leukaemic cells with monoclonal antibodies. In McMichael, A. J. and Fabre, J. W. (eds.) *Monoclonal Antibodies in Clinical Medicine*. pp. 129–165. (London: Academic Press)
35. Rheinwald, J. G. and Green, H. (1975). Serial cultivation of strains of human epidermal keratinocytes: the formation of keratinizing colonies from single cells. *Cell*, **6**, 331–344
36. Bennett, D. C., Peachey, L. A., Durbin, H. and Rudland, P. S. (1978). A possible mammary stem cell line. *Cell*, **15**, 283–298
37. Pierce, G. B., Nakane, P. K., Martinez-Hernandez, A. and Ward, J. M. (1977). Ultrastructural comparison of differentiation of stem cells of murine adenocarcinomas of colon and breast with their normal counterparts. *J. Natl. Cancer Inst.*, **58**, 1329–1345
38. Pierce, G. B. and Johnson, L. D. (1971). Differentiation and cancer. *In Vitro*, **7**, 140–145
39. Fialkow, P. J., Jacobson, R. J. and Papayannopoulou, T. (1977). Chronic myelocytic leukaemia: clonal origin in a stem cell common to the granulocyte, erythrocyte, platelet and monocyte/macrophage. *Am. J. Med.*, **63**, 125–130
40. Eaves, A. C. and Eaves, C. J. (1984). Erythropoiesis in culture. In McCulloch, E. A. (ed.) *Clinics in Haematology. Vol. 13:2 Cell Culture Techniques*. pp. 371–391. (Eastbourne: W. B. Saunders Co.)
41. Sachs, L. (1980). Constitutive uncoupling of pathways of gene expression that control growth and differentiation in myeloid leukaemia: a model for the origin and progression of malignancy. *Proc. Natl. Acad. Sci. USA*, **77**, 6152––6156
42. Dabelow, A. (1957). Die Milchdrüse. In von Möllendorff, W. (ed.) *Handbuch der mikroskopischen Anatomie des Menschen*. Vol. 3, part III/1, pp. 277–485. (Berlin: Springer-Verlag)
43. Salazar, H. and Tobon, H. (1974). Morphologic changes of the mammary gland during development, pregnancy and lactation. In Josimovich, J.B., Reynolds, M. and Cobo, E. (eds.) *Lactogenic Hormones, Fetal Nutrition and Lactation*. (New York: Wiley)
44. Ormerod, E. J. and Rudland, P. S. (1985). Isolation and differentiation of cloned epithelial cell lines from normal rat mammary glands. *In Vitro*, **21**, 143–153

45. Williams, J. M. and Daniel, C. W. (1983). Mammary ductal elongation: differentiation of myoepithelium and basal lamina during branching morphogenesis. *Dev. Biol.*, **97**, 274–290

46. Dulbecco, R., Unger, M., Armstrong, B., Bowman, M. and Syka, P. (1983). Epithelial cell types and their evolution in the rat mammary gland determined by immunological markers. *Proc. Natl. Acad. Sci. USA*, **80**, 1033–1037

47. Russo, J., Tay, L. K. and Russo, I. H. (1982). Differentiation of the mammary gland and susceptibility to carcinogenesis. *Breast Cancer Res. Treat.*, **2**, 5–75

48. Gusterson, B. A., Warburton, M. J., Mitchell, D., Ellison, M., Neville, A. M. and Rudland, P. S. (1982). Distribution of myoepithelial cells and basement membrane proteins in the normal breast and malignant breast diseases. *Cancer Res.*, **42**, 4763–4770

49. Bartek, J., Durban, E. M., Hallowes, R. C. and Taylor-Papadimitriou, J. (1985). A subclass of lumenal epithelial cells in the human mammary gland, defined by antibodies to cytokeratins. *J. Cell Sci.*, **75**, 17–33

50. Bartek, J., Taylor-Papidimitriou, J., Miller, N. and Millis, R. (1985). Patterns of expression of keratin 19 as detected with monoclonal antibodies in human breast tissues and tumours. *Int. J. Cancer*, **36**, 299–306

51. Chang, S. E. (1985). *In vitro* transformation of human breast epithelial cells. In Rich, M., Taylor-Papadimitriou, J. and Hager, J. (eds.) *Breast Cancer: on the Edge of Discovery.* (New York: Martinus Nijhoff) (In press)

52. Bennett, D. C. (1986). Instability and stabilization in melanoma cell differentiation. *Curr. Top. Dev. Biol.*, **20**, 333–344

53. Uriel, J. (1976). Cancer, retrodifferentiation and the myth of Faust. *Cancer Res.*, **36**, 4269–4275

54. Wyllie, A. H., Clayton, R. M. and Truman, D. E. S. (1982). Tumours, transposition and transdifferentiation. In Clayton, R. M. and Truman, D. E. S. (eds.) *Stability and Switching in Cellular Differentiation*. pp. 143–154. (New York: Plenum Press)

55. Bissell, M. J. (1981). The differentiated state of normal and malignant cells in culture. *Int. Rev. Cytol.*, **70**, 27–100

56. Fidler, I. J., Gerston, D. M. and Hart, I. R. (1978). The biology of cancer invasion and metastasis. *Adv. Cancer Res.*, **28**, 149–250

57. Fidler, I. J., Barnes, Z., Fogler, W. E., Kirsh, R., Bugelski, P. and Poste, G. (1982). Involvement of macrophages in the eradication of established metastases following intravenous injection of liposomes containing macrophage activators. *Cancer Res.*, **42**, 496–501

58. Nicholson, G. L. (1984). Tumor progression, oncogenes and the evolution of metastatic phenotypic diversity. *Clin. Exp. Metastasis*, **2**, 85–105

59. Bissell, M. J., Hall, H. G. and Parry, G. (1982). How does the extracellular matrix direct gene expression? *J. Theor. Biol.*, **99**, 31–68

60. Kratochwil, K. (1969). Organ specificity in mesenchymal induction demonstrated in the embryonic development of the mammary gland of the mouse. *Dev. Biol.*, **20**, 46–71

61. Sakakura, T., Nishizuka, Y. and Dawe, C. J. (1976). Mesenchyme-dependent morphogenesis and epithelium-specific cytodifferentiation in mouse mammary gland. *Science*, **194**, 1439–1441

62. Kallman, F. and Grobstein, C. (1965). Source of collagen at epitheliomesenchymal interfaces during inductive interaction. *Dev. Biol.*, **11**, 169–183

63. DeCosse, J. J., Gossens, C. L., Kuzma, J. F. and Unsworth, B. R. (1973). Breast cancer: induction of differentiation by embryonic tissue. *Science*, **181**, 1057–1058

64. Bennett, D. C. (1980). Morphogenesis of branching tubules in cultures of cloned mammary epithelial cells. *Nature*, **285**, 657–659

65. Ali, I. U., Mautner, V., Lanza, R. and Hynes, R. O. (1977). Restoration of normal morphology, adhesion and cytoskeleton in transformed cells by addition of a transformation-sensitive surface protein. *Cell*, **11**, 115–126

66. Marshall, C. J., Franks, L. M. and Carbonell, A.W. (1977). Markers of neoplastic transformation in epithelial cell lines derived from human carcinomas. *J. Natl. Cancer Inst.*, **58**, 1743–1751

67. Terranova, V. P., Williams, J. E., Liotta, L. A. and Martin, G. R. (1984). Modulation of the metastatic activity of melanoma cells by laminin and fibronectin. *Science*, **226**, 982–985

68. Paget, S. (1889). The distribution of secondary growths in cancer of the breast. *Lancet*, **i**, 571-573
69. Auerbach, R., Morrisey, L. W. and Sidky, Y. A. (1978). Gradients in tumour growth. *Nature*, **274**, 707-709
70. Levy, J. A., White, A. C. and McGrath, C. M. (1982). Growth and histology of a human mammary-carcinoma cell line at different sites in the athymic mouse. *Br. J. Cancer*, **45**, 375-383
71. Nicholson, G. L., Brunson, K. W. and Fidler, I. J. (1978). Specificity of arrest, survival and growth of selected metastatic variant cell lines. *Cancer Res.*, **38**, 4105-4111
72. Fidler, I. J. and Hart, I. R. (1982). Biological diversity in metastatic neoplasms: origins and implications. *Science*, **217**, 998-1003
73. Poste, G., Doll, J. and Fidler, I. (1981). Interactions among clonal subpopulations affect stability of the metastatic phenotype in polyclonal populations of B16 melanoma cells. *Proc. Natl. Acad. Sci. USA*, **78**, 6226-6230
74. Bennett, D. C., Dexter, T. J., Ormerod, E. J. and Hart, I. R. (1986). Increased experimental metastatic capacity of a murine melanoma following induction of differentiation. *Cancer Res.*, **46**, 3239-3244
75. Heppner, G. (1984). Tumour heterogeneity. *Cancer Res.*, **44**, 2259-2265
76. Brinster, R. L. (1974). The effects of cells transferred into the mouse blastocyst on subsequent development. *J. Exp. Med.*, **140**, 1049-1056
77. Illmensee, K. and Mintz, B. (1976). Totipotency and normal differentiation of single teratocarcinoma cells cloned by injection into blastocysts. *Proc. Natl. Acad. Sci. USA*, **73**, 549-553
78. Pierce, G. B., Pantazis, C. G., Caldwell, J. E. and Wells, R. S. (1982). Specificity of the control of tumor formation by the blastocyst. *Cancer Res.*, **42**, 1082-1087
79. Podesta, A. H., Mullins, J., Pierce, G. B. and Wells, R. S. (1984). The neurula stage mouse embryo in control of neuroblastoma. *Proc. Natl. Acad. Sci. USA*, **81**, 7608-7611
80. Gootwine, E., Webb., C. G. and Sachs, L. (1982). Participation of myeloid leukaemic cells injected into embryos in haematopoietic differentiation in adult mice. *Nature*, **299**, 63-65
81. Matioli, G. (1973). Friend leukemic mouse stem cell reversion to normal growth in irradiated hosts. *J. Reticuloendothel. Soc.*, **14**, 380-386
82. Smith, H. S., Wolman, S. R. and Hackett, A. J. (1984). The biology of breast cancer at the cellular level. *Biochim. Biophys. Acta*, **738**, 103--123
83. Bloch, A. (1984). Induced cell differentiation in cancer therapy. *Cancer Treat. Rep.*, **68**, 199-205
84. Gidlund, M., ⌐rn, A., Pattengale, P. K., Jansson, M., Wigzell, H. and Nilsson, K. (1981). Natural killer cells kill tumour cells at a given stage of differentiation. *Nature*, **292**, 848-850
85. Honma, Y., Kasukabe, T., Okabe, J. and Hozumi, M. (1979). Prolongation of survival time of mice inoculated with myeloid leukaemia cells by inducers of normal differentiation. *Cancer Res.*, **39**, 3167-3171
86. Strickland, S. and Sawey, M. J. (1980). Studies on the effects of retinoids on the differentiation of teratocarcinoma stem cells *in vitro* and *in vivo*. *Dev. Biol.*, **78**, 76-85

5
Concepts of territory and organization in normal tissue and their relation to neoplasia

C. TICKLE

INTRODUCTION

A critical feature that distinguishes malignant from benign tumours is invasiveness. In malignant tumours, cells locally invade adjacent tissues and may also spread to establish secondary growths in the process of metastasis. For example, breast carcinomas can give rise to secondary tumours in distant tissues, including brain and bone. In establishing this typical pattern of metastasis, the malignant cells leave the confines of the epithelium in which they originate and may invade the underlying connective tissues. They then invade lymph vessels in which they are disseminated. Later, they may leave the lymph vessels and invade foreign tissues in which they grow into secondary tumours. From this viewpoint, cancer can be considered to be a disease in which cells no longer respect tissue territories. Therefore, the rules that govern how tissues are established are basic to an understanding of malignant cell behaviour. During embryonic development, a single cell, the fertilized egg, gives rise to the complex, appropriately organized arrays of differentiated cells that form the tissues of the body. Furthermore, in the embryo, the development of specific tissues involves invasion. For instance, in the development of glands the epithelium invades the underlying mesenchyme. Likewise the formation of tissues derived from the neural crest involves extensive migration of cells. An understanding of the mechanisms involved in the invasiveness of embryonic cells and its control must surely be directly relevant to malignancy.

Tissues arise in a step-wise fashion

The development of the spatially organized arrays of specialized cells in adult tissues is the ultimate stage in a series of steps in which the parts of the body are progressively demarcated. At the cellular level, this involves the

83

commitment of cells to form a progressively restricted range of cell types. Thus, cells in the embryo become different long before the specialized proteins characteristic of a particular tissue type are synthesized. The way in which cells become progressively committed to form the different parts of the body is fundamental to an understanding of how tissue territories are assigned.

In the mouse, the first stages of development involve the commitment of cells to form either extra-embryonic tissues or the tissues of the adult. Up to the 8-cell stage, each of the cells appears to be capable of forming all the tissues of the embryo and the necessary extra-embryonic structures such as the protective membranes and part of the placenta[1]. By the 16-cell stage, the developmental potential of the cells has become restricted[2]. The cells on the outside of the mass give rise to extra-embryonic structures only. From the inside cells, the embryonic and ultimately the adult tissues will develop. However, a second step is required before cells embark on this course. This step takes place at the blastocyst stage. At this stage, a cavity has formed and the inside cells are now clustered at one end of the cavity (Figure 5.1). Within this cluster – the inner cell mass – cells adjacent to the cavity become different[3]. They will give rise to further extra-embryonic structures. The remaining cells within the inner cell mass will now form the tissues of the embryo proper.

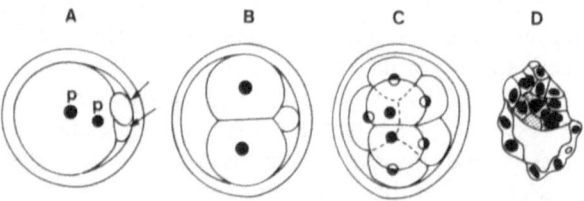

Figure 5.1 Early stages in mouse development. (A) A recently fertilized egg, with two pronuclei (p) and attached polar bodies (arrowed). (B) 2-cell-stage; about 24 h after fertilization. (C) 8-cell stage (the large cell on the left will divide to bring the total number of cells to 8); about 48 h after fertilization. (D) Blastocyst stage; the cluster of shaded cells is the inner cell mass; about 4 days after fertilization

Shortly after this stage, the body plan is drawn out in rough. Cells are assigned to one of the three main body layers: an outer cell layer – the ectoderm; a middle layer – the mesoderm; and an inner layer – the endoderm. These layers are brought into their appropriate positions during gastrulation. Cells in the ectoderm will give rise to the epidermis of the skin and the nervous system; cells in the mesoderm will give rise to muscle, connective tissues and blood; and the cells in the endoderm will give rise to the lining of the gut and associated glands and organs. An exception to this general scheme is that, in the head, the connective tissues are formed by cells of the neural crest that are derived from the ectoderm.

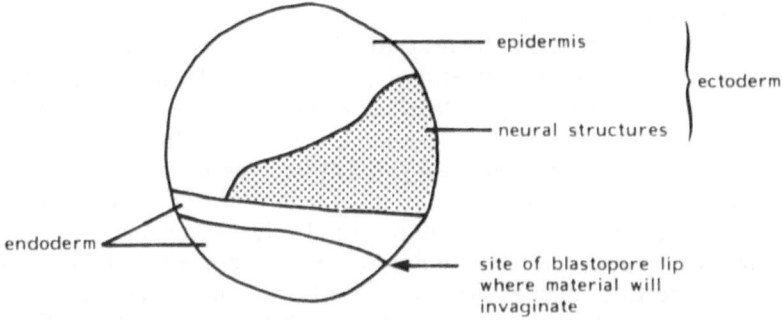

Figure 5.2 A diagram showing a fate map for *Xenopus*, an amphibian embryo, at the blastula stage. At this stage, the embryo consists of two layers of cells and the fate of cells in the outer layer is indicated. In the shaded region, this layer of cells will give rise to neural structures

In amphibian embryos, the regions of the cleaving egg that will give rise to the major parts of the body can be mapped using particles of dye. At the blastula stage, a region of the animal pole can be defined that will give rise to the neural tube (Figure 5.2). However, classical experiments by Spemann (reviewed[4]) have shown that if tissue from this region is grafted to the belly of a second embryo at the same stage of development, the graft does not develop into neural structures. Instead, it forms tissues appropriate to its new location. It is only when the same region of tissue is taken at the mid-gastrula stage, when the mesoderm has invaginated and come to lie beneath it, that the cells can be shown to be determined. Grafts to foreign sites then lead to the development of inappropriately positioned neural structures (Figure 5.3).

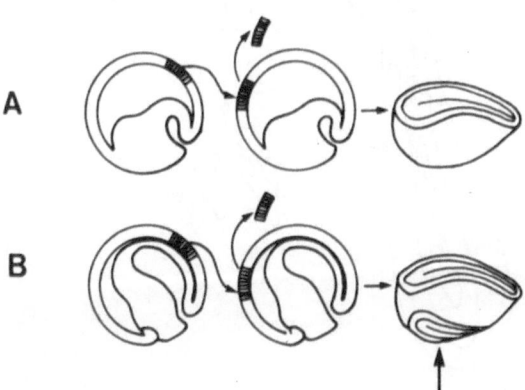

Figure 5.3 A diagram to illustrate the experiments of Spemann with newt embryos (reviewed[4]). (A) The presumptive neural tissue is taken from an embryo at the beginning of gastrulation and grafted to the region of presumptive belly epidermis in a second embryo at the same stage in development. The embryo that develops following this operation has a normal morphology and no misplaced neural structures develop. (B) The same operation performed at a later stage of development, when the mesoderm has been brought into place by the cell movements of gastrulation. In this case, the embryo that develops after the operation has an additional neural plate (arrowed) that will give rise to misplaced neural structures

Around the gastrula stage in vertebrates, regional differences are set up in the three tissue layers along the head to tail axis and probably the dorsal-ventral axis as well. The primary determinant is the establishment of a pattern in the mesoderm that then appears to be read off in a series of interactions with the other two layers[5]. For example, the interaction between the mesoderm and the ectoderm leads to spatial differences in the neural plate. At the head end of the embryo the brain is formed, while, at the tail end, the neural plate will form the spinal cord. It seems likely that regional differences in the mesoderm also lead to specialization of the endoderm and dictate the location of structures such as the lung and other organs associated with the gut. These regional differences may lead to the differentiation of specific cell types in appropriate positions. For example, some cells in the ectoderm ultimately differentiate into Purkinje cells in the brain, whereas endoderm will give rise to type II pneumocytes in the lung. Alternatively, different patterns of the same range of differentiated cell types may be generated in different positions. An example of this occurs in the development of the dorsal part of the mesoderm that will form the vertebral column. This part of the mesoderm breaks up into a series of blocks of tissue, the somites, on either

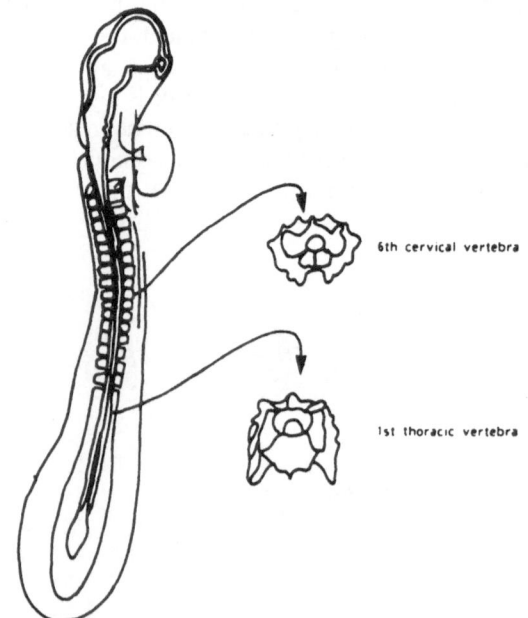

6th cervical vertebra

1st thoracic vertebra

Figure 5.4 A chick embryo at about 2 days of incubation (drawing on the left). Seventeen pairs of somites have formed dorsally on either side of the neural tube (the primitive spinal cord). The cells in posterior and anterior parts of adjacent somites in the region of somite 10 will differentiate into cartilage and form the 6th cervical vertebra. The 1st thoracic vertebra will develop by cartilage differentiation of cells from posterior and anterior parts of adjacent somites in the region of somite 19 (not yet formed from the somitic mesoderm in the diagram). The regionally distinctive patterns of cartilage will give rise to the individual forms of the vertebrae, as shown on the right for the two examples cited

side of the developing spinal cord. The development of the vertebral column involves the differentiation of cartilage and muscle cells. However, the pattern of cartilage, for example, will vary along the vertebral column and give rise to the defined sequence of morphologically distinct vertebrae in the appropriate positions (Figure 5.4).

Compartments in insect development

In insects such as *Drosophila*, the way in which parts of the body are constructed can be followed by tracing the lineage of cells. This can be done by taking advantage of genetic markers and using irradiation to cause mitotic recombination[6].

The way in which the wing of *Drosophila* is constructed has been followed using these techniques. The wing develops from an imaginal disk, a small nest of cells in the larval stages, that gives rise to the adult structure at metamorphosis. If, for example, larvae are irradiated, marked cells that end up in the wing disk can be generated at a low frequency by mitotic recombination. It can be arranged so that the progeny of these cells can be recognized in the wing of the adult by surface characteristics in the epidermis, for example, pigmentation or hair morphology. The clones formed by such genetically marked cells show striking localization patterns in the wing. If marked cells are produced in the first-stage larva, the clones that they give rise to are confined either to the anterior or to the posterior of the wing. The shapes of the clones show that there exists a boundary across the wing that does not correspond to any obvious tissue differences and is normally invisible[7] (Figure 5.5).

The regions of the wing separated by the boundary are known as compartments[8]. In addition to the anterior and posterior compartments, just described, dorsal and ventral compartments in the wing have been

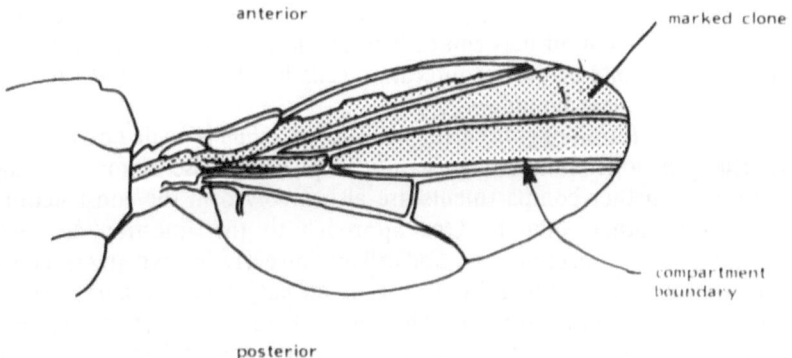

Figure 5.5 Diagram illustrating the distribution of a genetically marked clone in the wing of *Drosophila*. In this case, the genetically marked cells are produced in a background of cells homozygous for the mutation *Minute*. The genetically marked clone contains non-*Minute* cells that divide rapidly and so almost fill the compartment. The anterior-posterior compartment boundary is the straight line running almost down the centre of the wing blade

demonstrated by the same technique and appear to arise at a later stage in development[7]. Thus, the way in which the wing develops in *Drosophila* involves a series of commitments that assign groups of cells to particular regions of the wing that are not related to tissue type. The segments of the body of the insect are also made up of compartments and groups of cells are committed to the anterior or posterior compartment of each segment early in development[6].

The way in which compartments are delimited has obvious implications for an understanding of how tissue territories are maintained. At the compartment boundary, cells from neighbouring compartments abut. For example, in the wing, in contrast to the irregular outline of the clone elsewhere, there is a straight edge at the boundary and no intermingling of cells. This suggests that when cells are assigned to a compartment, this is accompanied by a change in their surface properties such that they preferentially adhere to other cells from the same compartment.

The distinctive behaviour of cells from anterior and posterior compartments is altered by mutation of the gene *engrailed*. For example, flies homozygous for a lethal *engrailed* mutation (en^{C2}) do not develop. However, clones of cells expressing *engrailed* mutations can be generated in flies by mitotic recombination. The mutant cells only lead to defects if they are in posterior compartments[9]. In the wing, mutant *engrailed* clones can straddle the compartment boundary[10,11]. This suggests that the expression of the normal *engrailed* gene is required for the commitment of cells to posterior compartments and the acquisition of the properties that distinguish them from anterior cells. Indeed, when cells dissociated from *engrailed* wing disks are mixed with normal wing cells, they remain associated with anterior cells and they do not associate with posterior cells[12]. The mechanisms that lead to the preferential associations between cells from the same compartments are not understood. However, a position-specific antigen has been detected that becomes confined to cells that occupy the dorsal compartment in the *Drosophila* wing disk[13] and this could be important in determining cell associations. Between segments, the boundary is marked by a reduction in cell-cell communication between cells in neighbouring compartments[14] and, in the wing, a zone of non-proliferating cells has been found at the dorso-ventral compartment boundary[15].

The demonstration of compartments in *Drosophila* is made possible by the powerful genetic techniques that can be applied in these animals. A major question is whether compartments are also involved in the construction of structures in other animals. One approach to this question as regards mammals involves injecting a marked cell into an early embryo and tracing the clones that develop. This is by no means an easy task compared with the mapping of clones in *Drosophila*. There appears to be considerable mixing of cells at later stages of mammalian embryonic development. Nevertheless, quite significant advances have been made in understanding how parts of the embryo are constructed. For example, in the development of the gut in mice, a single progenitor cell appears to give rise to each crypt in the small and large intestines[16].

Quite recently, investigations of the pattern of spinal nerve outgrowth in developing chick embryos have suggested that the somites are functionally divided into anterior and posterior halves. The nerves only traverse the anterior half of each somite and this pattern is maintained after operations in which the unsegmented somitic mesoderm has been rotated through 180° (ref. 17). This suggests a parallel with segmentation in the insect embryo, where, as we have discussed, each segment is constructed of an anterior and posterior compartment. However, at present it is not known how the differences in anterior and posterior somite cells arise in vertebrate embryos. If separate cell lineages gave rise to each cell population, the different parts of each somite would be analogous to compartments.

CELL DIFFERENTIATION AND DIFFERENTIAL GENE EXPRESSION

The differences that arise between cells in an embryo, leading to determination and ultimately the differentiation of cells of particular tissues, pose a problem of differential gene expression. This has been shown in a series of classical experiments with eggs of the frog, *Xenopus*[18]. If the nucleus from a blastula cell is injected into an enucleated egg, development may proceed. Even if the transplanted nucleus is taken from a specialized tissue cell, for example, an intestinal cell from a tadpole, the egg will in a small number of cases develop into a swimming tadpole. Thus, the nuclei of the cells of specialized tissues still contain all the information to make a new individual and the particular characteristics of specialized cells are due to specific patterns of gene expression. The central role of the genes and the way in which gene expression is controlled are fundamental concepts that are relevant to considerations of how tumours arise.

Gene expression in relation to cell commitment

The commitment of cells to particular parts of the body, for example the three main body layers in vertebrates, effectively limits the range of genes that are expressed. This commitment is presumably brought about by the action of genes, at present unidentified, that lead to the expression of a particular subset of genes appropriate to that particular body layer. Subsequent regionalisation will lead to the expression of cell-type specific genes (see, for example[19]). Likewise, genes must be selectively expressed when cells are committed to compartments in *Drosophila*. These genes do not appear to act by exclusively limiting the range of cell types that can differentiate. Instead they appear to affect the response of cells to subsequent signals, which then lead to the patterns of cellular differentiation appropriate to that part of that particular segment.

The *engrailed* gene in *Drosophila*, as we have already discussed, appears to be necessary for the commitment of cells to posterior compartments. Very recently, this gene has been cloned and hybridization probes have been constructed[20,21] which can be used to follow the expression of *engrailed* during development. The expression of *engrailed* is position-dependent and only expressed in the cells that will form the posterior compartments of segments[20,21] and imaginal disks, such as the wing disk[21].

The expression of the *fulzi tarazu* gene that is involved in constructing the basic plan of the insect body has been studied in the same way[22]. In the *fulzi tarazu* mutant, the fly has about half the normal number of segments. When the expression of the *fulzi tarazu* gene is mapped in normal embryos, it is found to be localized in a series of seven circular stripes at the cellular blastoderm stage (see later, Figure 5.7). These stripes do not correspond to the segments but are about one compartment (half a segment) out of register. Thus, the defect in the mutant appears to be due to the deletion of the posterior and anterior compartments of alternate segments. This pattern of gene expression together with other genetic and morphological data suggests that the posterior and anterior compartments that end up in neighbouring segments represent a basic building block in constructing the insect body. These blocks have been called parasegments[23]. The generation of the insect segments thus involves the commitment of cells to parasegments and compartments (Figure 5.6).

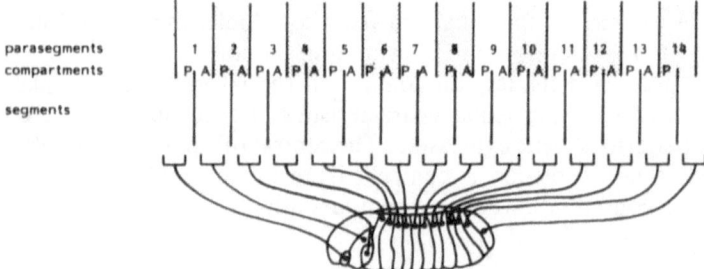

Figure 5.6 Diagram illustrating how the segments of the body of an insect are constructed. First, groups of cells are committed to parasegments. The *fulzi tarazu* gene is expressed in alternate parasegments (as indicated by shading) giving seven circular stripes. Second, groups of cells are committed to compartments, two compartments in each parasegment. The two compartments from each adjacent parasegment form a segment. The definition of compartments as anterior or posterior is made in relation to the segments

The cloning of *engrailed, fulzi tarazu* and other genes that control spatial organization has led to the identification of a common DNA sequence that codes for a highly conserved protein domain. This DNA sequence is about 180 bp long and has been called the homoeo box (reviewed[24]). The homoeo box sequence has been found in at least five genes in the *Antennapaedia* complex. This gene complex contains the *fulzi tarazu* gene together with genes that control spatial organization in the head and thorax, such as *Antennapaedia* itself. *Antennapaedia* is a homoeotic gene. In homoeotic mutants, structures are generated which are inappropriate to the segment in which they are formed. Thus, in the mutant *Antennapaedia*, the antennae of the fly are replaced by legs. The *Bithorax* complex is a cluster of homoeotic genes that control the spatial organization of the thorax and abdomen. Homoeo box sequences have been found in some of these genes too.

The homoeo box codes for a highly conserved basic protein domain whose predicted properties would be consistent with binding to DNA. The homoeo box may be essential for the functioning of a DNA-binding or chromatin protein that regulates gene expression. Even more remarkably, the homoeo box has been identified in DNA from *Xenopus*, mice and man[25]. These advances provide an exciting opportunity to identify for the first time genes controlling spatial organization in higher organisms. The expectation is that homoeotic genes with similar pattern controlling functions play an important role in vertebrate development. Homoeotic mutations that lead to obviously misplaced body structures are however uncommon in vertebrates. Slack[26] has recently analyzed the data on the occurrence of misplaced epithelial differentiation in human tissues and suggested that these may represent homoeotic mutations.

CONTROL MECHANISMS OF DIFFERENTIAL GENE EXPRESSION AND PATTERN FORMATION

The expression of, for example, the *engrailed* gene is position dependent, as we have just discussed. Likewise, the expression of other pattern controlling genes can be mapped to particular locations in the embryo. At later stages in development, cells in the appropriate positions differentiate and produce specialized products. This is the process of pattern formation and the mechanisms involved in the spatial control of gene expression are thus a major issue in considering how tissues arise.

From the viewpoint of positional information[27,28], pattern formation can be considered as a two-step process. In the first step, cells are informed of their position and in the second, they interpret this information in terms of their genome and their past history. There appear to be two major classes of mechanism that inform cells of their position within the embryo and lead to differential expression of controlling genes or those coding for tissue-specific characteristic proteins. One is an intracellular mechanism involving cytoplasmic factors that direct gene expression. The second involves cell interactions.

Intracellular control of gene expression

Cytoplasmic factors could serve to determine differential gene expression. This is easy to envisage at early stages in development when during cleavage the egg cytoplasm is partitioned between the daughter cells. Any asymmetries in the egg could lead to cytoplasmic differences between daughter cells.

Cytoplasmic factors appear to be involved in determining which cells will form the germ cells in *Drosophila*[29]. In the early development of *Drosophila*, division of the nucleus of the fertilized egg initially occurs without cleavage of

91

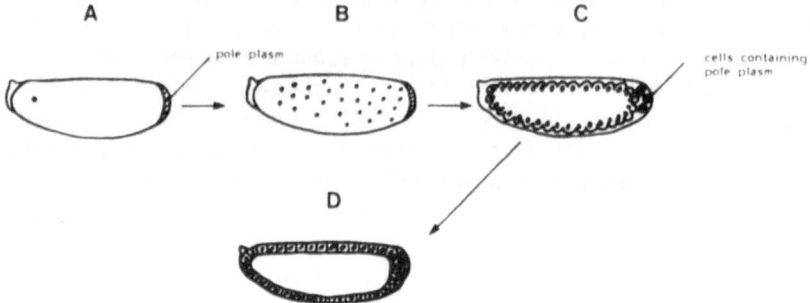

Figure 5.7 Diagram illustrating the early development of the *Drosophila* embryo. (A) At the posterior end of the fertilized egg, there is a specialized region of cytoplasm, the pole plasm. The first stages in the development of the fertilized egg involve the division of the nucleus without the accompanying formation of cells. (B) This gives rise to a syncytium with many nuclei. (C) The nuclei migrate to the periphery of the egg and cell boundaries begin to form. The cells formed at the posterior end enclose pole plasm and will form germ cells. (D) The formation of the cellular blastoderm is complete

the egg cytoplasm. After nine rounds of division, the nuclei migrate to the outer perimeter of the egg and cells are formed (Figure 5.7). The nuclei that migrate to the posterior end of the embryo and are enclosed in the cytoplasm there, the pole plasm, form the germ cells. If pole plasm is injected into the anterior end of an embryo, the cells that form there will now give rise to germ cells when grafted to a genetically distinguishable second host. Cytoplasmic differences could also lead to the position-dependent expression of early acting control genes in *Drosophila*. The expression of the *futzi tarazu* gene is localized even prior to the formation of cells[22].

Eggs of animals such as molluscs[30] and segmented worms have a highly invariant pattern of cleavage and this may serve to localize specific cytoplasmic constituents of the egg to particular daughter cells (Figure 5.8). Furthermore, some animals such as nematodes maintain such precise patterns of cell divisions well into development and invariant cell lineages are generated[31]. For example, the formation of the vulva in a nematode arises by a precise pattern of cell divisions from six precursor cells. These cells, in the region of the gonad, generate 22 vulval cells[32]. It is possible that during such divisions unequal division of the cytoplasm may lead to the differences in the subsequent cell lineages. However, the strict lineages may also lead to the ordered topography required for cell interactions. Laser ablation experiments have shown that the development of the vulva requires interaction with one specific cell in the gonad, the anchor cell[33].

Cell interactions lead to positional cues

The signals provided by other cells in the embryo may be required for cell commitment and determination. In early mouse development, the cells on the inside at the 16-cell stage are exposed to a different environment from that

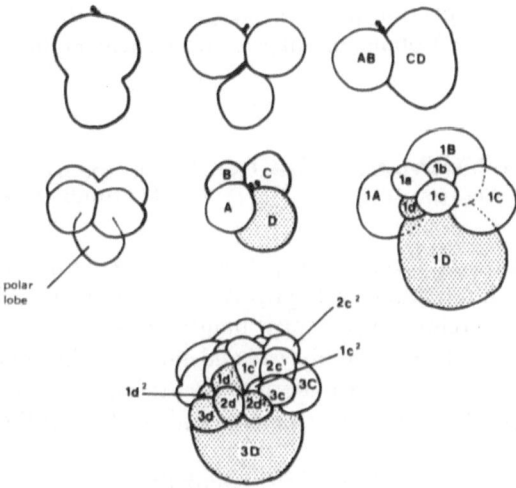

Figure 5.8 Diagram to show the pattern of cleavage in a mollusc, *Illyanassa*. The large bulge of cytoplasm, the polar lobe, becomes regularly incorporated into the D blastomere and the cell lineage is highly invariant. The descendants of the four blastomeres A, B, C and D are traced during two subsequent cleavage divisions. For simplicity, the descendants of the D and C blastomere only are shown in the last drawing. Polar lobe material is regularly apportioned to a specific group of cells

experienced by the cells on the outside. This is due to compaction, a process in which the outer cells broaden their contacts with each other, form tight junctions and seal off the inside cells from the external environment[34]. Further interactions between the inside cells lead to commitment of cells to form the embryo proper.

Particularly relevant to considerations of malignancy is the behaviour of embryonal carcinoma cells when injected into mouse embryos at the blastocyst stage[35]. Embryonal carcinoma cells are stem cells from malignant teratocarcinomas. These tumours can arise spontaneously from germ cells or be produced experimentally by grafting embryos to ectopic sites. The embryonal carcinoma cells can apparently respond to the signals in the normal embryo and participate in normal development. When cells from two different embryonal carcinoma cell lines were injected into blastocysts that were then implanted into foster mothers, the tumour cells were found to be present in many tissues in the resulting offspring. Experiments *in vitro* suggest that signals produced by the inner cell mass may serve to normalize the behaviour of the embryonal carcinoma cells[36].

Although the exact nature of cell interactions in early embryos and the signals involved are obscure, cell-cell communication via gap junctions is likely to play an important role. This has been demonstrated recently, for the first time, in early amphibian embryos[37]. An antibody to gap junction protein was injected into one of the cells at the 8-cell stage. When assayed at the

32-cell stage, communication between the progeny of the injected cell was inhibited. At later developmental stages, the treated embryos had severe localized defects.

EPITHELIAL-MESENCHYMAL INTERACTIONS AND POSITIONAL SIGNALLING IN PATTERN FORMATION IN DEVELOPING LIMBS

The development of vertebrate limbs provides a striking illustration of how the same range of differentiated cell types is generated in distinctive patterns. Limbs begin their development as small bulges of apparently homogeneous cells. As they grow out from the body wall and elongate, this small population of cells gives rise to the complex pattern of tissues characteristic of the limb. The same cell types differentiate in the arm and the leg but the patterns are different.

From the experimental analysis of chick limb development, the position of a cell within the developing limb appears to be specified by at least two different mechanisms[38]. To specify position along the proximo-distal axis (the axis running from the body wall to the tip of the limb), epithelial-mesenchymal interactions are involved, whereas position specification across the antero-posterior axis (the axis running for example, in the hand, from the thumb to little finger) involves a long range positional signal (Figure 5.9).

For the proximo-distal axis, cells are informed of their relative position by the time that they spend in the progress zone[39]. The progress zone is a region of undifferentiated cells that remains at the tip of the limb as it grows out.

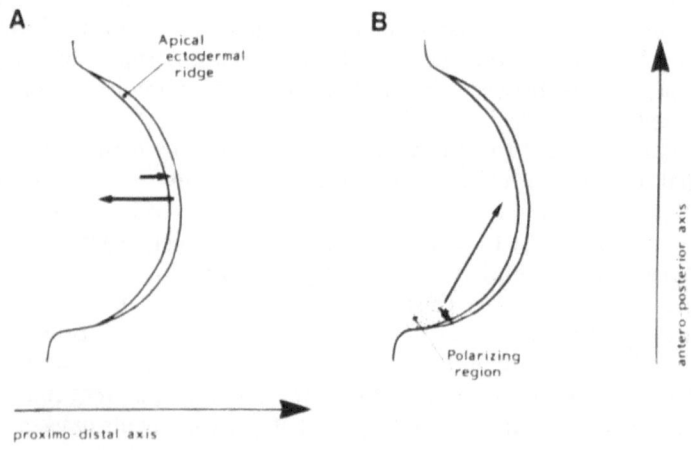

Figure 5.9 Diagram to show cell interactions in limb development. (A) For pattern formation along the proximo-distal axis, reciprocal interactions are required between the apical ectodermal ridge, the thickened epithelium at the tip of the early limb bud and the underlying mesenchyme. The undifferentiated region of mesenchyme near the ridge is maintained as the bud grows out and constitutes the progress zone. (B) For pattern formation across the antero-posterior axis, a long range positional signal is produced by the polarizing region, a small group of mesenchyme cells at the posterior margin of the bud

During bud outgrowth, cells are forced out of the progress zone. From the viewpoint of positional information, they can be considered to acquire positional values that they later interpret in terms of differentiation appropriate to that position. Cells that leave the progress zone early form proximal structures while cells leaving later form distal structures.

The progress zone is maintained by the apical ectodermal ridge, a thickened rim of epithelium at the bud tip. The apical ridge also mediates bud outgrowth (reviewed[40]). The nature of the signals generated by the apical ridge is unknown. Furthermore, there is a reciprocal interaction between cells of the progress zone and the ridge that is required to maintain the thickened epithelium. Again, the details of this set of interactions are at present obscure. However, quite recently it has been found, by investigating ridge maintenance in culture, that insulin is required[41]. This is a step towards analyzing the signals involved in the interplay between epithelium and mesenchyme.

The interaction between the progress zone and apical ridge is a specific example of the general class of epithelial-mesenchymal interactions that occur widely during development. Furthermore, epithelial-mesenchymal interactions also continue into adult life in organs such as the skin[42]. The basis for changes in epithelial cell behaviour may therefore be traced to a primary

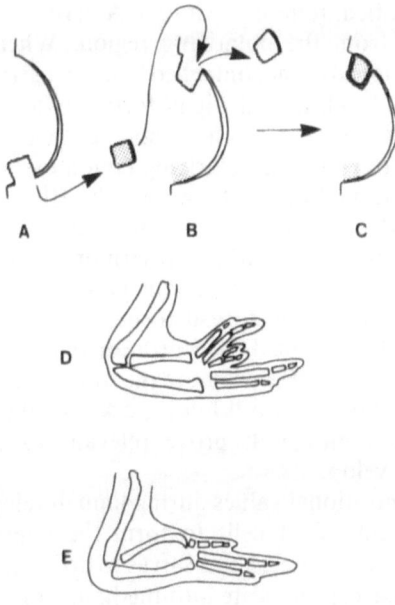

Figure 5.10 Diagram to illustrate an operation that demonstrates the signalling of the polarizing region. (A) The polarizing region is cut out of the posterior margin of one bud and then (B) grafted to an anterior site in a second bud. The bud now has polarizing region tissue at both anterior and posterior margins (C). The wing that develops (D) has a symmetrical pattern of cartilage elements, that is particularly clear in the digits. For comparison, a normal wing pattern is shown below (E)

lesion in the associated connective tissue and this may be particularly relevant when considering how carcinomas, tumours of epithelial origin, arise.

As regards the antero-posterior axis of the developing chick limb, cells are informed of their position by a signal from the polarizing region, a small group of mesenchyme cells at the posterior margin of the bud. The signal emanating from the polarizing region can be demonstrated by grafting an additional polarizing region to the anterior margin of a chick wing bud (Figure 5.10). The wing that develops possesses a duplicate set of structures in mirror-image symmetry with the normal set. For example[43], instead of the normal digit pattern of *234*, the digit pattern following the operation is *432234*. The additional structures arise almost entirely from the host bud in response to a signal from the graft. The response is graded, with cells nearest the polarizing region forming the posterior digit *4*, cells slightly farther away forming the middle digit *3*, and cells still farther away digit *2*, the anterior digit.

One model proposes that the signal from the polarizing region, which provides a measure of distance across the antero-posterior axis, is a diffusible morphogen[44]. The morphogen would be produced by the polarizing region cells and broken down in the bud mesenchyme so that a gradient is formed. The concentration of morphogen at any point would specify the positional value across the antero-posterior axis. Although the postulated morphogen has not yet been identified, retinoids (vitamin A derivatives) have been found to mimic the signal from the polarizing region. When retinoic acid, for example, is applied locally on controlled-release carriers to the anterior margin of a wing bud, additional digits form[45]. One explanation for the retinoid effect is that the cells in the immediate vicinity of the retinoid-releasing carrier are converted to polarizing region tissue which then signals the formation of additional digits. However, the effective concentration of retinoid in the bud tissue is in the nanomolar range and a gradient that is stable with time is soon established[45]. Furthermore, a graded distribution of retinoid is more effective in bringing about pattern changes than the same concentration of retinoid evenly spread throughout the bud tissue[46]. Thus, another possibility is that the local concentration of retinoid may itself assign positional values. Since retinoids promote the differentiation of tumour cells including embryonal carcinoma cell lines[47], a knowledge of how they bring about pattern changes may well prove relevant to understanding how malignant tumours develop.

The acquisition of positional values during limb development is postulated to direct the differentiation of cells to form the appropriate patterns of connective tissues. For the muscles, this serves to define the tissue boundaries. The prospective muscle cells migrate into the limb from the somites and are localised in the appropriate positions following the pattern of connective tissue sheaths[48]. The specific pattern of muscles is thus determined by connective tissue boundaries and the muscle cells themselves are all equivalent. If the somites opposite the developing wing are removed at an early stage in development and replaced by somites from another level along the body axis, a normal pattern of differentiated muscles is still obtained[49].

INVASION DURING DEVELOPMENT

Frequently during development cell rearrangements take place to mould the shape of the developing embryo. Furthermore, such relative movement involving migration and displacement of cells is required to bring together populations of cells that interact, as in the determination of the neural plate discussed above.

Neural crest

A consideration of the development of tissues derived from the neural crest is particularly relevant to understanding how tissue territories are established. The neural crest arises at the lateral borders of the neural plate, and during neural tube closure it is pinched off so that it comes to lie immediately alongside the neural tube beneath the ectoderm (Figure 5.11). The neural crest cells then invade adjacent tissues to take up appropriate positions and differentiate into a wide range of different cell types, including the neurones of the sympathetic and parasympathetic systems, Schwann cells, the pigment cells of the skin, some cells of the APUD system (cells in several tissues which

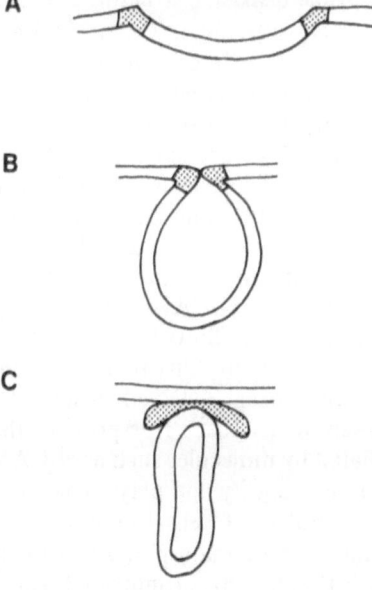

Figure 5.11 Schematic diagrams to show the origin of the neural crest. (A) The neural plate is shown in transverse section; the neural crest is the shaded region at each lateral edge. (B) The position of the neural crest as the neural plate folds to form the neural tube. Following closure of the neural tube and healing of the ectoderm, the neural crest comes to lie in a dorsal position (C). From this position neural crest cells migrate to form a wide range of tissues

have in common the properties of Amine Precursor Uptake and Decarboxylation) and the connective tissues in the head[50]. The proposed common origin of some of the APUD cells from the neural crest explains several related syndromes including forms of the so-called multiple endocrine tumours[51].

In general terms, there are two main ways in which the development of the neural crest could occur. The one envisages that the cells of the neural crest are determined before they start their migration and then take the appropriate pathways to localize in their correct positions. The second supposes that the cells in the crest are pluripotent and that their differentiation depends on the pathway that they take and the site in which they localize. These possibilities have been extensively investigated by exchanging regions of the crest before emigration occurs (see, for example,[52]). In the overwhelming majority of cases, the crest cells form structures appropriate to their new pathways and sites of localization. There does seem, however, to be an intrinsic difference between neural crest cells in the head and in the trunk. Trunk neural crest cells do not give rise to the appropriate connective tissues when transplanted to the head. Quite recently, a few other exceptions to the general rule (that neural crest cells are equivalent prior to migration) have been found. When stretches of neural crest are exchanged within the head of chick embryos, the neural crest that normally forms the connective tissues of the beak will still form these structures when implanted in place of the neural crest from more caudal levels. This results in ectopic beak-like structures developing in the neck[53].

From the viewpoint of considering how tissues are established, neural crest development raises a number of interesting questions. These concern how invasion by the neural crest is initiated, how the pathways of migration are determined and the way in which localization is controlled.

The initiation of migration is a crucial event in the development of tissues derived from the neural crest. The cells lose their associations and move into foreign tissue territories. The mechanisms involved may parallel those that lead to the invasiveness of tumours. The onset of neural crest cell invasiveness is correlated with changes in the cell surface. The cell adhesive molecule, Neural Cell-Adhesion Molecule (N-CAM), can no longer be detected[54]. It is possible that loss of this molecule allows the crest cells to dissociate from one another, and their latent inherent motility then comes into play. A decrease in surface N-CAM has also been detected when chick retinal cells are transformed by Rous sarcoma virus[55]. It is possible that changes in cell-cell adhesion systems mediated by molecules such as N-CAM[54] may be significant in the breakdown of tissue integrity and play a role in metastasis.

The pathways that neural crest cells follow as they invade the embryo appear to be well-defined[56]. One main pathway runs deep into the embryo and the neural crest cells that take this route will form derivatives such as the dorsal root ganglia and the ganglia of the sympathetic and parasympathetic nervous systems. The second pathway runs just beneath the ectoderm and cells that take this route will subsequently differentiate into the pigment cells of the skin. Their final localization involves invasion of the ectoderm. The way in which the neural crest cells enter the epithelial tissue territory is unknown but breaching of the basal lamina must occur. The mechanisms involved here could be particularly relevant to an understanding of carcinoma invasion where tumour cells cross the basal lamina to invade underlying connective tissues. Furthermore, in the dissemination and localization of tumour cells in metastases, the entry and exit from blood vessels may also involve crossing and recrossing the basal lamina of endothelia.

The way in which the neural crest pathways are defined may involve materials in the extracellular matrix. In a white strain of axolotls, the absence of pigmentation does not involve a defect in the differentiation of neural crest cells. Instead, a failure of neural crest migration appears to be involved. When ectoderm overlying the prospective pigment cell pathway is grafted from a dark axolotl, cells migrate from the neural crest and a patch of pigmented skin develops[57]. The promotion of crest cell migration appears to be brought about by the extracellular matrix supplied by the ectodermal graft. Inert carriers can be loaded with extracellular matrix components by placing them below the ectoderm in embryos of the dark strain. When these loaded carriers are subsequently grafted to embryos of the white strain, neural crest cell emigration is promoted[58].

At present, it is not clear which of the extracellular matrix components is of prime importance in defining the route of the neural crest invasion. In embryos of pigmented axolotl strains, oriented collagen fibrils appear to lie along the pathway followed by the prospective pigment cells[59]. However, in chick embryos, collagen fibrils appear to be aligned at right angles to the direction of neural crest migration[60]. Another component of the extracellular matrix that might be involved in neural crest cell migration is fibronectin. Fibronectin mediates the attachment of cells to collagen[61]. Neural crest cells do not appear to synthesise fibronectin[62]. However, the neural crest pathways are rich in fibronectin and the cells may preferentially accumulate in these fibronectin-rich regions[63,64]. Glycosaminoglycans in the extracellular matrix could also be important in defining the pathways taken by the neural crest cells. The presence of high levels of hyaluronic acid correlates both temporally and spatially with neural crest migration[65].

In general terms, the invasion routes of the neural crest show similarities to patterns of malignant invasion. A common feature is invasion along tissue interfaces such as that between the mesenchyme and the ectoderm, the pathway taken by the cells that will form the pigment in the skin. The idea that the pattern of invasion by the neural crest may be governed by the same factors as tumour cell invasion is reinforced by the behaviour of sarcoma 180 tumour cells[66]. When grafted adjacent to the neural tube in place of the neural crest, the tumour cells will disperse along the familiar pathways and some cells end up between the notochord and the dorsal aorta, the position where the chain of sympathetic ganglia normally forms. However, small latex beads when injected into the somites are also dispersed along the same routes[67]. This suggests that factors other than cell motility may be involved in translocation. Adhesion to extracellular matrix components appears to be important. Neural crest cells and other transplanted cells that invade, including sarcoma 180 cells, lack surface bound fibronectin. Furthermore, when beads pre-coated with fibronectin are injected into the somites, they do not translocate[67].

The factors that finally serve to localize the neural crest cells in appropriate positions are little understood. The mechanisms involved are central to an understanding of the establishment of the tissues derived from the crest. It appears that closure of the pathways may occur as development proceeds, rather than the crest cells acquiring new properties that cause them to stop moving. This has been shown by taking neural crest cells that have already localized and differentiated into parasympathetic ganglion cells and injecting them at the start of the migration route in younger embryos[68]. The transplanted cells will now migrate and follow pathways appropriate to the position in which they are grafted. The conclusion from these experiments is that the crest cells have a potential for invasion and this can be expressed if suitable environmental cues, presumably given by the extracellular matrix, are provided.

Gland development

The development of glands involves invasion of mesenchyme by an epithelium. This also occurs in the development of organs such as the liver. The development of the mammary gland involves an interaction between the ectoderm and the underlying mesenchyme. Regional differences in the mesenchyme may dictate the position where a gland forms. In this position, the ectoderm becomes locally thickened. The thickened epithelium enlarges and begins to penetrate the underlying mesenchyme. The epithelial sprout rapidly elongates and then branches to produce a ramifying system of cords of epithelial tissue. As the process of invasion is being completed, the epithelial cords develop a lumen. This involves polarization of the epithelial cells and soon the epithelial lining of the gland is established (Figure 5.12)[69].

The development of the mammary gland provides an attractive model for carcinoma invasion. A basic similarity lies in the penetration of a foreign tissue by epithelial cells, although during normal development this process is strictly controlled. The force for penetration during development appears to be generated by the expansion of the mammary epithelium brought about by cell proliferation in the sprout. In the developing salivary gland in the quail, which consists of a single epithelial sprout, cell proliferation is not localized. It has been proposed that the basal lamina of the developing gland may serve to direct expansion by constraining the sides of the sprout so as to allow penetration only at the tip[70]. This mechanism could apply to the morphogenesis of branching glands. Spatial differences in the composition of the basal lamina around the branching submandibular gland rudiments of mouse embryos provide some support for this proposal. Along the sides of the branches, the basal lamina is well organized and collagen type I is present whereas at the tips of the invading epithelial sprout, collagen is absent and there is a rapid turnover of glycosaminoglycans[71].

In epithelial tumours, the force for penetration of adjacent tissues may also be generated by proliferation. Another possible mechanism would involve active migration of the tumour cells[72]. To what extent these two mechanisms operate is controversial. There is no evidence that cell motility is involved in

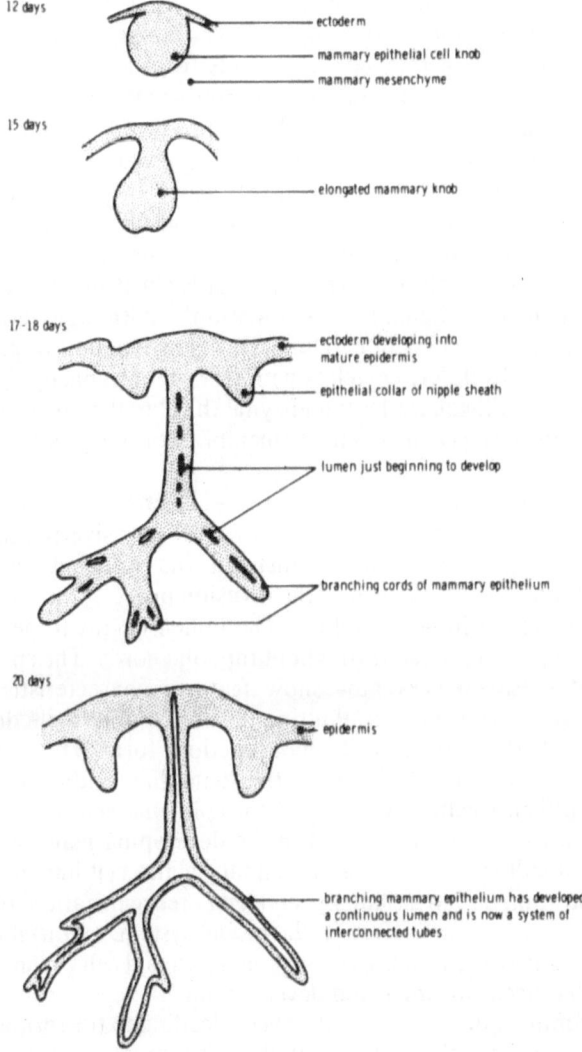

12 days

ectoderm

mammary epithelial cell knob

mammary mesenchyme

15 days

elongated mammary knob

17-18 days

ectoderm developing into
mature epidermis

epithelial collar of nipple sheath

lumen just beginning to develop

branching cords of mammary epithelium

20 days

epidermis

branching mammary epithelium has developed
a continuous lumen and is now a system of
interconnected tubes

Figure 5.12 Diagrams to illustrate the development of the mammary gland in female mouse embryos

the invasion by epithelial cells during gland development; thus if cell motility is of prime importance in malignant invasion, then the developing gland will not provide a good model. Furthermore, during gland development, although the basal lamina may be weaker at the tips of the invading epithelial cords, nevertheless a basal lamina appears totally to enclose the epithelial cells. Invading carcinoma cells may also be surrounded by basal lamina components. However, quite frequently breakdown of the basal lamina accompanies carcinoma invasion[73].

As the epithelium penetrates the mesenchyme during mammary gland development, changes in the mesenchyme must occur to accommodate the expanding epithelium. Some space appears to be created by the mesenchyme cells being pushed out of the way. This leads to a layer of flattened more tightly packed cells oriented around the invading sprout. Further space could be created if the mammary epithelium produced enzymes such as plasminogen activator, the enzyme which generates plasmin from plasminogen[74]. Plasmin is probably involved in the breakdown of the extracellular matrix. It directly attacks laminin and fibronectin (components of basement membranes) and may play a role in activating collagenases[75]. Enhanced production of plasminogen activator is a feature of many tumours and an early sign of malignant transformation[76]. Although thought to be important in the invasiveness of carcinomas, the production of plasminogen activator does not absolutely correlate with metastatic capacity. By contrast, the production of collagenase IV (an enzyme that breaks down the collagen type IV found exclusively in basement membranes) appears to be a better correlate[75].

The organization of the epithelial cells shows dramatic changes during the development of the mammary gland. During the invasive phase when the epithelial cords are penetrating the mesenchyme, the epithelial cells are tightly packed. However, towards the end of the invasion process, the epithelial cells start to polarize and a lumen develops. The lumen begins to develop when small crevices appear scattered throughout the solid cords. The epithelial cells that surround these crevices now show features characteristic of apical polarization. On the cell surfaces abutting the crevice microvilli develop and at the adjoining surfaces of the cells tight junctions form. The small crevices enlarge and join up to form the lumen of the gland that is now lined by a layer of polarized epithelial cells[69]. The trigger for epithelial cell polarization that leads to the start of lumen formation in the developing gland is unknown. However, when cultures of a mouse mammary gland cell line growing on a collagen substratum are overlain by collagen, reorganization of the cells occurs and a lumen appears. Thus, in the model system, extracellular matrix can provide a signal which leads to changes in epithelial cell organization that mimic those that occur during gland development[77].

In the development of the kidney, the events leading to the formation of the epithelia that will line the kidney tubules also involve a change in the association of cells, in this case derived from the mesoderm, so that they now form an epithelium. One of the earliest events is the appearance of the basal lamina component, laminin which can be detected by immunofluorescent tagged antibodies[78]. It appears that laminin may effect the polarization of the cells so that the apical and basal differences arise which are characteristic of cells of an epithelium but are lacking in mesenchymal cells. Thus basal lamina components can affect epithelial cell polarization and may also be instrumental in bringing about epithelial organization. This is particularly relevant when one considers the breakdown in epithelial organization that is a feature of carcinomas and points to the basal lamina as being of major importance.

The relationship between cell organization and invasion in the developing mammary gland may illustrate a general principle that also applies to carcinoma invasion. A feature of carcinomas is a loss of cell polarization and the invasion by cords or strands of cells. During the genesis of carcinomas of the breast, a characteristic cellular organization, a cribriform pattern, is sometimes seen[79]. In a cribriform pattern, the ducts of the gland are almost entirely filled with cells but there are holes scattered throughout. This pattern is reminiscent of the early stages in lumen formation during development of the gland. The loss of cell polarization appears to allow the formation of solid cords of cells. It appears that epithelial cells may require this type of organization to become invasive and penetrate surrounding tissue.

SUMMING UP

As we have seen, during the development of the fertilized egg into a new individual a limited number of fundamental processes are involved in constructing organs and tissues. In cell differentiation, cells become different. Ultimately this leads to the production of cells specialised for particular functions and characteristic of each tissue. In pattern formation, cell differentiation is spatially controlled and this leads to patterns of tissues. And in morphogenesis, cells become arranged to give appropriate shape and form to organs and tissues.

A fourth major process in development, one that we have not discussed in detail, is growth. A general feature of embryonic development is that differences arise in relatively small populations of cells as, for example, in the early mouse embryo and pattern formation in the limb[27]. The size of the cell population is probably limited by the range of positional signals and cell interactions. These cannot operate over large distances. Since the pattern of tissues is laid down when structures are very small, a large proportion of embryonic development is devoted to growth so that a reasonable size is attained by the time that the animal takes on an independent existence. During this growth phase, the tissues laid down enlarge and this must occur by faithful generation of cells of the same tissue type. In addition, the proliferation of tissues must be controlled so that the correct proportions are established and maintained. The control of growth processes in embryos may involve cellular oncogenes[80]. Furthermore, it has recently been found that the gene for insulin-like growth factor II is expressed in Wilms' tumours (embryonal nephroblastomas) at the high levels characteristic of fetal kidney tissues[81]. Thus, at the molecular level, the same mechanisms may operate in embryos and in tumour growth.

Only a small repertoire of cell activities are involved in developmental processes. Cells synthesise proteins and secrete them. Cells receive information from their environment and respond to it. Cells interact with other cells. Cells move, change shape and stick to other cells. Cells proliferate. Since malignant cells share this same repertoire of cell activities, it is the special way in which malignant cells call on this repertoire that marks the difference between them and normal cells.

Acknowledgements

I thank S. E. Wedden and Professor L. Wolpert for their helpful comments on the manuscript.

References

1. Kelly, S. J. (1977). Studies of the developmental potential of 4- and 8-cell stage mouse blastomeres. *J. Exp. Zool.*, **200**, 365-376
2. Hillman, N., Sherman, M. I. and Graham, C. (1972). The effect of spatial arrangement on cell determination during mouse development. *J. Embryol. Exp. Morphol.*, **28**, 263-278
3. Snell, G. D. and Stevens, L. C. (1966). Early embryology. In Green, E. L. (ed.) *Biology of the Laboratory Mouse*. 2nd edn. (New York: McGraw-Hill Book Coy)
4. Saxen, L. and Toivonen, S. (1962). *Primary Embryonic Induction*. (Gt. Britain: Logos Press)
5. Slack, J. M. W. (1983). *From Egg to Embryo*. (Cambridge: Cambridge University Press)
6. Garcia-Bellido, A., Lawrence, P. A. and Morata, G. (1979). Compartments in animal development. *Sci. Am.*, **241**, 90-98
7. Garcia-Bellido, A., Ripoll, P. and Morata, G. (1973). Developmental compartmentalization of the wing disk of *Drosophila. Nature, New Biol.*, **245**, 251-253
8. Crick, F. H. C. and Lawrence, P. A. (1975). Compartments and polyclones in insect development. *Science*, **189**, 340-347
9. Kornberg, T. (1981). *Engrailed*. A gene controlling compartment and segment formation in *Drosophila. Proc. Natl. Acad. Sci. USA*, **78**, 1095-1099
10. Morata, G. and Lawrence, P. A. (1975). Control of compartment development by the *engrailed* gene in *Drosophila. Nature*, **255**, 614-617
11. Lawrence, P. A. and Morata, G. (1976). Compartments in the wing of *Drosophila*: a study of the *engrailed* gene. *Dev. Biol.*, **50**, 321-338
12. Garcia-Bellido, A. and Santamaria, P. (1972). Developmental analysis of the wing disc in the mutant *engrailed* of *Drosophila melanogaster. Genetics*, **72**, 87-104
13. Wilcox, M., Brower, M. L. and Smith, R. J. (1981). A position-specific cell surface antigen in the *Drosophila* wing imaginal disc. *Cell*, **25**, 159 164
14. Warner, A. E. and Lawrence, P. A. (1982). Permeability of gap junctions at the segmental border in insect epidermis. *Cell*, **28**, 243-252
15. O'Brochta, D. A. and Bryant, P. J. (1985). A zone of non-proliferating cells at a lineage restriction boundary in *Drosophila. Nature*, **313**, 138-141
16. Ponder, B. A. J., Schmidt, G. H., Wilkinson, M. M., Wood, M. J., Monk, M. and Reid, A. (1985). Derivation of mouse intestinal crypts from single progenitor cells. *Nature*, **313**, 689-691
17. Keynes, R. J. and Stern, C. D. (1984). Segmentation in the vertebrate nervous system. *Nature*, **310**, 786-789
18. Gurdon, J. B. (1974). *The Control of Gene Expression in Animal Development*. (Oxford: Oxford University Press)
19. Mohun, T. J., Brennan, S., Dathan, N., Fairman, S. and Gurdon, J. B. (1984). Cell-type specific activation of actin genes in the early amphibian embryo. *Nature*, **311**, 716-721
20. Fjose, A., McGinnis, W. J., and Gehring, W. J. (1985). Isolation of a homoeo box-containing gene from the *engrailed* region of *Drosophila* and the spatial distribution of its transcripts. *Nature*, **313**, 284-289
21. Kornberg, T., Siden, I., O'Farrell, P. and Simon, M. (1985). The engrailed locus of *Drosophila*: In situ localization of transcripts reveals compartment-specific expression. *Cell*, **40**, 45-53
22. Hafen, E., Kuroiwa, A. and Gehring, W. J. (1984). Spatial distribution of transcripts from the segmentation gene *fushi tarazu* during *Drosophila* embryonic development. *Cell*, **37**, 833-841
23. Martinez-Arias, A. and Lawrence, P. A. (1985). Parasegments and compartments in the *Drosophila* embryo. *Nature*, **313**, 639-642

24. Gehring, W. J. (1985). The homoeo box: a key to the understanding of development? *Cell*, **40**, 3-5

25. McGinnis, W., Garber, R. L., Wirz, J., Kuroiwa, A. and Gehring, W. J. (1984). A homologous protein coding sequence in *Drosophila* homoeotic genes and its conservation in other metazoans. *Cell*, **37**, 403-408

26. Slack, J. M. W. (1985). Homoeotic transformations in man: implications for the mechanism of embryonic development and for the organization of epithelia. *J. Theor. Biol.*, **114**, 463-490

27. Wolpert, L. (1969). Positional information and the spatial pattern of cellular differentiation. *J. Theor. Biol.*, **25**, 1-47

28. Wolpert, L. (1971). Positional information and pattern formation. *Curr. Top. Dev. Biol.*, **6**, 183-223

29. Illmensee, K. and Mahowald, A. P. (1974). Transplantation of posterior polar plasm in *Drosophila*. Induction of germ cells at the anterior pole of the egg. *Proc. Natl. Acad. Sci. USA*, **71**, 1016-1020

30. Clement, A. C. (1952). Experimental studies on germinal localisation in *Ilyanassa*. I. The role of the polar lobe in determination of the cleavage pattern and its influence in later development. *J. Exp. Zool.*, **121**, 593-625

31. Sulston, J. E., Schierenberg, E., White, J. G., and Thomson, J. N. (1983). The embryonic cell lineage of the nematode *Caenorhabditis elegans*. *Dev. Biol.*, **100**, 64-119

32. Sulston, J. E. and Horvitz, H. R. (1977). Post-embryonic lineages of the nematode, *Caenorhabditis elegans*. *Dev. Biol.*, **56**, 110-156

33. Kimble, J. (1981). Alterations in cell lineage following laser ablation of cells in the somatic gonad of *Caenorhabditis elegans*. *Dev. Biol.*, **87**, 286-301

34. Ducibella, T., Albertini, D. F., Anderson, E. and Biggers, J. D. (1975). The preimplantation mammalian embryo: characterization of intercellular junctions and their appearance during development. *Dev. Biol.*, **45**, 231-250

35. Papaioannou, V. E., McBurney, M. W., Gardner, R. L. and Evans, M. J. (1975). Fate of teratocarcinoma cells injected into early mouse embryos. *Nature*, **258**, 70-73

36. Rossant, J. and Papaioannou, V. E. (1985). Outgrowth of embryonal carcinoma cells from injected blastocysts *in vitro* correlates with abnormal chimera development *in vivo*. *Exp. Cell Res.*, **156**, 213-220

37. Warner, A. E., Guthrie, S. C. and Gilula, N. B. (1984). Antibodies to gap junction protein selectively disrupt junctional communication in the early amphibian embryo. *Nature*, **311**, 127-131

38. Wolpert, L. (1978). Pattern formation in biological development. *Sci. Am.*, **239**, 154-164

39. Summerbell, D., Lewis, J. and Wolpert, L. (1973). Positional information in chick limb morphogenesis. *Nature*, **244**, 492-496

40. Saunders, J. W. (1977). The experimental analysis of chick limb development. In Ede, D. A., Hinchliffe, J. R. and Balls, M. (eds.) *Limb and Somite Morphogenesis*. pp. 1-24. (Cambridge: Cambridge University Press)

41. Boutin, E. L. and Fallon, J. F. (1984). An analysis of the fate of the chick wing bud apical ectodermal ridge in culture. *Dev. Biol.*, **104**, 111-117

42. Billingham, R. E. and Silvers, W. K. (1967). Studies on the conservation of epidermal specificities of the skin and certain mucosas in adult mammals. *J. Exp. Med.*, **125**, 429-446

43. Saunders, J. W. and Gasseling, M. T. (1968). Ectodermal-mesenchymal interactions in the origin of limb symmetry. In Fleischmajer, R. and Billingham, R. F. (eds.) *Epithelial-mesenchymal Interactions*. pp. 78-97. (Baltimore: Williams and Wilkins)

44. Tickle, C., Summerbell, D. and Wolpert, L. (1975). Positional signalling and specification of digits in chick wing morphogenesis. *Nature*, **254**, 199-202

45. Tickle, C., Lee, J. and Eichele, G. (1985). A quantitative analysis of the effect of all-*trans*-retinoic acid on the pattern of chick wing development. *Dev. Biol.*, **109**, 82-95

46. Eichele, G., Tickle, C. and Alberts, B. M. (1985). Studies on the mechanism of retinoid-induced pattern duplications in the early chick limb bud: temporal and spatial aspects. *J. Cell Biol.*, **101**, 1913 1920

47. Sporn, M. B. and Roberts, A. B. (1983). Role of retinoids in differentiation and carcinogenesis. *Cancer Res.*, **43**, 3034-3040

48. Chevallier, A., Kieny, M., Mauger, A. and Sengel, P. (1977). Developmental fate of the somitic mesoderm in the chick embryo. In Ede, D. A., Hinchliffe, J. R. and Balls, M. (eds.)

Vertebrate Limb and Somite Morphogenesis. (Cambridge: Cambridge University Press)

49. Chevallier, A., Kieny, M. and Mauger, A. (1977). Limb-somite relationship: origin of the limb musculature. *J. Embryol. Exp. Morphol.*, **41**, 245-258

50. Le Douarin, N. (1982). *The Neural Crest.* (Cambridge: Cambridge University Press)

51. Pearse, A. G. E. (1969). The cytochemistry and ultrastructure of polypeptide hormone producing cells of the APUD series and the embryologic, physiologic and pathologic implications of the concept. *J. Histochem. Cytochem.*, **17**, 303-313

52. Le Douarin, N. (1980). The ontogeny of the neural crest in avian embryo chimaeras. *Nature*, **286**, 663-669

53. Noden, D. M. (1983). The role of the neural crest in patterning of avian cranial skeletal connective and muscle tissues. *Dev. Biol.*, **96**, 144-165

54. Edelman, G. (1984). Cell adhesion and morphogenesis: the regulator hypothesis. *Proc. Natl. Acad. Sci. USA*, **81**, 1460-1464

55. Brackenbury, R., Greenberg, M. E. and Edelman, G. E. (1984). Phenotypic changes and loss of N-CAM-mediated adhesion in transformed embryonic chicken retinal cells. *J. Cell Biol.*, **99**, 1944-1955

56. Weston, J. A. (1970). The migration and differentiation of neural crest cells. *Adv. Morphog.*, **8**, 41-114

57. Keller, R. E., Lofberg, J. and Speith, J. (1982). Neural crest cell behaviour in white and dark embryos of *Ambystoma mexicanum*: epidermal inhibition of pigment cell migration in the white axolotl. *Dev. Biol.*, **89**, 179-196

58. Lofberg, J., Nynas-McCoy, A., Olsson, C., Jonsson, L. and Perris, R. (1985). Stimulation of initial neural crest cell migration in the axolotl embryo by tissue grafts and extracellular matrix transplanted on microcarriers. *Dev. Biol.*, **107**, 442-460

59. Lofberg, J. and Ahlfors, K. (1978). Extracellular matrix organization and early neural crest cell migration in the axolotl embryo. In Jacobson, C-O. and Ebendal, T. (eds.) *Formshaping Movements in Neurogenesis.* pp. 87-103. (Stockholm: Almquist and Wiksell International)

60. Tosney, K. W. (1982). The segregation and early migration of cranial neural crest cells in the avian embryo. *Dev. Biol.*, **89**, 13-25

61. Hynes, R. O. and Yamada, K. M. (1982). Fibronectins: multifunctional modular glycoproteins. *J. Cell Biol.*, **95**, 369-377

62. Newgreen, D. and Thiery, J-P. (1980). Fibronectin in early avian embryos: synthesis and distribution along the migration pathways. *Cell Tissue Res.*, **211**, 269-291

63. Duband, J. P. and Thiery, J.-P. (1982). Distribution of fibronectin in the early phase of avian cephalic neural crest cell migration. *Dev. Biol.*, **93**, 308-324

64. Thiery, J.-P., Duband, J. P. and Delouvee, A. (1982). Pathways and mechanisms of avian trunk neural crest cell migration and localization. *Dev. Biol.*, **93**, 324-344

65. Derby, M. A. (1978). Analysis of glycosaminoglycans within the extracellular environments encountered by migrating neural crest cells. *Dev. Biol.*, **66**, 321-336

66. Erickson, C. A., Tosney, K. W. and Weston, J. A. (1980). Analysis of migratory behaviour of neural crest and fibroblastic cells in embryonic tissues. *Dev. Biol.*, **77**, 142-156

67. Bronner-Fraser, M. (1982). Distribution of latex beads and retinal pigment epithelial cells along the ventral neural crest pathway. *Dev. Biol.*, **91**, 50-63

68. Le Douarin, N. M., Teillet, M. A., Ziller, C. and Smith, J. (1978). Adrenergic differentiation of cells of the cholinergic ciliary and Remak's ganglia in avian embryos after *in vivo* transplantation. *Proc. Natl. Acad. Sci. USA*, **75**, 2030-2034

69. Hogg, N. A. S., Harrison, C. J. and Tickle, C. (1983). Lumen formation in the developing mouse mammary gland. *J. Embryol. Exp. Morphol.*, **73**, 39-57

70. Nogawa, H. (1981). Analysis of elongating morphogenesis of quail anterior submaxillary gland: Absence of localized cell proliferation. *J. Embryol. Exp. Morphol.*, **62**, 229-239

71. Bernfield, M., Banerjee, S. D., Koda, J. E. and Rapraeger, A. C. (1984). Remodelling of the basement membrane: morphogenesis and maturation. In Porter, R. and Whelan, J. (eds.) *Basement Membranes and Cell Movement.* Ciba Foundation Symposium. No. 108, 179-192

72. Trinkaus, J. P. (1976). On the mechanism of metazoan cell movements. In Poste, G. and Nicolson, G. (eds.) *The Cell Surface in Animal Embryogenesis and Development. Cell Surface Review.* Vol. 1, pp. 225-329. (Amsterdam: North-Holland Publishing)

73. Liotta, L. A., Rao, C. N. and Barsky, S. H. (1983). Tumour invasion and the extracellular

106

matrix. *Lab. Invest.*, **49**, 636-649

74. Reich, E. (1973). Tumor-associated fibrinolysis. *Fed. Proc.*, **32**, 2174-2175

75. Salo, T., Liotta, L. A., Keski-Oja, J., Turpeenniemi-Hujanen, T. and Tryggvason, K. (1982). Secretion of basement membrane collagen degrading enzyme and plasminogen activator by transformed cells - role in metastasis. *Int. J. Cancer*, **30**, 669-673

76. Hince, T. A. and Roscoe, J. P. (1978). Fibrinolytic activity of cultured cells derived during ethylnitrosourea-induced carcinogenesis of rat brain. *Br. J. Cancer*, **37**, 424-433

77. Hall, H. G., Farson, D. A. and Bissell, M. J. (1982). Lumen formation by epithelial cell lines in response to collagen overlay: a morphogenetic model in culture. *Proc. Natl. Acad. Sci. USA*, **79**, 4672-4676

78. Ekblom, P., Alitalo, K., Vaheri, A., Timpl, R. and Saxen, L. (1980). Induction of a basement membrane glycoprotein in embryonic kidney: possible role of laminin in morphogenesis. *Proc. Natl. Acad. Sci. USA*, **77**, 485-489

79. Haagensen, C. D. (1971). *Diseases of the Breast*. 2nd edn. (Philadelphia, London and Ontario: W. B. Saunders Company)

80. Slamon, D. J. and Cline, M. J. (1984). Expression of cellular oncogenes during embryonic and fetal development of the mouse. *Proc. Natl. Acad. Sci. USA*, **81**, 7141-7145

81. Scott, J., Cowell, J., Robertson, M. E., Priestley, L. M., Wadey, R., Hopkins, B., Pritchard, J., Bell, G. I., Rall, L. B., Graham, C. F. and Knott, T. J. (1985). Insulin-like growth factor-II gene expression in Wilms' tumour and embryonic tissues. *Nature*, **317**, 260-262

6
Animal models of cancer

S. A. ECCLES

INTRODUCTION

A common approach to the analysis of complex phenomena is to develop a model which parallels the salient features of the subject of investigation, but which is more amenable to experimental dissection and manipulation. The International Union against Cancer (UICC) recognises over 200 distinct neoplastic diseases[1]; individuals vary enormously in their susceptibility to different types of cancer, in the rate of progression of their diseases, and in their responses to treatment. In the case of animal models of cancer(s) in man, therefore, a fundamental problem lies in the sheer diversity of phenomena which we wish to understand.

Until relatively recently it was assumed that cancers were an inevitable accompaniment of ageing[2]. Now it is accepted that 80–90% of cancers are associated with environmental risk factors[2-5], at least some of which have been identified, and could in theory, (unlike old age) be circumvented. Since this major conceptual breakthrough rapid progress has been and is being made in our understanding of the molecular and biochemical bases of malignancy, the mode of action of physical, viral and chemical carcinogens and the genetic and epigenetic processes involved in the evolution of a fully malignant cell.

Epidemiological data are invaluable but have obvious limitations[6]. (See also Chapter 7.) The studies are for expediency mostly retrospective, require large populations for analysis, and although able to establish the causal relationship between smoking and lung cancer[7,8] could not alone (without experimentation) identify or predict specific and co-operating risk factors, or the ultimate carcinogens or promoters in complex chemical mixtures. Further analysis, therefore, clearly requires model systems.

There is no doubt that most of the animal 'models' – either those devised in nature or in laboratories – do not mimic exactly any particular human cancer. The shortcomings of *in vitro* and *in vivo* assays of carcinogenicity, the multitude of inter-species differences in anatomy, physiology and metabolism, the differences between tissues, cells and even regions of DNA in response to viral and chemical carcinogens have exercised experimentalists and generated many critical reviews concerning their validity[9-16].

Available animal models fall roughly into two categories: naturally occurring cancers in wild or domesticated outbred stocks, and cancers induced in laboratory animals (commonly inbred rodents and occasionally other mammals including primates). In addition, *in vitro* systems of cell and organ culture are increasingly expanding our battery of available assays, and should also be considered. In the succeeding sections I intend to examine how relevant or useful such models are in furthering our understanding of the aetiology and pathology of human cancer.

CHEMICAL CARCINOGENESIS

Following the pioneering work of Kennaway and his colleagues in the 1930s, who showed that a pure chemical isolated from coal tar was carcinogenic in rodents[17], a wide variety of agents and protocols have been devised for inducing neoplasms in experimental animals. The problem is to determine which if any of these procedures best models the common human cancers.

Many of the classical concepts of multistage carcinogenesis have been derived from the mouse skin model, in which two stages of carcinogenesis, (initiation and promotion) have been clearly demonstrated[18-21]. The historical reasons for this approach are readily apparent: observations on scrotal skin cancer in chimney sweeps by Pott had led to the first deduction of a cause of cancer based on clinical and epidemiological data in the 18th century, and suspect substances could be applied to animal skin where the effects were easily observed. The 'skin painting' method has served not only in the identification, extraction and purification of agents which can contribute to the induction of cancer, but has allowed detailed analysis of a carcinogenic process and its potential for modification[22]. Some of the most notable successes of this system have been the isolation of 1,2,5,6-dibenzanthracene and 3,4-benzo(a)pyrene from coal tar, the identification of carcinogenic polycyclic aromatic hydrocarbons (PAH), nitrosamines, cocarcinogens and promoters in tobacco smoke[8], and the isolation of one of the most potent groups of promoters, the diterpene esters, from croton oil[23,24].

Nevertheless, the model is by no means without problems as a predictor of risk factors in human cancer. Marked differences exist in the susceptibility of skin to carcinogenesis, not only between species, but between strains of mice[25-27], and of course the relative sensitivity of different animals compared to man is unknown. The structure of rodent skin is quite different from that of man in terms of morphology, hair cycle and permeability to exogenous compounds[28]. Arsenic, a well-established carcinogen which can cause skin cancers in man, has repeatedly failed to do so in any animal system[15,29]. Tobin et al.[19] evaluated 51 chemicals with some evidence of carcinogenic potential in animals and/or man, and their survey showed that when tested in the skin painting protocol only 36/51 (71%) induced skin tumours. Some agents induced systemic tumours, but 7/20 chemicals were undetected as carcinogens when applied by the dermal route, although giving positive results by other routes. Since the skin is an effective barrier to penetration by harmful exogenous agents, a proportion of negative results is to be expected.

Another commonly employed assay for carcinogenic potential is a feeding test carried out for the lifetime of the animal. These long-term *in vivo* assays have been criticised for several reasons:

(a) the high 'spontaneous' tumour incidences in certain species and strains of animals originally employed[30] (although these have been considerably reduced);

(b) the necessary use of extremely high doses of compounds in order for carcinogenic potential to be manifest within the short lifespan of rodents[31];

(c) the known interspecies and interorgan differences in metabolism, carcinogen activation and inactivation[32,33], and susceptibility to carcinogens[34];

(d) the problem of extrapolating risk assessment and dose response curves from rodents to man[16,35,36]. (See also Chapter 6.)

Potential of animal models to detect human carcinogens

The IARC monographs list approximately 30 chemicals associated with the occurrence of cancer in man[15,37]. All but two of these (benzene and arsenic) were reported to be carcinogenic in at least one, and often more than one, animal species[9,14]. The consistent problem in modelling arsenic carcinogenesis is unexplained, but may yet be solved, since benzene is now known to produce leukaemias in mice[29]. For several chemical carcinogens carcinogenic potency in rodents approximates that in humans[14,16,26]. For some carcinogens the tissue specificity in rodents is the same as in humans, but this is not necessarily so[37,38]. Vinyl chloride induces angiosarcomas of liver, and asbestos causes mesotheliomas, in both mice and men. However, 2-naphthylamine (a human bladder carcinogen) is non-carcinogenic in rats, induces liver cancer in mice, but only in dogs, hamsters and monkeys is it associated with bladder cancer[9,29,39]. In contrast, 2-acetylaminofluorene, (2-AAF) is carcinogenic in the urinary bladder in rat, mouse and rabbit, but not guinea pigs[38]. Such factors clearly complicate current attempts to extrapolate data from animals to man, but they may yet provide the means by which the determinants of susceptibility will ultimately be deciphered. For example, by comparing susceptible and resistant cells, tissues and organ systems it may be possible to trace the metabolic pathways which determine the relative rate of production of active and inactive products of specific carcinogens. Already studies of 2-AAF have played an important role in the development of the electrophile theory of carcinogenesis[40], and have illustrated how the complete refractoriness of the guinea pig is due to a single metabolic difference (it does not N-hydroxylate 2-AAF) compared with susceptible species[41].

There are several well-documented examples of animal studies predicting the carcinogenicity of a compound before clinical/epidemiological data confirmed its effects in humans. Examples include melphalan, the production of vaginal cancers by transplacental diethylstilboestrol, the induction of bladder cancers by 4-aminobiphenyl, liver angiosarcomas by vinyl chloride, and lung cancer by bis-(chloromethyl)-ether[14]. Also, one of the most potent carcinogenic agents known, aflatoxin (which is still a major risk factor in human liver cancer in many countries)[42] was discovered following poultry poisoning due to *Aspergillus flavus* contamination, and was subsequently shown to be a hepatocarcinogen in many species[43]. More recently, compounds inducing cancers in animals have been withdrawn before their large-scale production (e.g. acetylaminofluorene) which means that for this, and many similar cases, we can never know if a potential human risk factor has been eliminated from our environment or not.

The way ahead would seem to be to analyse further the mechanism(s) of action of putative chemical carcinogens at the cellular and molecular level, to determine the biochemical bases of susceptibility and resistance, and thereby to provide a more rational interpretation of the results obtained in animal 'model' systems. The current dissatisfaction with *in vivo* carcinogenicity assays will not be overcome by the performance of more and more tests according to rigid protocols. New experimental designs[44] and improved models are constantly being developed, including short-term assays employing rodent and human cell and organ cultures for mutation and transformation tests[11,45,46], and modified Ames' tests (a test of mutation in bacteria) which detect more agents requiring metabolic activation than was previously possible[9,47]. Also, in recent years sensitive systems have been specifically designed to detect promoters, both *in vitro*[48-50] and *in vivo* in a variety of cell and tissue types[51-56].

It should be obvious that no single test or model will provide all the answers that we seek, but the intelligent choice of a range of assays and their continuing refinement should provide much information germane to the identification of potential human carcinogens in the thousands of new compounds developed by industry each year. The alternative is to allow man to be the experimental animal, and to determine retrospectively (as with cigarette smoking) and accurately the number of lethal cancers ascribable to carcinogen exposure.

Multistage carcinogenesis: the mouse skin model

The essential features of 'two-stage' carcinogenesis were described over 40 years ago in a mouse skin model which remains the paradigm for what is now considered to be a multistage continuum. Much evidence suggests that covalent binding of initiators (or their metabolites) to DNA is the critical event in initiation[18,57,58]. The process is permanent and irreversible, and thought to be due either to point mutations[59] or to gene amplifications and/or rearrangements[60-62]. The events involved in promotion are less well understood, and there is now evidence that the process(es) can be subdivided into at least two stages[18,63]. The first step can be induced by a single application of TPA, is irreversible, but can be blocked by the protease inhibitor tosyl phenylalanine chloromethyl ketone (TPCK). A second step can be accomplished by repeated applications of weak promoters (e.g. mezerein), is at first reversible, and although unaffected by TPCK can be specifically blocked by certain retinoids[64].

TPA, related phorbol ester tumour promoters and other classes of promoters such as indole alkaloids (e.g. teleocidin) and the polyacetate compound aplysiatoxin exert highly pleiotropic effects upon cells. Their primary site of action appears to be the cell membrane[60,65], and recent evidence suggests that binding of TPA (and the two unrelated classes of promoters mentioned above) to a 'phorboid receptor' is important in initiating the complex series of events which follow[66,67]. The relative ability of a series of phorbol esters to compete with a radiolabelled ligand for binding to the cell surface receptors is said to correlate well with their activities as promoters in the mouse skin model[61].

It was originally thought that phorbol ester promotion, while an interesting phenomenon, was applicable only to mouse skin and of little general relevance[20]. However, in several species and strains, phorbol and phorbol esters have been shown to promote tumours in liver, colon, lung, forestomach and mammary gland, and in some cases were capable of acting transplacentally[68-71]. Of particular interest are recent epidemiological data suggesting that diterpene-ester type promoters in *Euphorbeaceae* and *Thymelaceae* species may act as significant cocarcinogenic human risk factors[72]. The black and Creole populations of Curaçao have an extremely high incidence of oesophageal cancer which seems to be associated with the drinking of tea made from the leaves of *Croton flavens*. Soluble extracts of this plant contain several strong promoters of DMBA-tumorigenesis in mouse skin[72]. Initiators were postulated to have been provided by other commonly used plants on the island, and/or by contamination of the drinking water by petrol. Also, the recent demonstration of 'phorboid receptors' in diverse tissues and cell types in invertebrate, rodent, avian and human species[73,74], and the identification of the major receptor as a protein kinase C-phospholipid complex[75,76], suggest that future studies will yield valuable information concerning general mechanisms of cellular receptor response pathways. Of note are the parallels between the mode of action of peptide hormones, growth factors and the protein products of several oncogenic retroviruses[77,78] (discussed in detail in Chapter 3).

Critical events subsequent to promoter binding are difficult to elucidate, and the common pathway(s), if any, between different classes of chemicals and such diverse 'promoters' as wounding/surgery[79,80], infectious agents (viruses, parasites)[81,82], hormones[83], and even inert solid objects[84] remain obscure. One interesting possibility (recently reviewed by Trosko[85]) is that since intercellular communication plays a key role in regulating cell growth and differentiation, any condition which disrupts this process may allow the selective growth of abnormal cells, perhaps due to the loss of metabolic co-operation. Several observations are consistent with the hypothesis that tumour promotion involves inhibition of cellular communication by modulating Ca^{2+} and cAMP control of the genes (and their products) involved in differentiation[56,86]. Such pathways are likely to be well-conserved in vertebrate evolution, and thus encourage the view that, at the molecular level, there may be more similarities than differences in the ultimate activities of phorbol esters in mouse skin, and known and yet-to-be identified promoters of human carcinogenesis. Recently developed 'promoter-resistant' cell culture model systems (e.g. JB6)[87] will be helpful in discriminating which cellular responses are dissociable from, and which constitutive to promotion, and DNA transfection experiments should ultimately reveal the genes involved[88].

Multistage carcinogenesis in other tissues and organs – evidence from animal and human studies

In studies comparable to the 'initiation-promotion' regimen in mouse skin, many different tissues and organs have been tested for their susceptibility to carcinogenesis to determine if their responses would fit a generalised 'multistage' model. Although in some cases the experimental design was such that unequivocal proof of initiating or promoting activity could not be adduced, there is no doubt that in many systems the essence of a two-or-more stage process is readily discernible.

Liver

Following the observation of Peraino et al.[89] in the mid 1970s that liver tumorigenicity of 2-AAF in rats could be enhanced by phenobarbital, DDT, and other compounds, and that the essential features paralleled the classical mouse skin model, a variety of multistage hepatocarcinogenesis regimens have been developed. Further studies have led to the identification of a series of morphologically and/or biochemically identifiable preneoplastic lesions, at least some of which may physically represent the five or six stages mathematically calculated to be required for full liver (and skin) carcinogenesis[90-92] (and see Chapter 1). Farber et al.[93] have suggested that one class of initiated liver cell is a hepatocyte that has acquired resistance to the inhibitory effects of carcinogens on cell proliferation (the 'resistant hepatocyte' (RH) model). Forty diverse chemical carcinogens were shown to induce 'resistant hepatocytes' during initiation, and some of the subsequent early steps which were identified proved remarkably similar in seven quite different hepatocarcinogenesis models examined[51,52].

The discovery of liver tumour promoters has increased the sensitivity of the system such that certain compounds previously thought to have no hepatocarcinogenic potential are now identifiable as initiators (e.g. BP, DMBA, and 2-methyl-4-dimethylaminoazobenzene)[94]. Other known liver tumour initiators are aromatic amines, nitrosamines, nitrosamides and PAHs. Promoters include phenobarbital, 1,1,1-trichlorobenzo-p-dioxin, polychlorinated biphenyls, 5-azacytidine, as well as regimes of orotic acid supplemented/low methionine diets. 2-AAF appears to be able to act as an 'early-stage' carcinogen for mouse liver, whereas the main effect of DDT appears to be on late-stage transitions[95]. These observations, based not on initiation-promotion protocols, but on the effect of cessation of treatment on tumour incidence, again suggest that in hepatocarcinogenesis, different agents can affect different stages of the process.

Two carcinogens in particular have been shown to be preferentially associated with cancers of the liver in animals and man: vinyl chloride (mentioned earlier) and aflatoxin. Aflatoxin (AFB_1) has been shown to induce cancers in trout, fowl, rodents and non-human primates[29,96]. Human liver cells contain the enzymes required to produce the epoxymetabolites (especially AFB_1-8,9-epoxide) thought to be the ultimate carcinogens, and the incidence of liver cancer in Thailand, Singapore, Kenya, Swaziland, Mozambique and China is related to the levels of dietary aflatoxin[42]. The level of binding of AFB_1 to liver DNA *in vivo* correlates with trends in carcinogenesis in different species, and the major DNA adducts formed are generally the same (as is the case for active derivatives of BP and certain nitrosamines)[60,97,98]. In addition to its role as an initiator, there is evidence that AFB_1 can act as a promoter/cocarcinogen in hepatitis B virus (HBV)-infected cells[99].

In high incidence areas of human liver cancer, hepatomas and chronic liver disease are also prevalent in ducks[100]. Ducks are highly susceptible to AFB_1, and if the young are fed with local aflatoxin-contaminated corn, hepatic cancers occur at high frequency. Another interesting parallel in human and animal hepatocellular carcinoma (HCC) occurs in the age and sex distribution of the disease. In man, there is an early onset in high incidence areas and it occurs predominantly in males. In animal models also, young animals, and males in particular, are most susceptible to the carcinogenic effects of AFB_1[98]. The similarities in AFB_1-associated HCC in both domestic animal populations and man have provided an almost unique opportunity to study a recognised human carcinogen. Clearly the removal of this risk factor (identified first in animal model systems) is feasible, and together with immunisation against HBV may yield a significant reduction in incidence of HCC, mortalities associated with which are currently over 250 000 per year.

In certain countries alcohol is considered to be a significant factor in hepatic cancer (and is also thought to be related to the incidence of cancers of the upper digestive tract)[15,98]. Although ethanol was reported to be non-carcinogenic in laboratory animals[101], it has been shown to enhance the metabolism of certain carcinogens by rat liver microsomes[102], and to act as a cocarcinogen by virtue of its hepatotoxicity[103]. In this instance, a significant risk factor, acting neither as a classical 'initiator' nor 'promoter' was undetected in standard two-stage protocols. This example cautions against the assumption that all potentially carcinogenic agents will fall neatly into place in a multistage model; some do not, and therefore alternative strategies for their testing must be devised.

Urinary bladder

Classical two-stage carcinogenesis has been shown to be applicable to the urinary bladder in a variety of animal models[104,105]. In 1975 Hicks was successful in demonstrating the promoting activities of sodium saccharin and cyclamate in rats receiving subthreshold doses of N-methyl-N-nitrosourea (MNU)[106]. Subsequently, experiments with the nitrofuran N-[4-(5 nitro-2-furyl)-2-thiazolyl]-formamide (FANFT) and the nitrosamine N-butyl-N-(4-hydroxybutyl)-nitrosamine (BBN) as initiators and tryptophan and phenacetin as promoters were equally successful in rats, mice and dogs[107-109]. The promoters alone induced only very low incidences or no bladder cancers. As in the case of hepatic carcinogenesis, sequential morphological changes could be observed in the urothelium suggestive of critical stages in the evolution of invasive carcinomas[110].

The aromatic amine 2-AAF has long been recognised as a bladder (and liver) carcinogen. Interestingly, although predominantly a first stage (or initiating) carcinogen for the liver[95], in the bladder 2-AAF appears to have mainly promoting activity[111]. Saccharin, the most effective promoter of bladder carcinogenesis, evokes cellular responses similar to those produced in skin by phorbol esters. It may be significant that it also interferes with intercellular communication[112], and inhibits the binding of EGF to cultured cells[113].

In man, cancer of the lower urinary tract has been aetiologically associated with exposure to chemicals since Rehn observed a high incidence of bladder cancers in workers in the aniline dye industry in the 19th century. Huepper and colleagues subsequently demonstrated that one of the carcinogens involved was 2-aminonaphthalene, based on its ability to produce bladder cancers in dogs. Since then, a variety of chemicals have been recognised as human bladder carcinogens including benzidine, 4-aminobiphenyl and cyclophosphamide[114]. Several aromatic amines and amides are carcinogenic in animal species, but with varying organ specificities which seem to be related to differences in metabolism[115]. In all cases their predominant action seems to be on early stage transitions. Cyclophosphamide is reported to be non-carcinogenic for rat bladder, but capable of promoting tumours in animals initiated with FANFT, and to act as a cocarcinogen in mouse bladder[113]. The infrequency of human case histories precludes analysis of its mode of action in bladder carcinogenesis in man.

Much debate has centred on the relative roles of urine, urinary calculi and bladder parasites in experimental and human bladder cancer, which will not be discussed here (for reviews see 105,113,115-117). It is clear that unwanted parasitic infection of rodents (e.g. by *T. crassicauda*) should be excluded, and newer methods of inducing bladder cancer which do not involve the intravesicular implantation of pellets avoid the possible artefactual stimulus of a foreign body. The osmolality and pH of urine in rodents differ from man, and since urine may act as a carrier of carcinogens and may have endogenous promoting activity, further work on interspecies differences is required[115].

Respiratory tract

Most of the studies on experimental respiratory tract carcinogenesis have, not surprisingly, concentrated on tobacco smoke condensates as carcinogens and promoters, many of which have been shown to be active in the mouse skin assay[118]. Animal models have not been very successful in determining the potential of inhaled chemical carcinogens to produce lung cancer. Animals are (sensibly!) reluctant to inhale cigarette smoke, and anatomical features protect the bronchial tree from airborne particles. Benign and malignant laryngeal tumours have been produced in hamsters, and bronchogenic carcinomas in other species on occasion[8]. Urethane and PAHs have been identified as potent initiators of lung tumours in mice, and butylated hydroxytoluene (BHT) and phorbol as promoters[119]. Animal and human tracheobronchial organ culture systems are proving useful in analysing multistage carcinogenesis *in vitro*, and in studying both metabolic activation of potential respiratory tract carcinogens and the action of promoters and antipromoters[120-122].

In man, cigarette smoking has been unequivocally associated with increased risk of bronchial carcinoma[7,8]. Cigarette smoke contains a plethora of complete carcinogens, directly and indirectly acting initiators, promoters, cocarcinogens and mutagens, and epidemiological data suggest excellent conformity with multistage model theory[6]. The age-related incidences, and effects of cessation of smoking, are consistent with an effect on early stage transitions, and a further effect at a penultimate stage[95]. The cocarcinogenic effect of uranium or asbestos exposure on bronchial carcinoma suggests that these agents act at different, as yet undefined, stages. The age incidence of mesothelioma following asbestos exposure also fits a quadratic equation, and may indicate the effect of an early-stage carcinogen[95]. Tumours of the lung and nasal sinuses associated with exposure to nickel refining processes prior to 1930 appear consistent with major effects at a late stage of carcinogenesis. These examples provide convincing evidence that a variety of tumours of the human respiratory tract arise as a result of exposure to agents capable of acting at different stages in a multistage process.

Further sites

In addition to the detailed examples cited above, multistage carcinogenesis has been adequately (though less exhaustively) demonstrated in animal models of cancer in the fore-stomach[70], colon[123,124] and breast[68,125]. Breast and colon cancers account for a significant proportion of human neoplasias, and although risk factors have been identified or suggested for both, no specific 'causes' acting at defined rate-limiting steps have been conclusively documented. Experimental data suggest that large bowel contents may contain initiating and promoting agents, that dietary fat is an important factor, and that bile acids may act as promoters in colon carcinogenesis. The available information suggests that it is probable that these considerations may apply to man[124,126].

Breast cancer is interesting since, unlike most human cancers of epithelial origin, its age-related incidence does not fit the Armitage-Doll model (i.e. a linear relationship between logarithms of death rate and age) but rather increases until the menopause and then inflects[127,128]. However, Moolgavkar *et al.*[129] have extended the two-stage model to allow for the growth, shedding and replenishment of target tissue, and the curves obtained approximate closely to those obtained in human populations, again suggesting a modified multistage process. (See Chapter 1.) Certain hormones have been shown to be of cardinal importance in the development of breast (and other) cancers in animals and humans[127], and have been suggested to act as promoters, i.e. to increase the rate of late stage events[125]. Ionizing radiation is the only known initiator in human breast cancer[130], but other known 'risk factors' such as age at first birth, parity, age at menarche and menopause can be accommodated in the Moolgavkar model.

This section has examined carcinogenesis in animal models, and the aetiology of certain animal and human tumours where chemical 'risk factors' are involved. The simple 'two-stage' initiation-promotion model described in mouse skin carcinogenesis seems to extend in essence to the majority of the epithelial cancers considered[131]. Obviously the rigid application of two or more precise 'stages' is not appropriate, but should merely be taken as an operational definition to simplify analysis of a complex continuum of phenotypic changes which culminate in an invasive carcinoma. Less than 10% of fatal human cancers are non-carcinomas (i.e. sarcomas and lympho-reticular neoplasias) and unlike the epithelial cancers there is considerable heterogeneity in their age-related incidences. These patterns suggest that their aetiological determinants differ from those of carcinomas, and from each other; and these have not been discussed.

Use of animal models to screen anticarcinogenic agents

Although prevention of human exposure to environmental carcinogenic risk factors is theoretically the ideal way to decrease cancer incidence, it is the least practical. An optimistic outlook is that if human carcinogenesis is a prolonged, multistage process, a variety of interventions may be possible, with those aimed at inhibiting penultimate or ultimate events yielding the most rapid decline in cancer incidence[95].

Compounds belonging to over 20 different classes of chemicals (including vitamins, protease inhibitors, flavones, anti-oxidants and anti-inflammatory steroids) have been reported to inhibit complete carcinogenesis in animals, but more instructive have been specific studies of potential inhibitors of the initiation and promotion phases in two-stage models[120,132,133]. In experimental systems, substances have been described which can prevent the formation of active carcinogens from their precursors, can exert a 'barrier' function between the carcinogen and its target tissue, and can suppress the expression of neoplasia in cells previously exposed to a carcinogen[134]. Agents are also known which are able specifically to inhibit early and/or late stages of promotion (e.g. TPCK and some retinoids)[120]. Many of these compounds are naturally occurring constituents of food, and it has been suggested that their inclusion in the diet may exert a protective effect against cancer in man. Inverse correlations between consumption of certain vegetables and colon and stomach cancer have been reported[135,136], and between serum β-carotene levels or vitamin A intake and lung cancer[137,138].

The relationship between vitamin A and cancer has attracted much interest since the linking of its deficiency in the diet to the development of stomach cancer in rodents. (For recent reviews see[139-143]). Since then there have been many reports of retinoids (vitamin A analogues) inhibiting carcinogenesis induced by PAH, aromatic amines, nitrosamines, azo dyes, radiation and viruses in such diverse tissues as skin, breast, colon, bladder and respiratory tract[140]. Some retinoids have been shown not only to prevent, but to reverse certain pre-malignant lesions (e.g. of epidermis and prostate)[144] and are being seriously considered for the chemoprophylaxis of neoplasia in various 'at risk' human populations, e.g. patients with recurrent superficial bladder cancers, cervical and oesophageal dysplasias, polyposis coli, and smokers with bronchial mucosa metaplasia[145-147]. However, it must be appreciated that both naturally occurring and synthetic retinoids vary enormously in their biological properties. Experimental studies are beginning to reveal how modification of the hydrocarbon ring, side chain, or polar terminal group of retinoic acid analogues can differentially influence their tissue distribution, toxicity and anticarcinogenic potential. For example, retinyl acetate is effective in preventing rat mammary tumour development, but not two-stage skin carcinogenesis in mice; 13-cis-retinoic acid is an effective inhibitor of phorbol ester-induced tumour promotion in skin, and of MNU or BBN induced bladder cancer in rats, but is ineffective in rat mammary gland. In terms of toxicity, although both retinyl acetate and 4-hydroxyphenylret- inamide (HPR) are effective in preventing experimental breast cancer, dietary intake of the latter results in higher levels of retinoid in the mammary gland, with relatively little liver accumulation and hepatotoxicity compared with the former compound[148]. Several retinoids are already used in the treatment of skin disorders in man, and data on their relative efficacy, toxicity and suitable dosage schedules are available to determine comparability in pharmacokinetic parameters. It is possible that further analysis of structure–activity relationships and interspecies comparisons will (as in analogous studies of chemical carcinogens) reveal the as yet unknown molecular and biochemical basis of the mechanism(s) of action of retinoids in vivo.

We are then left with the not inconsiderable problem of defining a human population at risk of developing cancer in which a particular retinoid may be appropriately tested as a chemopreventive agent. Even heavy cigarette smokers have a lifetime expectancy of developing invasive lung cancer of less than 10%[149], and, because of the difficulty in generating animal models of lung carcinoma, the potential of retinoids to influence the process has not been experimentally explored. The majority of animal studies have utilized the chemical induction of tumours in the skin, mammary gland and urinary bladder. No chemical carcinogenic risk factors have been identified for human breast cancer, and it is possible that, even within the 'high risk' groups which have so far been defined, the probability of developing mammary cancer is insufficient to justify intervention. Nevertheless, a randomised trial using HPR (the most effective analogue against mammary carcinoma in rats) is planned in Milan, to examine its effects on the incidence of second tumours in the other breast[147]. Clearly trials of this type will be important not only to provide empirical data in man, but also to evaluate the predictive potential of animal studies.

In urinary bladder cancer there is good evidence for chemical risk factors in many cases, and the probability of developing subsequent lesions following treatment of an initial superficial cancer is between 40 and 80%. Several plausible animal models of both squamous cell and transitional cell urinary bladder cancer exist, which have been shown to be susceptible to a variety of retinoids[104,113,150]. For these reasons this disease may be one of the most suitable for retinoid intervention trials[77] and, indeed, several are already underway[145,147].

Basic biological principles which have emerged from animal studies may be of value in the design and evaluation of human intervention studies. It is clear that retinoids are generally more effective as 'anti-promoters' than as therapeutic agents for the established cancer, and their effects are reversible on cessation of treatment in some systems. The implications of these observations are threefold. Firstly, there may exist in the treatment population lesions which, although undetectable, represent a stage of tumour progression beyond that at which a retinoid may exert its effects. Such lesions would be expected to progress to frank carcinomas early in the course of treatment, and perhaps result in premature termination of the trial before any effects on early stage transitions could become apparent. Secondly, long-term treatment must be anticipated as continual exposure is required to maintain the anticarcinogenic effect. The attendant risks and toxicity of such regimes must therefore be minimised to obtain any potential benefit. Thirdly, it must be expected that retinoid prophylaxis, even if effective, will at best only delay, rather than prevent, the development of neoplastic disease. However, an extension of symptom-free life would benefit any patient, and in older individuals of limited life-expectancy delay in development of cancer could be equivalent to a cure. On the other hand, in view of the potential teratogenic and toxic effects of most of the current generation of retinoids, their prophylactic use in young individuals at the reproductive stage of life must be seriously questioned[147]. Further work is required to clarify the mechanism(s) of action of retinoids, to understand and exploit their apparent tissue specificities, and to develop more effective and less toxic analogues[151].

VIRAL CARCINOGENESIS

In 1911 Rous showed that avian leukaemia and sarcoma could be transmitted by cell-free filtrates, and in 1951 the first mammalian retrovirus (murine leukaemia virus) was isolated by Gross. Subsequent investigations showing that both natural and experimental infection with viruses could lead to the development of malignant tumours in many species increased the expectation that at least some human tumours may have a viral aetiology. (For recent comprehensive reviews see references[152-154].)

DNA tumour viruses associated with cancers in animals and man

All DNA virus families with the exception of parvoviruses have been associated with cancers in animals and/or man[152].

Herpesviruses

Two herpesviruses (Lucké herpesvirus (LHV) and Marek's disease virus (MDV)) are of interest as the only DNA viruses unequivocally associated with naturally occurring animal cancers: LHV induces renal adenocarcinomas in the leopard frog *Rana pipiens*, and MDV is associated with a contagious lymphoproliferative disease in fowl. Causal relationships were established by introducing the viruses into normal animals and recovering the organisms from lesions in the experimentally-infected hosts.

Of more immediate relevance to human oncogenesis have been studies with T- and B-cell tropic viruses of primates. Herpesvirus saimiri (HVS) and herpesvirus ateles (HVA) are indigenous in certain types of monkey, and are capable of inducing T cell lymphomas and of transforming lymphocytes in culture. B-cell tropic viruses are found in human and Old World primates, Epstein-Barr virus being the prototype.

Of the five known herpesviruses, four are associated with malignant disease: Epstein-Barr virus (EBV), herpes simplex types 1 and 2 (HSV-1, HSV-2) and cytomegalovirus (CMV). EBV is the causative agent of infectious mononucleosis, and is closely linked to the development of two chronic neoplastic diseases: Burkitt's lymphoma (BL) in Africa, and undifferentiated nasopharyngeal carcinoma (NPC). Burkitt tumours do not contain virions, but EBV particles which are shed in tissue culture can transform normal human lymphocytes, and induce multifocal lymphomas very similar to BL in owl monkeys or cotton top marmosets[155]. It has been suggested that immunocompromised hosts are more susceptible to EBV-induced diseases[156]. This factor may explain the prevalence of BL in areas where malaria is endemic, and the particular sensitivity of cotton top marmosets which show delayed allograft rejection and lower antibody titres compared with related species[154]. EBV is very similar to several B-cell tropic viruses of Old World monkeys and apes, in terms of both antigenicity and DNA sequence homology[157]. Herpesvirus papio (HVP), isolated from hamadryas baboons, seems to be strongly associated with an endemically high incidence of spontaneous lymphomas in a research colony of animals at Sukhuri in the USSR. An EBV-related virus is prevalent in the colony, the clinical disease histologically resembles lymphoblastic lymphosarcomas of the BL type and prolymphocytic lymphosarcomas, and there is a degree of associated immunosuppression[158]. This natural 'experiment' would seem to be an ideal situation in which to study factors determining the expression of different lymphoid neoplasias, and the possible prophylactic or therapeutic effects of vaccination against EBV-related membrane antigens.

EBV-associated malignancies can readily be interpreted in terms of multistage carcinogenesis. In BL pathogenesis, it has been suggested that early EBV infection may act as an initiating event, with malaria acting as a permissive or enhancing factor in the expansion of malignant clones. In NPC it is proposed that EBV may rather be associated with a late stage event, with, for example, nitrosamine-containing salted fish providing an initiating stimulus in Chinese populations, and the habit of eating *Euphorbeaceae* plants adding promotion[159]. HSV-1 and HSV-2 are associated with a variety of human cancers, but the most suggestive (although by no means conclusive) evidence is for a causal relationship between HSV-2 and cervical carcinomas. The oncogenic potential of the human virus has been shown by its capacity to transform rodent cells in culture, to induce sarcomas at the site of inoculation in hamsters, and by direct genital infection of rodents to produce cervical lesions almost identical to atypia, carcinoma *in situ* and malignant tumours of women[160,161].

CMV has recently been implicated in human prostatic cancer and Kaposi sarcoma[162]. Studies are hampered by the fact that this virus can only be propagated in human cells. However, it has been shown to transform hamster cells and human embryo fibroblasts, and following passage *in vitro* such lines are tumorigenic in immune deprived hosts[151]. Molecular biological techniques are now being applied to detection of herpesvirus genomes in tumour tissue, and the identification of regions responsible for induction and/or maintenance of the malignant phenotype. Such approaches will finally elucidate the role of these and other viral genes in human cancer, and their isolation and the delineation of susceptible target cells will expand the *in vitro* and *in vivo* model systems available.

Hepatitis B virus

Substantial evidence suggests that hepatitis B virus (HBV) is a significant risk factor in human hepatocellular carcinoma (HCC) in many areas of Africa and S.E. Asia. The study of this virus has been facilitated by the cloning and transfection of HBV DNA into mammalian cells, and by the discovery, since 1978, of HBV-like viruses in woodchucks (WHV), ground squirrels (GSHV) and ducks (DHBV)[163]. HBVC and the three related 'Hepadna' viruses share unique ultrastructural, molecular and antigenic features[164]. In two colonies of woodchucks in the USA, about 30% of animals infected with WHV develop hepatocellular carcinoma per year; the disease is absent from uninfected animals[164]. In contrast, GSHV infected squirrels develop little or no hepatitis and no HCC, and although viral particles have been isolated from duck hepatomas in areas with a high incidence of human HCC, the relationship of DHBV to the duck HCC is not yet clear. The differences in liver diseases (including neoplasias) associated with infection of the Hepadna viruses would appear to provide ideal model systems in which to identify the role of genetic and environmental factors critical to the pathogenesis of HCC. As with BL, the existence of naturally 'at risk' animal populations may be used to monitor the effectiveness of vaccination, or of other interventions in the primary prevention of HCC[165].

Advances in *in vitro* techniques, particularly the development of human fetal liver cell cultures which can metabolically activate aflatoxins and other carcinogens, and retain the HBV receptor, will allow analysis of mechanisms of action of co-operating risk factors such as these at the biochemical and molecular level.

Papovaviruses

The first association between the papilloma subgroup viruses and cancer was made by Shope in 1932 using rabbits. Most papilloma viruses (except bovine strains) are host specific, and in most cases, in animals and man, cancer induction requires co-operation with other carcinogenic agents[166]. For example in cattle, bracken fern, which contains a potent carcinogen, induces oesophageal and bladder cancers in association with the virus. In man, benign skin warts induced by HPV-5 can undergo malignant conversion if exposed to sunlight and X-irradiation in genetically susceptible individuals. At least 24 different HPVs have been identified, and since no permissive cell system for virus replication has so far been established, their association in various tumours has been sought using DNA sequence analysis. Using these methods two hitherto unknown human papillomaviruses, HPV 16 and HPV 18, were identified in 44% of carcinomata *in situ* and 57% of cervical cancers[167]. Such approaches would seem to be the most suitable for the further investigation of human risk due to the species specificity and tissue specificity of this heterogeneous group of viruses.

The polyoma subgroup of papovaviruses was only discovered to include human viruses in 1971[168], whereas the related simian virus 40 (SV40)[169] has been extensively studied, completely sequenced, and the transforming region identified. The two human polyoma viruses so far described, JCV and BKV, seem to be ubiquitous in the human population but, like their animal counterparts, only become 'activated' in immunologically compromised individuals. Inoculation of either virus induces central nervous system and other tumours in hamsters, and JCV has been shown to induce gliomas and astrocytomas in New World primates[169,170]. The involvement, if any, of these viruses in human cancer is under investigation, but currently available data are inconclusive. Similarly, although various adenovirus serotypes are tumorigenic in newborn hamsters, and can transform cells *in vitro*, this family is not thought to be associated with human cancer.

RNA tumour viruses associated with cancers in animals and man

A vast literature on the tumorigenic properties of acute transforming retroviruses and their associated oncogenes (reviewed[171-176]) attests to the significance of recent developments in this field. Here I merely intend to outline some of the interesting parallels that are emerging between members of all classes of retrovirus in animal and human studies.

RNA viruses (retroviruses) associated with cancer are generally type C, the only B type of interest being the mouse mammary tumour virus MuMTV, of which the most familiar is the 'milk factor' described by Bittner. This virus has been studied for over 40 years as a murine curiosity, but recently sequences homologous to the RNA of MuMTV, particles containing the appropriate 70s RNA (reverse transcriptase), and antigens related to the viral core and envelope gp52 have been detected in human breast cancers[177,178]. These intriguing findings may or may not have aetiological implications, and suggestions that they could lead to the development of sensitive assays for the detection of occult breast cancer remain to be evaluated. The oncogenic potential of MuMTV seems to depend on proviral insertion and activation of one or two new cellular oncogenes, Int 1 and Int 2[179]. Sequences homologous to Int 1 have been conserved in evolution, being present in the genome of *Drosophila*, fish, birds and mammals including man[180]. It is thought that these genes are not equivalent to the closely-related transforming genes found to be activated in a human mammary tumour cell line and in chemically induced and MuMTV-associated murine mammary tumours[181].

C type retroviruses are classically divided into two groups. The chronic transforming viruses, when inoculated into susceptible animals, generate primarily leukaemias following a long latency; whereas the acute transforming viruses induce a variety of tumours within weeks, and, unlike the former, can transform cells *in vitro*. It is now apparent that the viral oncogenes (v-*onc*) of the acutely-transforming retroviruses are derived from normal cellular genes (c-*onc*) which have been transduced by the viruses and which, when under the control of their transcriptional promoters, are responsible for induction and/or maintenance of the transformed state (see Chapter 1). The remarkable evolutionary conservation of c-*onc* genes[174], and the revelation that many of their protein products are key factors in the control of cell growth and differentiation (see Chapter 3) may indicate a unifying hypothesis for the mechanism of action of chemical, viral and physical carcinogens, and many tumour promoters[172].

Slowly transforming retroviruses lack oncogenes and, in spite of the fact that, unlike the acutely transforming viruses, they have long been associated with naturally occurring cancers (especially lymphomas and leukaemias) in mice, chickens, cats, cattle and gibbon apes[182], evidence for human counterparts has only recently emerged. In several models, especially avian and murine systems, extensive virus replication precedes leukaemia, and virus particles are associated with the neoplastic cells. This is not the case for feline leukaemia virus (FeLV) and bovine leukaemia virus (BLV), and the latter in particular shows remarkable parallels with the first human retrovirus to be discovered, HTLV-I[183-185].

Early searches for viral aetiologies of human cancers were discouraged by the lack of viremia or C type particles associated with neoplasia, and the failure to detect antigens cross-reactive with known animal retroviruses. BLV was then isolated and found not to be expressed in primary tumours, nor to be detectable using nucleic acid probes from other leukaemia viruses, but to be expressed *in vitro* after prolonged cell culture. Once the growth of mature human T-cells in long-term culture was accomplished using T-cell growth factor (interleukin-2), it was not long before HTLV-I was isolated and found to be associated with adult T-cell leukaemia/lymphoma (ATLL). Two further members of the HTLV family have since been described: HTLV-II, which, although isolated from a patient with hairy cell leukaemia, has not been linked to any specific disease[186], and HTLV-III, the cause of Acquired Immune Deficiency Syndrome (AIDS)[185]. Retroviruses closely related to HTLV-I have now been identified in subhuman primates: one is linked with the occurrence of lymphoma in macaques[183], and characteristics of its reverse transcriptase,

direction other than towards cancer[206]. It is clear that not all papillomas are equal, and some are more equal than others in the development of malignant progeny. Burns[207] has discriminated between promoter-dependent 'conditional' papillomas, and a minority (<5%) of 'autonomous' papillomas which can persist following cessation of TPA treatment. Repeated low doses of initiators preferentially yield autonomous papillomas and a higher rate of carcinomas. Autonomous papillomas, therefore, probably represent a pre-neoplastic stage, but this may not be obligatory. Single high doses of DMBA induce carcinomas without prior evidence of palpable papillomas[208], but it is possible that microscopic 'autonomous clones' provide an analogous pathway. On the other hand, evidence that papillomas induced by DMBA+ TPA can be inhibited by retinoic acid, whereas tumours induced by DMBA alone are refractory[209] suggests that the lesions are different biological entities. The conversion of papillomas to carcinomas can be significantly increased by re-exposure to initiating agents[210], suggesting that further genetic change(s) may be required for their progression. Since promoters such as phorbol ester are now known to be able, indirectly, to damage DNA[211] it is possible that under initiation-promotion regimes, also, sequential genetic (rather than epigenetic) events, although occurring at lower frequency, are responsible for the few carcinomas that eventually ensue.

In liver carcinogenesis, many morphologically and biochemically distinct pre-neoplastic stages have been described. In some instances, the occurrence of frank hepatocellular carcinomas arising entirely within 'persistent' nodules is suggestive of their intimate relationship[212]. Similar sequences, while not usually detectable in human HCC which develops in cirrhotic liver, are readily observed in non-cirrhotic livers in which the occurrence of HCC is linked to the use of contraceptive or anabolic steroids. Also, three agents (vinyl chloride, inorganic arsenicals and Thorotrast) produce a sequence of histological and morphological changes in man which have been duplicated in rodents[213]. In induced and 'spontaneous' HCC in rodents, as in man, a high level of serum α-fetoprotein (AFP) has proved a useful marker for pre-malignant or occult disease[98]. Metastasis of human HCC is found in about 60% of patients, and although the frequency of metastasis of chemically induced HCC in the rat is lower, the routes of spread are identical[98].

In man, clinical experience has led to the discrimination of benign lesions that are considered 'pre-malignant' from those where such a risk is negligible (e.g. lipomas)[214,215]. In the colon three histological classes of adenomas can be ranked according to their malignant potential: small adenocarcinomas are found within 5% of tubular adenomas and 41% of villous adenomas, with the mixed villo-tubular adenomas giving an intermediate value of 22%. These data are consistent with an adenoma-to-carcinoma progression[216]. It is of interest that the ability of cultured cells from these three types of lesion to respond to TPA by plasminogen activator secretion is related to their potential for malignant conversion[217].

Other examples of conditions predisposing to malignancy which can be found in humans and experimental animals are papillomas in bladder, atypical hyperplasia/metaplasia in cervix and bronchus, and some classes of benign hyperplasias in breast. The regression of certain of these lesions in man has been documented, which again parallels observations on skin papillomas and liver nodules. However, although the histological lesions may disappear, preneoplastic cells may persist[218].

In summary, the available evidence seems to suggest that the 'benign' lesions discussed are a gross manifestation of an underlying malignant process which may be progressing in subclones of cells within the discernible foci. Until the resolution of biochemical and molecular genetic techniques extends to the level of individual cells, the phenotype(s) of the malignant progenitors may remain obscured by those surrounding cells destined to remain benign. In vitro also, only a minority of cells respond to chemical and viral carcinogens by expressing full tumorigenic potential. We need to know whether this is the result of random events, or whether certain special properties predispose individual cells in apparently homogeneous populations to respond.

Of greatest biological significance, in terms of tumour progression, is the acquisition by neoplastic cells of the capacity to metastasize, as it is disseminated disease which is responsible for most therapeutic failures in man. Animal tumour models have been criticised for their supposed failure to metastasize as readily as human cancers, but such criticisms are not always valid. Certain tumours, e.g. those induced by high doses of PHA or by viruses such as SV40, express strongly immunogenic cell surface antigens. Such tumours remain localised, and may regress in immunocompetent hosts. However, when grown in immunodeprived animals, their intrinsic ability to disseminate can be revealed. In many studies, primary tumours are allowed to grow until they kill the host, when gross metastases may not be evident (although detectable histologically[219] or by bioassay)[220]. In some cases, extirpation of the primary tumour to extend the lifespan of the host (as practised clinically) is all that is required to allow time for development of overt secondary disease[221]. Nevertheless, there remain examples of experimental tumours which rarely metastasize under these conditions. Given the long latency calculated for most human cancers, it should not surprise us that some tumours arising relatively rapidly in short-lived species may appear to represent fairly 'immature' neoplasms.

At its first manifestation a tumour may be at any stage of progression, and (even in man) this process may not reach an endpoint within the lifetime of the host. In a series of mouse squamous cell carcinomas and mammary adenocarcinomas, we found primary tumours ranging from benign to highly malignant, irrespective of whether they were induced by chemical carcinogens, endogenous virus or were of 'spontaneous' origin[221]. (I personally do not share the view that 'spontaneous' tumours in animals necessarily represent a better model of human malignant diseases than induced tumours[222,223].) The more that is learnt about carcinogenic processes the clearer it becomes that all tumours are 'caused' by interactions between genetic, chemical, viral, dietary, hormonal and other risk factors. Spontaneity, therefore, is not a virtue but merely an unidentified aetiological principle).

The benign tumours in our (and other) studies, if their lifespans were extended by serial transplantation in syngeneic hosts, progressed at variable rates towards a more malignant phenotype (increased growth rate, decreased differentiation, increased metastatic capacity)[221,224]. Also, benign tumours may contain within them minor clones of cells which when isolated can express metastatic potential[225,226]. Such observations have been taken as experimental proof of Nowell's hypothesis that progression represents the sequential selection of variant subpopulations produced as a consequence of genetic instability. Other studies have suggested either that the minority of cells successfully seeding secondary sites are random survivors of those released from the primary tumour, or that metastatic phenotypes arise in response to adaptive or inductive stimuli provided by the host environment[227,228]. There is currently no consensus (although much debate) concerning the relative importance of these alternatives in experimental and human metastasis, and it is probable that they are by no means mutually exclusive.

In conclusion, although the phenomenology of tumour progression and metastasis has been extensively described, the critical underlying genetic and/or epigenetic tumour and host factors are still largely undefined. It is not possible to select a particular animal tumour (or even a human one) as representative of neoplasia in man. However, the careful choice of appropriate models for the studies in question, and a recognition of their particular limitations, coupled with the use of human tumour cell culture and xenograft systems, should broaden our understanding of these complex and interesting processes.

Acknowledgement

I am indebted to Mrs Pat Usher for her skilful typing of the manuscript.

References

1. International Union Against Cancer (1965). *Illustrated Tumour Nomenclature.* (Berlin: Springer-Verlag)
2. Doll, R. (1977). Strategy for detection of cancer hazards to man. *Nature (London)*, **265**, 589-596
3. Higginson, J. (1979). Environmental carcinogenesis: a global perspective. In Emmelot, P. and Kreik, E. (eds.) *Environmental Carcinogenesis*. pp. 9-24. (Amsterdam: Elsevier/North-Holland)
4. Doll, R. and Peto, R. (1981). The causes of cancer: quantitative estimates of avoidable risks of cancer in the United States today. *J. Natl. Cancer Inst.*, **66**, 1193-1308
5. Epstein, S. (1974). Environmental determinants of human cancer. *Cancer Res.*, **34**, 2425-2435
6. Peto, R. (1978). Epidemiology, multistage models and short-term mutagenicity tests. In Hiatt, H.H., Watson, J.D. and Winsten, J.A. (eds.) *Origins of Human Cancer*. pp. 1403-1428. (New York: Cold Spring Harbor)
7. Doll, R. and Peto, R. (1976). Mortality in relation to smoking: 20 years observations on male British doctors. *Br. Med. J.*, **2**, 1525-1536
8. Loeb, L. A., Ernster, V. L., Warner, K. E., Abbots, J. and Laszlo, J. (1984). Smoking and lung cancer: an overview. *Cancer Res.*, **44**, 5940-5958

9. Weinstein, I. B. (1981). The scientific basis for carcinogen detection and primary cancer prevention. *Cancer*, **47**, 1133-1141

10. Ashby, J. (1983). The unique role of rodents in the detection of possible human carcinogens and mutagens. *Mutat. Res.*, **115**, 177-213

11. Ashby, J., De Serres, F. J., Draper, M., Ishidate, M., Margolin, B. H., Matter, B. E., and Shelby, M. D. (eds.) (1985). Evaluation of short-term tests for carcinogenesis. *Prog. Mutat. Res.* Vol. 5. (Amsterdam: Elsevier)

12. Salsburg, D. (1983). The lifetime feeding study in mice and rats - an examination of its validity as a bioassay for human carcinogens. *Fundam. Appl. Toxicol.*, **3**, 63-67

13. Hogan, M. D. (1983). Extrapolation of animal carcinogenicity data: limitations and pitfalls. *Environ. Health Perspect.*, **47**, 333-337

14. Tomatis, L. (1979). The predictive value of rodent carcinogenicity tests in the evaluation of human risks. *Annu. Rev. Pharmacol. Toxicol.*, **19**, 511-530

15. *IARC Monographs* (on the evaluation of carcinogenic risk of chemicals to humans) (1971-1985). Nos. 1-20 (Lyon: IARC)

16. Rall, D.P. (1979). Validity of extrapolation of results of animal studies to man. *Ann. N.Y. Acad. Sci. USA*, **329**, 85-91

17. Kennaway, E. (1955). The identification of a carcinogenic compound in coal tar. *Br. Med. J.*, **2**, 749-752

18. Slaga, T. J., Fischer, S. M., Weeks, C. E. and Klein-Szanto, A. J. P. (1980). Multistage chemical carcinogenesis in mouse skin. *Curr. Probl. Dermatol.*, **10**, 193-218

19. Tobin, P. S., Kornhauser, A. and Schleuplein, R. J. (1982). An evaluation of skin painting studies as determinants of tumorigenesis potential following skin contact with carcinogens. *Regul. Toxicol. Pharmacol.*, **2**, 22-37

20. Boutwell, R. K., Verma, A. K. Ashendel, C. L. and Astrup, E. (1982). Mouse skin: a useful model system for studying the mechanism of chemical carcinogenesis. In Hecker, E., Fusenig, N. E., Kunz, W. and Marks, F. (eds.) *Carcinogenesis.* Vol. 7, pp. 1-12. (New York: Raven Press)

21. Berenblum, I. (1974). *Carcinogenesis as a Biological Problem.* (Amsterdam: Elsevier/North Holland)

22. Homburger, F. (ed) (1983). Skin painting techniques and *in vivo* carcinogenesis bioassays. *Prog. Exp. Tumour Res.*, **26**

23. Hecker, E. (1967). Phorbol esters from croton oil: Chemical nature and biological activities. *Naturwissenschaften*, **11**, 282-284

24. Hecker, E. (1981). Co-carcinogens and tumour promoters of the diterpene-ester type as possible carcinogenic risk factors. *J. Cancer Res. Clin. Oncol.*, **99**, 103-124

25. Wheldrake, J. F., Marshall, J., Ramli, J. and Murray, A. W. (1982). Skin carcinogenesis and promoter binding characteristics in different mouse strains. *Carcinogenesis*, **3**, 805-807

26. Rall, D. P. (1977). Species differences in carcinogenesis testing. In Hiatt, H. H., Watson, J. D. and Winsten, J. A. (eds.) *Origins of Human Cancer.* pp. 1383-1390. (New York: Cold Spring Harbour)

27. Stenbach, F. (1980). Skin carcinogenesis as a model system: observations on species, strain and tissue sensitivity to 7, 12- dimethylbenz(a)anthracene with or without promotion from croton oil. *Acta Pharmacol. Toxicol.*, **46**, 89-97

28. Bock, F. G. (1983). Comparative anatomy and function of skin as related to experimental chemical carcinogenesis. *Prog. Exp. Tumor Res.*, **26**, 5-17

29. Highland, J. (1983). The use of *in vivo* carcinogenesis bioassay data in the development of policies aimed at protecting public health. *Prog. Exp. Tumor Res.*, **26**, 292-300

30. Homburger, F. (1983). Introduction: carcinogenesis bioassay in historical perspective. *Prog. Exp. Tumor Res.*, **26**, 182-186

31. Dolan, W. D. (1983). The AMA's position on carcinogenesis bioassays. *Prog. Exp. Tumor Res.*, **26**, 301-310

32. Selkirk, J. K., Macleod, M. C., Moore, C. J., Mansfield, B. K., Nikbakht, A. and Dearstone, K. (1982). Species variance in the metabolic activation of polycyclic hydrocarbons. In Harris, C. C. and Cerutti, P. A. (eds.) *Mechanisms of Chemical Carcinogenesis.* pp. 331-349. (New York: Alan R. Liss)

33. Merletti, F., Heseltine, E., Saracci, R., Simonata, L., Vainio, H. and Wilbourn, J. (1984). Target organs for carcinogenicity of chemicals and industrial exposure of humans: A review

of results in the IARC Monographs on the evaluation of carcinogenic risk of chemicals to humans. *Cancer Res.*, **44**, 2244-2250

34. Purchase, I. F. H. (1980). Interspecies comparisons of carcinogenicity. *Br. J. Cancer*, **41**, 454-468

35. Mantel, N. and Schneiderman, M. A. (1975). Estimating "safe" levels, a hazardous undertaking. *Cancer Res.*, **35**, 1379-1386

36. Gehring, P. J. and Blau, G. E. (1979). Mechanisms of carcinogenesis: The dose response. *Cancer Bull.*, **29**, 152-161

37. Tomatis, L., Agthe, C., Bartsch, H., Huff, J., Montesanto, R., Saraci, R., Walker, E. and Wilbourne, E. (1978). Evaluation of the carcinogenicity of chemicals, a review of the monograph programme of the International Agency on Cancer (1971-1977). *Cancer Res.*, **38**, 877-885

38. Langenbach, R., Nesnow, S. and Rice, J. M. (eds.) (1983). Organ and species specificity in chemical carcinogenesis. *Basic Life Sciences*. Vol. 24. (New York: Plenum Press).

39. Clayson, D. B. (1977). Principles underlying testing of carcinogenicity. *Cancer Bull.*, **29**, 161-166

40. Miller, E. C. and Miller, J. A. (1976). The metabolism of chemical carcinogens to reactive electrophiles and their possible mechanisms of action in carcinogenesis. In Searle, C. E. (ed.) *Chemical Carcinogens*. ACS Monograph 173. pp. 737-762. (Washington, D.C.: American Chemical Society)

41. Miller, E. C., Miller, J. A. and Enomoto, M. (1964). The comparative carcinogenicities of 2 acetyl aminofluorene and its N-hydroxymetabolite in mice, hamsters and guinea pigs. *Cancer Res.*, **24**, 2018-2031

42. Peers, F. G., Gilman, G. A. and Linsell, C. A. (1976). Dietary aflatoxins and human liver cancer. *Int. J. Cancer*, **17**, 167-176

43. Wogan, G. N. (1973). Aflatoxin carcinogenesis. *Methods Cancer Res.*, **7**, 309-344

44. Portier, C. J. and Hoel, D. G. (1984). Design of animal carcinogenicity studies for goodness-of-fit of multistage models. *Fundam. Appl. Toxicol.*, **4**, 949-959

45. Heidelberger, C. (1982). Relationship between carcinogenesis and transformation of cell cultures. In Harris, C.C. and Cerutti, P.A. (eds.) *Mechanisms of Chemical Carcinogenesis*. pp. 563-573. (New York: Alan Liss).

46. Pienta, R. J. (1980). Transformation of Syrian hamster embryo cells by diverse chemicals and correlation with their reported carcinogenic and mutagenic activities. In De Serres, F.F. and Hollaender, A. (eds.) *Chemical Mutagens*. Vol. VI, pp. 175-202. (New York: Plenum)

47. Ames, B. N. (1982). Mutagens, carcinogens and anti-carcinogens. *Basic Life Sci.*, **21**, 499-508

48. Parkinson, E. K., Pera, M. F., Emmerson, A. and Gorman, P. A. (1984). Differential effects of complete and second-stage tumour promoters in normal but not transformed human and mouse keratinocytes. *Carcinogenesis*, **5**, 1071-1077

49. Okhawa, Y., Iwata, K., Shibuya, H., Fujiki, H. and Inui, N. (1984). A rapid simple screening method for skin tumor promoters using mouse peritoneal macrophages *in vitro*. *Cancer Lett.*, **21**, 253-260

50. Bohrman, J. S. (1983). Identification and assessment of tumour-promoting and co-carcinogenic agents: state-of-the-art *in vitro* methods. *CRC Crit. Rev. Toxicol.*, **11**, 121-167

51. Farber, E. (1984). The multistep nature of cancer development. *Cancer Res.*, **44**, 4217-4223

52. Farber, E. (1984). Cellular biochemistry of the stepwise development of cancer with chemicals. *Cancer Res.*, **44**, 5463-5474

53. Shubik, P. (1984). Progression and promotion. *J. Natl. Cancer Inst.*, **5**, 1005-1011

54. Sivak, A. (1982). An evaluation of assay procedures for detection of tumour promoters. *Mutat. Res.*, **98**, 377-387

55. Garner, H., Schor, S. and Kinsella, A. R. (1984). Susceptibility of skin fibroblasts from individuals genetically predisposed to cancer to transformation by the tumour promoter 12-0-tetradecanoylphorbol-13-acetate. *Int. J. Cancer*, **34**, 349-357

56. Trosko, J. E., Jone, C. and Chang, C. C. (1984). The use of *in vitro* assays to study and to detect tumour promoters. In Borzsonyi, M., Day, N. E., Lapis, K. and Yamasaki, H. (eds.) *Models Mechanisms and Etiology of Tumour Promotion*. IARC Publications. No. 56, pp. 239-252. (Lyon: IARC)

57. Weinstein, I. B., Yamasaki, H., Wigler, M., Lee, L. S., Fisher, P. B., Jeffrey, A. Grunberger, D. (1979). Molecular and cellular events associated with the action of initiating carcinogens and tumour promoters. In Griffin, A. C. and Shaw, C. R. (eds.) *Carcinogens: Identification and Mechanisms of Action.* pp. 399-418. (New York: Raven Press)

58. Brookes, P. and Lawley, P. D. (1964). Evidence for the binding of polynuclear aromatic hydrocarbons to the nucleic acids of mouse skin. Relation between carcinogenic power of hydrocarbons and their binding to deoxyribonucleic acid. *Nature (London)*, **202**, 781-784

59. Harvey, R. G. (1982). Polycyclic hydrocarbons and cancer. *Am. Sci.*, **70**, 386-392

60. Weinstein, I. B. (1981). Current concepts and controversies in chemical carcinogenesis. *J. Supramol. Struct. Cell. Biochem.*, **17**, 99-120

61. Weinstein, I. B., Horowitz, A., Jeffrey, A. and Ivanovic, V. (1983). Cellular events in multistage carcinogenesis. In Weinstein, I. B. and Vogel, H. J. (eds.) *Genes and Proteins in Oncogenesis.* pp. 99-110. (New York: Academic Press)

62. Cairns, J. (1981). The origin of human cancers. *Nature (London)*, **289**, 353-357

63. Slaga, T. J. (1983). Overview of tumor promotion in animals. *Environ. Health Perspect.*, **50**, 3-14

64. Slaga, T. J., Fischer, S. M., Weeks, C. E., Nelson, K., Mamrack, M. and Klein-Szanto, A. J. P. (1982). Specificity and mechanism(s) of promoter inhibitors in multistage promotion. In Hecker, E., Fusenig, N. E., Kunz, W., Marks, F. and Thielmann, H. W. (eds.) *Carcinogenesis: A Comprehensive Survey.* Vol. 7. *Cocarcinogenesis and Biological Effects of Tumor Promoters.* pp. 19-34. (New York: Raven Press).

65. Blumberg, P. M. (1981). *In vitro* studies on the mode of action of phorbol esters, potent tumour promoters. *CRC Crit. Rev. Toxicol.*, **9**, 199-234

66. Blumberg, P. M., Dunn, J. A., Jaken, S., Jeng, A. Y., Leach, K. L., Sharkey, N. A. and Yen, H. (1984). Specific receptors for phorbol ester tumour promoters and their involvement in biological responses. In Slaga, T. J. (ed.) *Mechanisms of Tumour Promotion 3. Tumour Promotion and Co-carcinogenesis in vitro.* pp. 143-184. (Boca Raton: CRC Press)

67. Horowitz, A., Fujiki, H., Weinstein, I. B., Jeffrey, A., Oken, E., Moore, R. E. and Sugimura, T. (1983). Comparative effects of aplysiatoxin, debromoaplysiatoxin and teleocidin on receptor binding and phospholipid metabolism. *Cancer Res.*, **43**, 1529-1535

68. Armuth, V. and Berenblum, I. (1974). Promotion of mammary carcinogenesis and leukaemogenic action by phorbol in virgin female Wistar rats. *Cancer Res.*, **34**, 2704-2707

69. Armuth, V. and Berenblum, I. (1972). Systemic promoting action of phorbol in liver and lung carcinogenesis in AKR mice. *Cancer Res.*, **32**, 2259-2262

70. Goerrtler, K., Loehrke, H., Schweizer, J. and Hesse, B. (1979). Systemic 2-stage carcinogenesis in the epithelium of the forestomach of mice using 7, 12-dimethylbenz(a) anthracene as initiator and the phorbol ester 12-0-tetradecanoylphorbol-13-acetate as promoter. *Cancer Res.*, **39**, 1293-1297

71. Czuka, O., Szentirmay, Z. and Sugar, J. (1984). The effect of promoters on 1, 2 dimethylhydrazine-induced colon carcinogenesis. In Börzsönyi, M., Day, N. E., Lapis, K. and Yamasaki, H. (eds.) *Models, Mechanisms and Etiology of Tumour Promotion.* IARC Publications. No. 56, pp. 129-136. (Lyon: IARC)

72. Hecker, E. (1984). Co-carcinogens of the tumour-promoter type as potential risk factors of cancer in man. In Börzönyi, M., Day, N. E., Lapis, K. and Yamasaki, H. (eds.) *Models, Mechanisms and Etiology of Tumour Promotion.* IARC Publications. No. 56, pp. 441-463. (Lyon: IARC)

73. Blumberg, P. M., Declos, K. B. and Jaken, S. (1981). Tissue and species specificity for phorbol ester receptors. In Langenbach, R., Nesnow, S. and Rice, J. M. (eds.) *Organ and Species Specificity in Chemical Carcinogenesis.* pp. 201-230. (New York: Plenum Press)

74. Horowitz, A. D., Greenbaum, E. and Weinstein, I. B. (1981). Identification of receptors for phorbol ester tumour promoters in intact mammalian cells and of an inhibitor of receptor binding in biologic fluids. *Proc. Natl. Acad. Sci. USA*, **78**, 2315-2319

75. Neidel, J. E., Kuhn, L. J. and Vandenbark, G. R. (1983). Phorbol diester receptor co-purifies with protein kinase C. *Proc. Natl. Acad. Sci. USA*, **80**, 36-40

76. Ashendel, C. L., Staller, J. M. and Boutwell, R. K. (1983). Identification of a calcium- and phospholipid-dependent phorbol ester binding activity in the soluble fraction of mouse tissues. *Biochem. Biophys. Res. Commun.*, **111**, 340-345

77. Ponder, B. A. J. (1984). Clinical implications of current studies in carcinogenesis. *J. Cancer Res. Clin. Oncol.*, **108**, 264-273

78. Weinstein, I. B., Horowitz, A. D., Mufson, R. A., Fisher, P. B., Ivanovic, V. and Greenbaum, E. (1982). Results and speculations related to recent studies on mechanisms of tumour promotion. In Hecker, E., Fusenig, N. E., Kunz, W., Marks, F. and Thielmann, H. W. (eds.) *Carcinogenesis. A Comprehensive Survey*. Vol. 7. *Cocarcinogenesis and Biological Effects of Tumour Promoters*. pp. 599-616. (New York: Raven Press).

79. Frei, J. V. (1976). Some mechanisms operative in carcinogenesis: a review. *Chem. Biol. Interact.*, **12**, 1-25

80. Argyris, T. S., Slaga, T. J. (1981). Promotion of carcinomas by repeated abrasion in initiated skin of mice. *Cancer Res.*, **4**, 5193-5195

81. Coursaget, P., Maupas, P., Goudean, A., Chiron, J-P., Drucker, J., Denis, F., Diop-Mar, I. (1980). Primary hepatocellular carcinoma in intertropical Africa: relationship between age and hepatitis B virus etiology. *J. Natl. Cancer Inst.*, **65**, 687-690

82. Brand, K. G. (1979). Schistosomiasis-cancer. Etiological considerations. *Acta Trop*, **36**, 203-214

83. Yager, J. D., Jager, R. (1980). Oral contraceptive steroids as promoters of hepatocarcinogenesis in female Sprague-Dawley rats. *Cancer Res.*, **40**, 3680-3685

84. Ryan, W. L., Stenback, F. and Curtis, G. L. (1981). Tumor promotion by foreign bodies (I.U.D.). *Cancer Lett.*, **13**, 299-302

85. Trosko, J. E., Chang, C., Medcalf, A. (1983). Mechanisms of tumour promotion: potential role of intercellular communication. *Cancer Invest.*, **1**, 511-526

86. Yamasaki, H. (1984). Modulation of cell differentiation by tumour promoters. In Slaga, T.J. (ed.) *Mechanisms of Tumour Promotion*. 4. *Cellular Responses to Tumour Promoters*. pp. 1-26. (Boca Raton: CRC Press)

87. Colburn, N. H., Srinivas, L., Hegamyer, G. A., Dion, L. D., Wendel, E. J., Cohen, M. and Gindhart, T. D. (1984). Role of specific membrane and genetic changes in the mechanism of tumour promotion. Studies with promoter-resistant variants. In Börzsönyi, M., Day, N. E., Lapis, K. and Yamasaki, H. (eds.) *Models, Mechanisms and Etiology of Tumour Promotion*. IARC Scientific Publications. No. 56 (Lyon: IARC)

88. Colburn, N. H., Talmadge, C. B. and Gindhart, T. D. (1983). Transfer of sensitivity to tumour promoters by transfection of DNA from sensitive into insensitive mouse JB6 epidermal cells. *Mol. Cell. Biol.*, **3**, 1182-1186

89. Peraino, C., Fry, R. J., Staffeldt, E. E. and Christopher, J. P. (1975). Comparative enhancing effects of phenobarbital, amobarbital, diphenylhydantoin and dichloro-diphenyltrichloroethane and 2-acetylaminofluorene-induced hepatic tumorigenesis in the rat. *Cancer Res.*, **35**, 2284-2289

90. Ito, N., Tatematsu, M., Imaida, K., Hasegawa, R., Murasaki, G. (1980). Effects of various promoters on the induction of hyperplastic nodules in rat liver. *Gann*, **71**, 415-416

91. Scherer, E. and Emmelot, P. (1976). Kinetics of induction and growth of enzyme-deficient islands involved in hepatocarcinogenesis. *Cancer Res.*, **36**, 2544-2554

92. Becker, F. F. (1976). Sequential phenotypic and biochemical alterations during chemical hepatogenesis. *Cancer Res.*, **36**, 2563-2566

93. Solt, D. B. and Farber, E. (1976). New principle for the analysis of chemical carcinogenesis. *Nature (London)*, **263**, 702-703

94. Stevens, F. J. and Peraino, C. (1983). Liver as a model system for analysing mechanisms of tumour initiation and promotion. In Langenbach, R., Nesnow, S. and Rice, J.M. (eds.) *Organ and Species Specificity in Chemical Carcinogenesis*. pp. 231-252. (New York: Plenum Press)

95. Day, N. E. and Brown, C. C. (1980). Multistage models and primary prevention of cancer. *J. Natl. Cancer Inst.*, **64**, 977-989

96. Croy, R. G., Essigmann, J. M. and Wogan, G. N. (1983). Aflatoxin B_1: correlations of patterns of metabolism and DNA modification with biological effects. In Langenbach, R., Nesnow, S. and Rice, J. M. (eds.) *Organ and Species Specificity in Chemical Carcinogenesis*. pp. 49-62. (New York: Plenum Press)

97. Booth, S. C., Bosenberg, H., Garner, R. C., Hertzog, P. J., and Norpoth, K. (1981). The activation of aflatoxin B_1 in liver slices and in bacterial mutagenicity assays using livers from different species including man. *Carcinogenesis*, **2**, 1063-1068

98. Okuda, K. and Mackay, I. (eds.) (1982). *Hepatocellular carcinoma*. (Geneva: UICC Technical Report series volume 74)

99. Ayoola, E. A. (1984). Synergism between HBV and aflatoxin in hepatocellular carcinoma. In Williams, A. O., O'Connor, G. T., De-the, G. B. and Johnson, C. A. (eds.) *Virus-associated Cancers in Africa*. pp. 167-179 (Lyon: IARC Scientific Publications no. 63)

100. Tsung-Tang, S. and Neng-Jin, W. (1983). Studies on human liver carcinogenesis. In Harris, C.C. and Autrup, H.N. (eds.) *Human carcinogenesis*. pp. 757-780. (New York: Academic Press)

101. Kuratsune, M., Kohchi, S., Horie, A. and Nishizumi, M. (1971). Test of alcohol beverages and ethanol solutions for carcinogenicity and tumour-promoting activity. *Gann*, **62**, 395-405

102. Schwartz, M., Appel, K. E., Schrenk, D. and Kunz, W. (1980). Effect of ethanol on microsomal metabolism of dimethylnitrosamine. *J. Cancer Res. Clin. Oncol.*, **97**, 233-240

103. Schwartz, M., Buchmann, A., Moore, M. and Kunz, W. (1984). The mechanism of co-carcinogenic action of ethanol in rat liver. In Börzsönyi, M., Day, N. E., Lapis, K. and Yamasaki, H. (eds.) *Models, Mechanisms and Etiology of Tumour Promotion*. IARC Scientific Publications. No. 56, pp. 83-92 (Lyon: IARC)

104. Hicks, R. M. (1980). Multistage carcinogenesis in the urinary bladder. *Br. Med. Bull.*, **36**, 39-46

105. Cohen, S. M., Hasegawa, R., Greenfield, R. and Ellwein, L. B. (1984). Urinary bladder carcinogenesis. In Börzsönyi, M., Day, N. E., Lapis, K. and Yamasaki, H. (eds.) *Models, Mechanisms and Etiology of Tumour Promotion*. IARC Scientific Publications. No. 56, pp. 93-108. (Lyon: IARC)

106. Hicks, R.M., Wakefield, J. and Chowaniec, J. (1975). Evaluation of a new model to detect bladder carcinogens or co-carcinogens. Results obtained with saccharin, cyclamate and cyclophosphamide. *Chem. Biol. Interact.*, **11**, 225-233

107. Nakanishi, K., Fukushima, S., Shibata, M., Shirai, T., Ogiso, T. and Ito, N. (1978). Effect of phenacetin and caffeine on the urinary bladder of rats treated with N-butyl-N-(4-hydroxybutyl) nitrosamine. *Gann*, **69**, 395

108. Matsushima, M. (1977). The role of the promoter L-tryptophan on tumorigenicity in the urinary bladder. 2. Urinary bladder carcinogenesis of FANFT (initiating factor) in mice. *Jpn. J. Urol.*, **68**, 731-736

109. Radomski, J. L., Radomski, T. and McDonald, W. E. (1977). Cocarcinogenic interaction between D, L tryptophan and 4-aminobiphenyl or 2-naphthylamine in dogs. *J. Natl. Cancer Inst.*, **58**, 1831-1834

110. Cohen, S. M. (1979). Urinary bladder carcinogenesis: initiation-promotion. *Semin. Oncol.*, **6**, 157-160

111. Littlefield, N. A., Greenman, D. L., Farmer, J. H. and Sheldon, W. G. (1980). Effects of continuous and discontinued exposure to 2-AAF on urinary bladder hyperplasia and neoplasia. *J. Environ. Pathol. Toxicol.*, **3**, 35-53

112. Trosko, J. E., Dawson, B., Yotti, L. P. and Chang, C. C. (1980). Saccharin may act as a tumor promoter by inhibiting metabolic co-operation between cells. *Nature (London)*, **285**, 109-110

113. Hicks, R. M. (1982). Promotion in bladder cancer. In Hecker, E., Fusenig, N. E., Kunz, W., Marks, F. and Thielmann, H. W. (eds.) *Carcinogenesis - a Comprehensive Survey*. Vol. 7, pp. 139-153. (New York: Raven Press)

114. Price, J. M. (1971). Etiology of bladder cancer. In Maltry, E. (ed.) *Benign and Malignant Tumours of Urinary Bladder*. pp. 189-251. (New York: Medical Examination Publication Co.)

115. Cohen, S. M. (1983). Promotion of urinary bladder carcinogenesis. In Langenbach, R., Nesnow, S. and Rice, J. M. (eds.) *Organ and Species Specificity in Chemical Carcinogenesis*. pp. 253-270. (New York: Plenum Press)

116. Hicks, R. M. (1983). Effect of promoters on incidence of bladder cancer in experimental animal models. *Environ. Health Perspect.*, **50**, 37-49

117. Clayson, D. B. (1974). Bladder carcinogenesis in rats and mice: possibility of artefacts. *J. Natl. Cancer Inst.*, **52**, 1685-1689

118. Van Duuren, B. L. and Goldschmidt, B. M. (1976). Co-carcinogens and tumour-promoting agents in tobacco carcinogenesis. *J. Natl. Cancer Inst.*, **56**, 1237-1242

119. Witschi, H. P. (1983). Promotion of lung tumors in mice. *Environ. Health Perspect.*, **50**, 267-273

120. Slaga, T. J. (1984). Can tumour promotion be effectively inhibited? In Börzsönyi, M., Day, N. E., Lapis, K. and Yamasaki, H. (eds.) *Models, Mechanisms and Etiology of Tumour Promotion.* IARC Scientific Publications. No. 56, pp. 497-506. (Lyon: IARC)

121. Autrup, H., Grafstrom, R. C. and Harris, C. C. (1983). Metabolism of chemical carcinogens by tracheobronchial tissues. In Langenbach, R., Nesnow, S. and Rice, J. M. (eds.) *Organ and Species Specificity in Chemical Carcinogenesis.* pp. 473-492. (New York: Plenum Press)

122. Nettesheim, P., Barret, J. C., Mass, M. J., Steele, V. E. and Gray, T. E. (1984). Studies on the action of tumour promoters and antipromoters on respiratory tract epithelium. In Börzsönyi, M., Day, N. E., Lapis, K. and Yamasaki, H. (eds.) *Models, Mechanisms and Etiology of Tumour Promotion.* IARC Scientific Publications. No. 56, pp. 109-127. (Lyon: IARC)

123. Pollard, M. and Luckert, P. H. (1979). Promotional effect of sodium barbiturate on intestinal tumours induced in rats by dimethylhydrazine. *J. Natl. Cancer Inst.*, **63**, 1089-1092

124. Reddy, B. S., Weisburger, J. H. and Wynder, E. L. (1978). Colon cancer: bile salts as tumour promoters. In Slaga T.J., Sivak, A. and Boutwell, R.K. (eds.) *Carcinogenesis: a Comprehensive Survey.* Vol. 2, pp. 453-464. (New York: Raven Press)

125. Dao, T. L. and Chan, P. (1983). Hormones and dietary fat as promoters in mammary carcinogenesis. *Environ. Health Perspect.*, **50**, 219-225

126. Weisburger, J. H., Reddy, B. S., Barnes, W. S. and Wynder, E. L. (1983). Bile acids but not neutral sterols are tumor promoters in the colon in man and in rodents. *Environ. Health Perspect.*, **50**, 101-107

127. Bulbrook, R. D., Moore, J. W., Wang, D. Y. and Clark, G. M. G. (1984). Oestrogens and the etiology and clinical course of breast cancer. In Börzsönyi, M., Day, N. E., Lapis, K. and Yamasaki, H. (eds.) *Models, Mechanisms and Etiology of Tumour Promotion.* IARC Scientific Publications. No. 56, pp. 385-395. (Lyon: IARC)

128. Day, N. E. (1982). Epidemiological evidence of promoting effects - the example of breast cancer. In Hecker, E., Fusenig, N. E., Kunz, W., Marks, F. and Thielmann, H. W. (eds.) *Carcinogenesis - a Comprehensive Survey* Vol. 7, pp. 183-199. (New York: Raven Press)

129. Moolgavkar, S. H., Day, N. E. and Stevens, R. G. (1980). Two-stage model for carcinogenesis. Epidemiology of breast cancer in females. *J. Natl. Cancer Inst.*, **65**, 559-569

130. Thomas, D. B. (1983). Factors that promote the development of human breast cancer. *Environ. Health Perspect.*, **50**, 209-218

131. Greenbaum, E. and Weinstein, I. B. (1981). Relevance of the concept of tumor promotion to the causation of human cancer. In Fenoglio, C. M. and Wolff, M. (eds.) *Progress in Surgical Pathology.* pp. 27-43. (New York: Masson)

132. Slaga, T. J. (1983). Host factors in the susceptibility of mice to tumour initiating and promoting agents. In Turusov, V. and Montesano, R. (eds.) *Modulators of Experimental Carcinogenesis.* IARC Scientific Publications. No. 51 (Lyon: IARC)

133. Wattenberg, L. W. (1985). Chemoprevention of cancer. *Cancer Res.*, **45**, 1-8

134. Wattenberg, L. W. (1980). Inhibitors of chemical carcinogenesis. *J. Environ. Pathol. Toxicol.*, **3**, 35-52

135. Graham, S., Dayai, H., Swanson, M., Mittleman, A. and Wilkinson, G. (1978). Diet in the epidemiology of cancer of the colon and rectum. *J. Natl. Cancer Inst.*, **61**, 709-714

136. Haenszel, W., Kurihara, M., Segi, M. and Lee, R. K. C. (1972). Stomach cancer among Japanese in Hawaii. *J. Natl. Cancer Inst.*, **49**, 969-988

137. Nomura, A., Slemmermann, G. N., Heilbrun, L. K., Salkeld, R. M. and Virilleumier, J. P. (1985). Serum Vitamin A levels and the risk of cancer of specific sites in men of Japanese ancestry in Hawaii. *Cancer Res.*, **45**, 2369-2372

138. Peto, R., Doll, R., Buckley, J.D. and Sporn, M.B. (1981). Can dietary beta-carotene materially reduce human cancer rates? *Nature (London)*, **290**, 201-208

139. Kummet, T., Moon, T. E., Meyskens, F. L. (1983). Vitamin A: Evidence for its preventive role in human cancer. *Nutr. Cancer.* **5**, 96-106

140. Blunck, J. M. (1984). Modification of neoplastic processes by Vitamin A and retinoids. In Briggs, M.H. (ed.) *Recent Vitamin Research.* pp. 104-125. (Boca Raton: CRC Press Inc.)

141. Sporn, M. B. and Roberts, A. B. (1983). Role of retinoids in differentiation and carcinogenesis. *Cancer Res.*, **43**, 3034-3040
142. Bollag, W. and Hartmann, H. R. (1983). Prevention and therapy of cancer with retinoids in animals and man. *Cancer Surv.*, **2**, 293-314
143. Nugent, J. and Clark, S. (eds). (1985). *Retinoids, differentiation and disease*. Ciba Foundation Symposium 113. (London: Pitman)
144. Bollag, W. (1974). Theraupeutic effects of an aromatic retinoic acid analog. *Chemotherapy*, **21**, 236-247
145. Alfthan, D., Tarlkanen, J., Gorhn, P., Heinonen, E., Pyrhonen, S. and Saila, K. (1983). Tigason (Etretinate) in prevention of recurrence of superficial bladder tumours. *Eur. Urol.*, **9**, 6-9
146. Meyskens, F. L., Gilmartin, E., Alberts, D. S., Levine, N. S., Brooks, R., Salmon, S. E., Surwit, E. A. (1983). Activity of isotretinoin against squamous cell cancers and pre-neoplastic lesions. *Cancer Treat. Rep.*, **66**, 1315-1319
147. Rustin, G. J. S. and Eccles, S. A. (1985). The potential clinical use of retinoids in oncology. (Meeting Report). *Br. J. Cancer.* **51**, 443-445
148. Moon, R. C., McCormick, D. L. and Mehta, R. G. (1983). Inhibition of carcinogenesis by retinoids. *Cancer Res.* (Suppl.), **43**, 2469s-2475s
149. Sporn, M. B. (1980). Retinoids and Cancer Prevention. *In* Slaga, T. J. (ed.) *Carcinogenesis*. Volume 5. *Modifiers of Chemical Carcinogenesis*. (New York: Raven Press)
150. Sporn, M. B., Squire, R. A., Brown, C. C., Smith, J. M., Wenk, M. L. and Springer, S. (1977). 13-*cis*-Retinoic acid: inhibition of bladder carcinogenesis in the rat. *Science*, **195**, 487-489
151. Eccles, S. A. (1985). Effects of retinoids on growth and dissemination of malignant tumours: immunological considerations. *Biochem. Pharmacol.*, **34**, 1599-1610
152. Rapp, F. (1983). Viral carcinogenesis. *Int. J. Cytol.*, **15**, Suppl. **15**, 203-244
153. Wyke, J. and Weiss, R. A. (1984). The contribution of tumour viruses to human and experimental oncology. *Cancer Surv.*, **3**, 1-24
154. Gilden, R. V. amd Rabin, H. (1982). Mechanisms of viral tumorigenesis. *Adv. Virus Res.*, **27**, 281-334
155. Ernberg, I. and Kallin, B. (1984). Epstein-Barr virus and its association with human malignant diseases. *Cancer Surv.*, **3**, 51-89
156. Purtilo, D. T. and Klein, G. (1981). Introduction to Epstein-Barr virus and lymphoproliferative diseases in immunodeficient individuals. *Cancer Res.*, **41**, 4209-4304
157. Heller, M. and Keiff, E. (1981). Colinearity between the DNA's of Epstein-Barr virus and herpesvirus papio. *J. Virol.*, **37**, 821-826
158. Yohn, D. S., Lapin, B. A. and Blakeslee, J. R. (eds.) (1980). *Advances in Comparative Leukaemia Research*. (Amsterdam: Elsevier)
159. De Thé, G. (1980). Multistep carcinogenesis, Epstein-Barr virus and human malignancies. In Essex, M., Todara, G., Zur Hausen, H. (eds.) *Viruses in Naturally-Occurring Cancers*. pp. 11-21. (New York: Cold Spring Harbor Laboratory)
160. Munoz, N. (1973). Effect of herpes-virus type 2 and hormonal imbalance on the uterine cervix of the mouse. *Cancer Res.*, **33**, 1504-1508
161. Wenz, W. B., Reagen, J. W., Heggie, A. D., Fu, Y. and Anthony, D. D. (1981). Induction of uterine cancer with inactivated Herpes simplex virus types 1 and 2. *Cancer*, **48**, 1783-1790
162. Giraldo, G., Beth, E. and Huang, E. S. (1980). Kaposi's sarcoma and its relationship to cytomegalovirus (CMV). III. CMV DNA and CMV-early antigens in Kaposi's sarcoma. *Int. J. Cancer*, **26**, 23-29
163. Summers, J. A., Smolec, J. M. and Snyder, R. (1978). A virus similar to human hepatitis B virus associated with hepatitis and hepatoma in Woodchucks. *Proc. Natl. Acad. Sci., USA*, **75**, 4533-4537
164. Marion, P. L. and Robinson, W. S. (1983). Hepadna viruses: hepatitis B and related viruses. *Curr. Top. Microbiol. Immunol.*, **105**, 99-121
165. Blumberg, B. S. and London, W. T. (1985). Hepatitis B virus and the prevention of primary cancer of the liver. *J. Natl. Cancer Inst.*, **74**, 267-273
166. Pfister, H. (1984). Biology and biochemistry of papilloma viruses. *Rev. Physiol. Biochem. Pharmacol.*, **99**, 111-181
167. Gissmann, L. (1984). Papilloma viruses and their association with cancer in animals and in man. *Cancer Surv.*, **3**, 161-181

168. Gardner, S. D., Field, A. M., Coleman, D. V. and Hulme, B. (1971). New human papovavirus (BK) isolated from urine after renal transplantation. *Lancet*, i, 1253-1257

169. Takemoto, K. K. (1980). Human polyoma viruses: evaluation of their possible role in human cancer. In Essex, M., Todaro, G., Zur Hausen, H. (eds.) *Viruses in Naturally-occurring Cancers*. pp. 311-318. (New York: Cold Spring Harbor Laboratories)

170. Houff, S. A., London, W. T., Zu Rhein, G. M., Padgett, B. L., Walker, D. L. and Sever, J. G. (1983). New World primates as a model of virus-induced astrocytomas. *Prog. Clin. Biol. Res.*, **105**, 223-226

171. Aaronson, S. A. Reddy, E., Robbins, K., Devare, S., Swan, D., Pierce, J. H. and Tronick, S. R. (1983). Retroviruses, *onc* genes and human cancer. In Harris, C. C. and Autrup, H. N. (eds.) *Human Carcinogenesis*. pp. 609 630. (New York: Academic Press)

172. Bishop, J. M. (1983). Cellular oncogenes and retroviruses. *Annu. Rev. Biochem.*, **52**, 301-354

173. Gilden, R. W. and Rice, N. R. (1983). Oncogenes. *Carcinogenesis*, **4**, 791-794

174. Varmus, H. E. (1985). Viruses genes and cancer. 1. The discovery of cellular oncogenes and their role in neoplasia. *Cancer*, **55**, 2324-2333

175. Land, H., Parada, L. F. and Weinberg, R. A. (1983). Cellular oncogenes and multistep carcinogenesis. *Science*, **222**, 771-778

176. Furmanski, P., Hager, J. C. and Rich, M. A. (eds.) (1985). *RNA Tumor Viruses, Oncogenes, Human Cancer and Aids: On the Frontiers of Understanding*. (The Hague: Martinus Nijhoff)

177. Spiegelman, S., Mesa-Tejada, R., Ohno, T., Ramanarayanan, M., Nayak, R., Bausch, J. and Fenoglio, C. (1980). The presence and clinical implications of a virus-related protein in human breast cancer. In Essex, M., Todaro, G., Zur Hausen, H. (eds.) *Viruses in Naturally Occurring Cancers*. pp. 1149-1170. (New York: Cold Spring Harbor Laboratories)

178. Schlom, J., Colcher, D., Drohan, W. and Kettman, R. (1978). The use of molecular hybridisation to track the mode of transmission and distribution of murine mammary tumour viruses: a model for etiological studies of human breast cancer. *Prog. Exp. Tumour Res.*, **21**, 140-158

179. Peters, G., Kozac, C. and Dickson, C. (1984). Mouse mammary tumor virus integration regions Int 1 and Int 2 map on different mouse chromosomes. *Mol. Cell. Biol.*, **4**, 375-378

180. Nusse, R., Van Ooyen, A., Cox, D., Fung, Y., and Varmus, H. (1984). Mode of proviral activation of a putative mammary oncogene (Int 1) on mouse chromosome 15. *Nature*, **307**, 131-136

181. Lane, M., Sainten, A. and Cooper, G. M. (1981). Activation of related transforming genes in mouse and human mammary carcinomas. *Proc. Natl. Acad. Sci. USA*, **78**, 5185-5189

182. Wong-Stahl, F. and Gallo, R. C. (1982). Retroviruses and leukaemia. In Gunz, F. and Henderson, E. (eds.) *Leukaemia*. Edition 4, pp. 329-358. (New York: Grune and Stratton)

183. Shaw, G. M., Broders, S., Essex, M. and Gallo, R. C. (1984). Human T-cell leukaemia virus: its discovery and role in leukaemogenesis and immunosuppression. *Adv. Intern. Med.*, **30**, 1-27

184. Ferrer, J. F., Cabradilla, C. and Gupta, P. (1980). Bovine leukaemia: a model for viral carcinogenesis. In Essex, M., Todaro, G. and Zur Hausen, H. (eds.) *Viruses in Naturally Occurring Cancers*. pp. 887-899. (New York: Cold Spring Harbor Laboratories)

185. Gallo, R. C. (1985). Human T cell leukaemia (lymphotropic) retroviruses and their causative role in T-cell malignancies and acquired immune deficiency syndrome. *Cancer*, **55**, 2317-2323

186. Kalyanaraman, V. S., Sarngadharan, M. G., Robert-Guroff, M., Miyoshi, I., Blayney, D., Golde, D. and Gallo, R. C. (1982). A new subtype of human T-cell leukaemia virus (HTLV-II) associated with a T cell variant of hairy cell leukaemia. *Science*, **218**, 571-573

187. Reif, A. E. (1984). Synergism in carcinogenesis. *J. Natl. Cancer Inst.*, **73**, 25-39

188. Zarbl, H., Sukumar, S., Arthur, A. V., Martin-Zanca, D. and Barbacid, M. (1985). Direct mutagenesis of Ha-ras-1 oncogenes by N-nitroso-N-methyl urea during initiation of mammary carcinogenesis. *Nature (London)*, **315**, 382-385

189. Balmain, A., Ramsden, M., Bowden, G. T. and Smith, J. (1984). Activation of the mouse cellular Harvey-*ras* gene in chemically induced benign skin papillomas. *Nature (London)*, **307**, 658-660

190. Klein, G. and Klein, E. (1985). Evolution of tumours and the impact of molecular biology. *Nature (London)*, **315**, 190 195

191. Johnson, F. B. (1982). Chemical interactions with herpes simplex type 2 virus: enhancement of transformation by selected chemical carcinogens and pro-carcinogens. *Carcinogenesis*, **3**, 1235-1240

192. McCarter, J. A. and Ball, J. K. (1974). Studies on the combined effects of oncornaviruses and chemical carcinogens in mice. In Ts'o, P. and Di Paolo, J. (eds.) *Chemical Carcinogenesis*. pp. 631-638. (New York: Marcel Dekker Inc.)

193. Tennant, R. W. and Rascati, R. J. (1980). Mechanisms of co-carcinogenesis involving endogenous retroviruses. In Slaga, T.J. (ed.) *Carcinogenesis: A Comprehensive Survey*. Vol. 5, pp. 185-205. (New York: Raven Press)

194. Yamamoto, N. (1984). Interaction of viruses with tumour promoters. *Rev. Physiol. Biochem. Pharmacol.*, **101**, 111-159

195. Hsiao, W., Gattoni-Celli, S. and Weinstein, I. B. (1984). Oncogene-induced transformation of C_3H 10 T½ cells is enhanced by tumour promoters. *Science*, **226**, 552-556

196. Arya, S. K. (1980). Phorbol ester mediated stimulation of the synthesis of mouse mammary tumour virus. *Nature*, **284**, 71-73

197. Land, H., Parada, L. F. and Weinberg, R. A. (1983). Tumorigenic conversion of primary embryo fibroblasts requires at least two co-operating oncogenes. *Nature (London)*, **304**, 596-602

198. Newbold, R. F. and Overell, R. W. (1983). Fibroblast immortalisation is a pre-requisite for transformation by EJ C-H-*ras* oncogene. *Nature*, **304**, 648-651

199. Marshall, C. J. and Rigby, P. (1984). Viral and cellular genes involved in oncogenesis. *Cancer Surv.*, **3**, 183-214

200. Thomassen, D. G., Gilmer, T. M., Annab, L. A. and Barrett, J. C. (1985). Evidence for multiple steps in neoplastic transformation of normal and preneoplastic syrian hamster embryo cells following transfection with Harvey Murine sarcoma virus oncogene (v-Ha-ras). *Cancer Res.*, **45**, 726-732

201. Thorgeirsson, U. P., Turpeenniemi-Hujanen, T., Williams, J. E., Westin, E. H., Heilman, C. A., Talmadge, J. E. and Liotta, L. A. (1985). NIH/3T3 cells transfected with human tumor DNA containing activated *ras* oncogenes express the metastatic phenotype in nude mice. *Mol. Cell. Biol.*, **5**, 259-262

202. Eccles, S. A., Marshall, C. J., Vousden, K. and Purvies, H. P. (1985). Enhanced spontaneous metastatic capacity of mouse mammary carcinoma cells transfected with H-ras. In Hellmann, K. and Eccles, S. A. (eds.) *Treatment of Metastasis: Problems and Prospects*. pp. 385-88. (Basingstoke, UK: Taylor and Francis)

203. Turusov, V. S. (ed.) (1973, 1979, 1982). *Pathology of Tumours in Laboratory Animals*. Volumes I-III. (Lyon: IARC Publications nos. 5, 23 and 34)

204. Zweiten, M. J. van (1984). *The Rat as Animal Model in Breast Cancer Research*. (The Hague: Martinus Nijhoff)

205. Reddy, A. L. and Fialkow, P. J. (1983). Papillomas induced by initiation-promotion differ from those produced by carcinogen alone. *Nature (London)*, **283**, 397-398

206. Scribner, J. D. and Scribner, N. K. (1982). Is the initiation-promotion regimen in mouse skin relevant to complete carcinogenesis? In Hecker, E., Fusenig, N. E., Kunz, W., Marks, F. and Thielmann, H. W. (eds.) *Carcinogenesis: A Comprehensive Survey*. Vol. 7, pp. 13-17. (New York: Raven Press)

207. Burns, F. J., Vanderlaan, M., Snyder, G. and Albert, R.E. (1978). Induction and progression kinetics of mouse skin papillomas. In Slaga, T.J., Sivak, A. and Boutwell, R.K. (eds.) *Carcinogenesis: A Comprehensive Survey*. Vol. 2, pp. 91-96. (New York: Raven Press)

208. Turusov, V., Day, N., Andrianov, L. and Jain, D. (1971). Influence of dose on skin tumours induced in mice by single application of 7, 12 dimethylbenz (a) anthracene. *J. Natl. Cancer Inst.*, **47**, 105-111

209. Verma, A. K., Conrad, E. A. and Boutwell, R. K. (1982). Differential effects on retinoic acid and 7, 8 benzoflavone on the induction of mouse skin tumours by the complete carcinogenesis process and by the initiation-promotion regimen. *Cancer Res.*, **42**, 3519-3525

210. Hennings, H., Shores, R., Wenk, M. L., Splangler, E. F., Tarone, R. and Yuspa, S. H. (1983). Malignant conversion of mouse skin tumours is increased by tumour initiators and unaffected by tumour promoters. *Nature (London)*, **304**, 67-69

211. Marx, J. L. (1983). Do tumor promoters affect DNA after all? *Science*, **219**, 158–159
212. Solt, D. B., Medline, A. and Farber, E. (1977). Rapid emergence of carcinogen-induced hyperplastic lesions in a new model for the sequential analysis of liver carcinogenesis. *Am. J. Pathol.*, **85**, 595–618
213. Popper, H. and Selikoff, I. J. (1977). Comparison of neoplastic hepatic lesions in man and experimental animals. In Hiatt, H. H., Watson, J. D. and Winsten, J. A. (eds.) *Origins of Human Cancer.* pp. 1359–1382. (New York: Cold Spring Harbor Laboratories)
214. De Cosse, J. J. (ed.) (1983). Precancer. *Cancer Surv.*, **2** no. 3. (London: Oxford University Press)
215. Carter, R. L. (ed.) (1984). *Precancerous States.* (London: Oxford University Press)
216. Muto, T., Bussey, H. J. R. and Morson, B. C. (1975). The evolution of cancer of the colon and rectum. *Cancer*, **36**, 2251–2270
217. Friedman, E., Urmacher, C. and Winawer, S. (1984). A model for human colon carcinoma evolution based on the differential response of cultured pre-neoplastic, pre-malignant and malignant cells to 12-0-tetradecanoylphorbol-13-acetate. *Cancer Res.*, **44**, 1568–1578
218. Harris, C. C. (1985). Concluding remarks: role of carcinogens, cocarcinogens and host factors in cancer risk. In Harris, C. C. and Autrup, H. N. (eds.) *Human Carcinogenesis*, pp. 941–970 (New York: Academic Press)
219. Lee, A. E., Pang, L. S. C., Rogers, L. A. and Jeffery, R. E. (1983). Metastasis of mammary tumours in mice: relationship with morphology of primary tumours and reproductive background of host. *Clin. Exp. Metastasis*, **1**, 223–227
220. Anderson, J. C., Fugmann, R. A., Stolfi, R. L. and Martin, D. S. (1974). Metastatic incidence of a spontaneous murine mammary adenocarcinoma. *Cancer Res.*, **34**, 1916–1920
221. Eccles, S. A. (1983). Differentiation and neoplasia. Invasion and metastasis; experimental systems. *J. Pathol.*, **141**, 333–353
222. Hewitt, H. B. (1980). Animal tumour models: the intrusion of artefacts. In Hellmann, K., Hilgard, P. and Eccles, S. (eds.) *Metastasis: Clinical and Experimental Aspects.* pp. 18–22. (The Hague: Martinus Nijhoff)
223. Schirrmacher, V. (1984). Cancer metastasis and the use of animal model systems. *Behring Inst. Mitt.*, **74**, 195–200
224. Barnett, S. C. and Eccles, S. A. (1984). Studies of mammary carcinoma metastasis in a mouse model system. I. Derivation and characterisation of cells with different metastatic properties during tumour progression *in vivo. Clin. Exp. Metastasis*, **2**, 15–36
225. Lollini, P.-L., Giovanni, C. D. E., Eusebi, V., Nicoletti, G., Prodi, G. and Nanni, P. (1984). High-metastatic clones selected *in vitro* from a recent spontaneous BALB/C mammary adenocarcinoma cell line. *Clin. Exp. Metastasis*, **2**, 251–259
226. Kripke, M. L., Gruys, E. and Fidler, I. J. (1978). Metastatic heterogeneity of cells from an ultraviolet-light-induced murine fibrosarcoma of recent origin. *Cancer Res.*, **38**, 2962–2967
227. Weiss, L. (1983). Random and non-random processes in metastasis and metastatic inefficiency. *Invasion Metastasis*, **3**, 193–207
228. Schirrmacher, V. (1980). Shifts in tumor cell phenotypes induced by signals from the microenvironment. Relevance for the immunobiology of cancer. *Immunobiology*, **157**, 89–98

7
Environmental causes of cancer in man

R. MONTESANO, D. M. PARKIN AND L. TOMATIS

INTRODUCTION

While screening programmes can reduce mortality from cervical cancer, and to a lesser extent, that from breast cancer[1], the early detection of other cancers and the treatment of established disease are likely to have a rather limited impact in reducing mortality due to the major human cancers. It has been estimated, for example, that, while modern surgery is effective in significantly decreasing cancer mortality, use of additional types of treatment (e.g., X-ray, chemotherapy) after surgery could result in no more than a 5% reduction in the number of deaths from cancer each year[2]. These considerations emphasize the importance of primary prevention of cancer, which involves the identification of the causes of human cancers.

The burden of cancer world-wide

In order to bring about reductions in the overall burden of cancer morbidity and mortality, priorities must be formulated taking into consideration the frequencies of cancer not only in industrialized countries but also on a worldwide basis. It is therefore important to have information on the relative importance of different cancers in each region or country of the world. This information cannot be substituted by extrapolations from one country to another, and, in particular, from a highly industrialized to a less developed country. Parkin et al.[3] (1984) estimated the numbers of new cases of cancer at twelve common sites and of all cancers that occurred in 1975 in 24 areas of the world. The total number of new cases of cancer was estimated conservatively to be 5.9 million; the distributions of cancers at eight principal sites are shown in Table 7.1. In men, lung and stomach are the most frequent cancers followed by colon and rectum, mouth and pharynx, prostate and oesophagus; in women, breast and cervix are the most frequent, followed by stomach, colon/rectum, lung, mouth and pharynx and oesophagus. It should be noted that cancer of the breast is the most frequent cancer in a single sex. These estimates are based on the size and age structure of the world population in 1975 and will certainly change, given the present rapid increase of the world population and, in many areas, the increase in the proportion of the elderly, who are at higher risk of developing cancer. Thus, even if there were no change in current incidence rates, the anticipated number of new cases by the year 2000 would be about 10 million. Broad estimates of the changing incidence rates of certain cancers suggest there may be a considerable shift in the 1975 rankings. It can be expected that lung cancer will become, globally, the most common tumour within a few years, possibly before the end of the century, if of course no measures are taken to reduce sharply the use of tobacco. The different relative importance of tumours arising at sites other than the lung, however, is very likely to persist; and in certain regions of the world, cancer at sites other than the lung will continue to be the most important.

Table 7.1 Worldwide frequency of occurrence of cancer at major sites in 1975 with rank order in parentheses (ref. 3)

Site	Males	Females
Lung	464 000 (1)	127 000 (5)
Stomach	422 000 (2)	261 000 (3)
Colon/rectum	251 000 (3)	256 000 (4)
Mouth/pharynx	233 000 (4)	107 000 (6)
Prostate	198 000 (5)	—
Oesophagus	194 000 (6)	102 000 (7)
Cervix	—	459 000 (2)
Breast	—	541 000 (1)

Descriptive epidemiological studies have shown that there are enormous variations in the risks of certain cancers in different parts of the world. For example, the incidence of oesophageal cancer is very high in parts of China, Southern Africa and in Normandy (France), while that of cervical cancer is very low in the countries of the Middle East. These variations suggest the importance of environmental factors in cancer causation; genetic variation can account for only a small proportion of the differences, and the changes in incidence over time (e.g., the decline in the incidence of stomach cancer in Japan and increases in lung cancer in many populations) are far too rapid to be explained in this way. Figure 7.1 shows time trends in mortality rates over a 50-year period in the USA; there is a striking increase in the death rates from lung cancer and a decrease in rates for stomach cancer, with smaller changes for colon and rectum. Studies of migrant populations show that their cancer patterns become similar to those of the inhabitants of their new environment within one or two generations[4-6]. Such population comparisons and evidence from epidemiological and experimental studies (discussed below) suggest that as much as 80-90% of human cancer is environmentally determined and thus, in theory at least, preventable[7-9]. However, although the environment as a whole may be inculpated in the causation of human cancer, the precise agents or exposures responsible, which might be the target of preventive action, are frequently difficult to define.

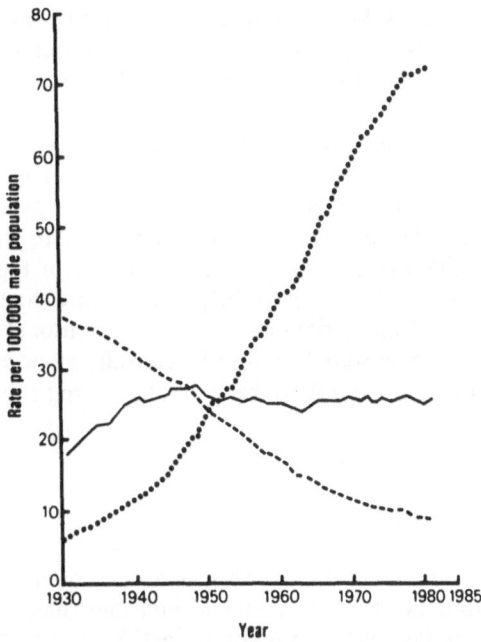

Figure 7.1 Age-adjusted death rates for cancers of the lung (...), stomach (---) and colon and rectum (___) in males (USA, 1930-1981; from ref. 125)

IDENTIFICATION OF ENVIRONMENTAL CARCINOGENS

The epidemiologist is concerned with identifying environmental exposures which are associated with an increased (or decreased) risk of a particular cancer, and accepts these as 'causative' if they meet certain criteria[10]. Thus, certain discrete environmental exposures such as tobacco smoke, alcohol, ionising radiation and industrial processes can be clearly linked to human cancer. Some of these exposures have been linked to the 'lifestyle' of individuals; however, it should be stressed, as Terris[11] has pointed out, that "... individual health behaviour, like all other behaviour, does not occur in a vacuum; it is conditioned by past history, by the entire economic, social and political structure of the society". Nevertheless, for many of the major cancers (e.g., breast, stomach, prostate) such discrete causes are not evident, and the major associations identified are with less easily quantifiable aspects of lifestyle or diet. The role of diet in particular has received much attention recently[12-14]. Because it is a ubiquitous exposure, it is clearly likely to be of major importance. However, there is little doubt not only that the roles played by the major foodstuffs or nutrients in the process of carcinogenesis are complex, but also that the classical methods of epidemiology, which investigate single factors producing large excess risks of certain cancers, are not well suited to their elucidation[15].

Some of the evidence linking certain environmental exposures to human cancers is presented below. The main source of information used in this paper derives from a programme that the International Agency for Research on Cancer (IARC) developed in 1970 on the evaluation of the carcinogenic risk of chemicals to humans, which is focused on the production of monographs[16,17], in which, with the help of groups of experts, available information on uses and exposures as well as all the epidemiological and experimental data on certain environmental chemicals are analysed, and the evidence for a possible association between chemicals or types of exposure and human cancer is evaluated. Up to the present, more than 700 chemicals, groups of chemicals and industrial processes or occupational exposures have been evaluated; 39 of these were found to be causally associated with cancer in humans, and 14 were found to be probably carcinogenic to humans (see[16,18,19]).

Occupational carcinogens

The occurrence of cancer among workers as a consequence of exposure to carcinogenic substances through their occupations has been recognized historically ever since Percival Pott reported in 1775 that soot was a cause of scrotal cancer among chimney-sweeps. Although it would appear that cancers of the skin, lung and bladder are those most frequently associated with occupational exposures, such cancers can in fact occur at a variety of sites[20]. Early in this century, cancer of the skin described in cotton-mill spinners was found to be due to exposure to mineral oils[21]. An increased incidence of lung cancer among miners in Schneeberg and Jachymow in Europe and in Colorado, USA, due to exposure to radiation, was also described at the beginning of this century, although a disease of the lung in Schneeberg miners[22] attributed to inhalation of dust had already been described 300 years earlier by Paracelsus and Agricola. Rehn[23] was the first to provide evidence of a risk of bladder cancer among workers engaged in the manufacture of magenta, and the International Labour Office[24] indicated in 1921 that 2-naphthylamine and benzidine were the responsible carcinogens. The comprehensive epidemiological studies carried out by Case[25] in 1954 showing an enormously increased risk of bladder cancer in workers in the UK exposed to 2-naphthylamine, benzidine or 1-naphthylamine resulted in the passing of legislation banning the use of these carcinogens and in the recognition of this type of cancer as a professional disease entitled to compensation. The most rewarding result of studies of occupational carcinogenesis is that, once the carcinogen(s) have been identified, measures can be taken to avoid or control exposure. Generally, even very small risks in the workplace are considered to be unacceptable[18]. However, it is not possible to ignore the fact that 2-naphthylamine and benzidine were still in use, in Italy and France for example, up to the 1970s and 1980s, and they are probably still used in various developing countries.

Many occupational carcinogens (see Tables 7.2 and 7.3) were identified through epidemiological studies; however, in some instances evidence of

Table 7.2 Industrial processes and occupational exposures causally associated with cancer in man. (Refs. 17, 21 and 123)

Exposure	Target organs[a]
Auramine manufacture	Bladder
Boot and shoe manufacture and repair (certain occupations)	Leukaemia, nasal sinus (bladder)
Coal gasification (older processes)	Skin, lung (bladder)
Coke production	Skin, lung (kidney)
Furniture manufacture (wood dusts)	Nasal sinus
Isopropyl alcohol manufacture (strong acid process)	Nasal sinus (larynx)
Nickel refining	Nasal sinus, lung (larynx)
Rubber industry (certain occupations)	Bladder, leukaemia (stomach, lung, skin)
Underground haematite mining (with exposure to radon)	Lung

[a]Suspected associations are indicated in parentheses.

Table 7.3 Chemicals and groups of chemicals causally associated with cancer in man and for which the main type of exposure is of occupational origin. (Refs. 17, 20, 21, 123 and 124)

Exposure	Target organs[a]
4-Aminobiphenyl	Bladder
Arsenic and certain arsenic compounds	Skin, lung (liver, haematopoietic system)
Asbestos	Lung, pleura, peritoneum (gastrointestinal tract, larynx)
Benzene	Leukaemia
Benzidine	Bladder
Bis (chloromethyl) ether	Lung
Chromium and certain chromium compounds	Lung (nasal cavity, gastrointestinal tract)
Coal-tars (and iatrogenic exposures)	Skin
Coal-tar pitches	Skin (larynx, lung, oral cavity, bladder)
Mineral oils (certain)	Skin (respiratory tract, bladder, gastrointestinal tract)
Mustard gas	Lung (larynx, pharynx)
2-Naphthylamine	Bladder
Shale-oils	Skin (colon)
Soots	Skin, lung
Vinyl chloride	Liver (lung, brain, lymphatic and haematopoietic system, gastrointestinal tract)

[a]Suspected associations are indicated in parentheses.

carcinogenicity in experimental animals preceded such evidence in man. 4-Aminobiphenyl was shown to be carcinogenic in rats and dogs[26] and for this reason was not manufactured in the UK. However, in the USA, this was not the case, and cancer of the bladder was observed in 18% of 171 workers involved in the manufacture of this carcinogen[27].

Asbestos has long been known to be carcinogenic[28]. The results of animal experiments show that inhalation and intrapleural, intratracheal and intraperitoneal administration of these fibres produce tumour types (mesotheliomas and lung cancers) identical to those seen in the majority of occupational exposures. Further, mesotheliomas have occurred in persons living in the vicinity of asbestos factories and mines, or even living in the same house as an asbestos worker. Partly because of its valuable insulation properties and widespread use in the past, reduction in the use of and exposure to asbestos has been a slow process.

These observations were made mainly in the past and based mainly on epidemiological investigations. A comparative analysis of carcinogenicity data in man and in experimental animals shows that experimental data have a high predictive value[29], which should be taken into account in the implementation of primary prevention of occupational cancer.

Table 7.4 Drugs causally associated with cancer in man (Ref. 17)

Exposure	Target organs[a]
Analgesic mixtures containing phenacetin	Renal pelvis (ureter, bladder)
Azathioprine	Lymphoma (leukaemia, skin, thyroid, lung hepato-biliary system, bladder)
Certain combined chemotherapy regimes (MOPP)	Leukaemia (lymphomas)
Chlorambucil	Leukaemia
Chlornaphazine	Bladder
Conjugated oestrogens	Endometrium (breast, ovary, testis)
Cyclophosphamide	Bladder (lymphatic and haematopoietic system, skin)
Diethylstilboestrol	Cervix, vagina
Melphalan	Leukaemia
Methoxsalen with UVA therapy	Skin
Myleran	Leukaemia
Treosulfan	Leukaemia

[a]Suspected associations are indicated in parentheses.

Iatrogenic carcinogens

The majority of drugs found to be carcinogenic to humans (Table 7.4), or strongly suspected of being associated with the development of cancer in man[29], are chemotherapeutic agents that are used in cancer therapy alone or following surgery; the cancer most frequently observed as an unwanted side-effect of the use of cytostatic drugs is non-lymphocytic leukaemia. Since the association was demonstrated by Reimer et al.[30] in 1977 between the occurrence of non-lymphocytic leukaemia and alkylating agent therapy in patients with ovarian cancer, various epidemiological studies have shown similar associations in patients treated for other types of cancer. Recently, Boice et al.[31] reported that among 2067 patients who received methyl-CCNU, as adjuvant therapy following surgery for gastrointestinal cancer, the relative risk of leukaemia was 12.4 as compared to those receiving other forms of therapy, with a six-year cumulative risk of 4.0%. These groups of alkylating agents produce, in addition to a long-lasting and cumulative myelo-suppression, alkylating intermediates which result in cross-linking of DNA via the formation of O^6-methylguanine[32]. From the present knowledge of the mechanisms of action of carcinogenic nitrosoureas and their carcinogenic effect in experimental animals, these observations in man are not unexpected. Furthermore, a carefully randomized study of patients with colon cancer showed that various forms of adjuvant chemotherapy (which included methyl-CCNU) did not result in increased survival over that of a group treated with surgery alone[33,34]. These observations indicate that caution should be exercised in the use of chemotherapy, avoiding the use of certain drugs, as well as unnecessarily high doses, given for too long a time.

Chlornaphazine, [N,N-bis(2-chloroethyl)-2-naphthylamine] was used in combination with ^{32}P to treat polycythaemia vera, but induced bladder cancer in 10 of 61 patients in one study. The major metabolite of chlornaphazine produced in the body is 2-naphthylamine, which is a well-known carcinogen for the human bladder (see Table 7.3).

The mechanisms of action of carcinogenic hormones are much less well understood, and there is no good evidence that they can directly damage DNA. Continuous administration of conjugated oestrogens results in the induction of adenocarcinoma of the endometrium; evidence for increased incidence of tumours of breast, ovary and testis is less convincing. Diethyl-stilboestrol causes carcinoma of the vagina in women exposed in utero. There is also some epidemiological evidence of carcinogenic activity for combined or sequential oral contraceptives and for oxymethalone; in addition, various oestrogens and progestins have been shown to be carcinogens in experimental animals[17,35].

Tobacco and tobacco smoke

It was calculated[3] that in 1975 some 117000 new cases of cancer of the mouth and pharynx occurred in Middle South Asia, where they accounted for one-quarter of new cases of cancer in males. The leading cause of this type of cancer is the habit of chewing tobacco and/or betel quid or taking snuff[36]. These habits are not confined to that region of the world: it was estimated that in 1979 at least 200 million people worldwide practised the chewing habit, and in Sweden there are 700000 to 800000 snuff users[36]. Thus, the cancer risk due to these habits is an important public health problem. Since the combination of smoking and chewing multiplies the risk of oral cancer[37], the situation is likely to become worse in developing countries where cigarette smoking is increasing.

There is overwhelming evidence that tobacco smoking is the major cause of lung cancer and is responsible for the rapid increase in mortality due to lung cancer observed during the last few decades in developed countries[38]. The risk of lung cancer in uranium[39] or asbestos[40] workers is substantially increased by

Table 7.5 Cultural and socio-economic determinants causally associated with human cancer

Exposure	Target organs[a]	Reference
Betel-quid chewing	Oral cavity (pharynx, larynx, oesophagus)	36
Smokeless tobacco use (chewing and oral snuff)	Oral cavity (pharynx, oesophagus)	36
Tobacco smoke	Lung, bladder, oral cavity, larynx, pharynx, oesophagus, pancreas, renal pelvis (stomach, liver, cervix)	38
Schistosoma haematobium	Bladder	44
Clonorchis sinensis	Liver (cholangiocarcinoma)	47
Hepatitis B virus infection	Liver	62
Aflatoxins	Liver	74
Sexual promiscuity (papilloma virus)	Cervix uteri	91
Human T-cell leukaemia virus	T-cell leukaemia	89

[a]Suspected associations are indicated in parentheses.

cigarette smoking; smoking also gives rise to a multiplicative effect with alcohol on the risk of oral cancer[41] and oesophageal cancer[42]. There is evidence for a causal association between tobacco smoking and cancers of the oral cavity, larynx, pharynx, oesophagus, pancreas, renal pelvis and bladder; the association with cancers of the stomach, liver and cervix uteri is less convincing (see Table 7.5). It has been calculated that smoking is responsible for one-third of all cancer incidence in the USA[43].

Parasites

Although infection with *Schistosoma haematobium* has been associated with squamous-cell carcinoma of the bladder in Egypt and in some other areas of Africa and the Middle East[44], the nature of this association is not understood. In the past, chronic irritation due to the presence of schistosome eggs in the bladder was suggested to be a critical factor in the development of cancer. More recently, other aetiological hypotheses have been proposed:

(a) production of carcinogenic toxins by miracidia or worms;

(b) alteration of liver function by the hepatic schistosomiasis, leading to urinary excretion of carcinogenic tryptophan metabolites; and

(c) formation of nitrosamines by the secondary bacterial infections that frequently complicate urinary schistosomiasis[45].

This last hypothesis has received some support from experimental evidence indicating that low levels of nitrosamines can occur in the urine of young Egyptian men, and that concomitant exposure of baboons to low doses of *N*-butyl-*n*-butanolnitrosamine and infection with *S. haematobium* results in papillary tumours and some carcinomas that were not present, or present to a lesser extent in corresponding controls[46].

There is a close correlation between infection with liver flukes (*Clonorchis sinensis* and *Opisthorchis viverrini*) and the occurrence of cholangio-carcinoma in southern China and other parts of South-east Asia[47]. The mechanism of action is obscure but probably depends not only on the length and severity of infection and the immune response to it, but also upon interaction with other carcinogens, possibly dietary in origin.

Radiation

The mutagenic and carcinogenic properties of ionizing radiation have been recognized for many decades. The major interest in the subject now relates to the possible effects of small doses of radiation on large numbers of the population (e.g., as a consequence of occupation, or through exposure to products of nuclear industries or to diagnostic radiation) and the information that can be provided by radiation-induced cancers about mechanisms of carcinogenesis.

Because radiation is a relatively weak carcinogen and induces cancers that are indistinguishable from those resulting from other exposures, even if very large populations (over a million, say) exposed to low doses were studied, the

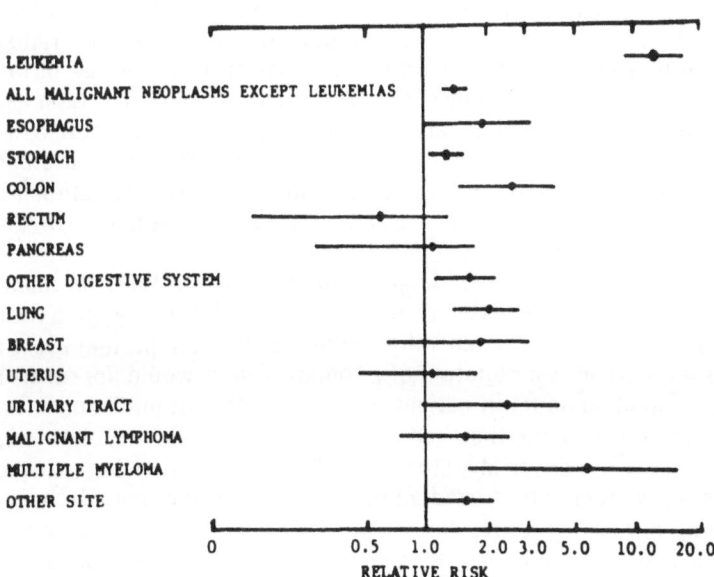

Figure 7.2 Relative risks (and 90 per cent confidence intervals) of dying from specific types of cancer after exposure to up to 200+ rad (Kerma). Hiroshima and Nagasaki data combined, 1950–1978 (reproduced from Kato and Schull[51])

chance of detecting the excess of cancers consistent with current estimates of risk is small[48]. Risk estimates have been derived from studies of special groups exposed to much higher doses of radiation (e.g. atomic bomb survivors, persons irradiated as a consequence of medical investigation or treatment). Reviews of these studies have recently been published[49,50].

The relative risks of dying from specific types of cancer, based on follow up of atomic bomb survivors between 1950 and 1978, are shown in Figure 7.2[51]. The highest relative risk is seen for leukaemia – however, both the relative risk and excess risk for leukaemia appear to fall with increasing time since exposure to radiation. This is not the case for other cancers, and the increased risk seen 15 years and more after exposure appears to persist for at least 30 years. Another group that has yielded a great deal of information are the 14000 patients with ankylosing spondylitis treated with X-rays between 1935 and 1954 and followed up for periods as long as 25 years[52]. These patients showed an excess of leukaemia deaths and an excess of other cancers at sites likely to have been heavily irradiated. The timing for the increased risk of leukaemia was broadly the same as that in atomic bomb survivors; the increased risk for other cancers occurred at about 10 years, and then persisted unchanged[53].

Because of the difficulty in measuring the risk of cancer due to low doses, the possible effects have been deduced by extrapolation from high doses. Yet, there is no evidence that the dose-response curve is linear – with very high levels of radiation, cell killing may reduce the number of cells in which mutations can take place, and so many fewer cancers may occur than predicted. It is therefore possible that at low doses the effect is less than that implied by extrapolation. The UN report on the effects of radiation[54] estimated that exposure of one million persons each to one rad of ionizing radiation may ultimately induce 20 leukaemias and 100 other fatal cancers. The usual exposure of individuals to radiation is lower than this. In Sweden it has been estimated[54] that the average *per capita* exposure from diagnostic X-rays is 110 mrad per annum (the dose from a barium examination is about 440 mrad). It is unlikely that even as few as 3% of cancers in the USA can be attributed to radiation[55].

The evidence from epidemiological studies suggests that the manner in which ionizing radiation acts may be very different depending upon the target tissue. Thus, although it is generally assumed that the important event at the cellular level involves a mutation of a somatic cell, it would appear from the studies of solid tumours in patients exposed to the atomic bomb (or with ankylosing spondylitis) that radiation acts at a relatively late stage in carcinogenesis[56]. Conversely, studies of the excess risk of breast cancer in cohorts of women after irradiation[57] show that the risk declines with increasing age at exposure, consistent with an effect at an early stage of carcinogenesis. It should also be remembered that the effect of radiation is probably multiplicative with that of other carcinogens, e.g., tobacco smoke (*vide supra*).

The importance of ultraviolet radiation, specifically from sunlight, in the genesis of skin cancer has also long been recognized[58]. The risk to individuals depends upon the level of skin pigmentation, and fair complexioned individuals of Celtic ancestry are at particularly high risk. Geographic and occupational risks are also a function of associated exposure to sunlight, modified by the skin pigmentation of the population concerned. The current fashion for a suntanned skin has undoubtedly been responsible for increasing the incidence of skin cancer[17]. This is particularly evident with regard to malignant melanoma, the incidence of which is increasing markedly in successive generations in North America, Northern Europe and Australia[59]. Furthermore, the progressive change in sub-site distribution, with increased frequencies of tumours of the legs and trunk, is in keeping with increasing recreational exposure to sunlight, even though this does not entirely explain the observed increase.

Viruses (see also chapter 6)

Hepatitis B

The incidence of hepatocellular carcinoma in some parts of the world (e.g., Taiwan, Japan, China, Republic of Korea, Greece, and large areas of Africa) is associated with the prevalence of the hepatitis B surface antigen (HBsAg) carrier state[60]. Numerous case-control studies in different populations have shown that the relative risk of incurring hepatocellular carcinoma in subjects with evidence of active infection with hepatitis B virus (HBV) (usually carriers of HBsAg) is some 10-30 times that of non-infected individuals[61]. In a prospective study in Taiwan[62], almost 23000 male civil servants were followed up, and the incidence rate of hepatocellular carcinoma was over 200 times higher in HBsAg carriers than in non-carriers. Further evidence implicating HBV is the finding that woodchucks (*Marmota monax*) infected with a hepatitis virus that has 60-70% nucleotide homology with the human HBV have a greater incidence of hepatocellular carcinoma than non-infected animals[63]. The mechanism by which HBV could bring about malignant transformation of hepatic cells is completely unknown, although various hypotheses have been formulated on the basis of experimental evidence[64-69]. In general terms, moderate to high incidences of liver cancer are almost always found in association with a carriage rate of HBsAg in excess of 2-5%. However, the correlation of incidence to carriage rate is not perfect, and there are areas where high carriage rates coexist with apparently low incidences of hepatocellular carcinoma, e.g., Greenland[70], Central and Western Asia[71] and within China[72]. In a recent study, no serological marker of hepatitis B infection was detected in 44 patients with hepatocellular carcinoma and HBV DNA integration into tumour cell DNA was observed in only three of these patients[73]. HBV is thus probably not a sufficient cause for cancer and other factors are presumably involved. In view of their known hepatocarcinogenicity in animals, aflatoxins have received considerable attention[74]. There is some evidence that the incidence of hepatocellular carcinoma correlates with aflatoxin contamination of foodstuffs in areas with presumably constant levels of HbsAg carriage[72,75,76].

Epstein-Barr virus

Since the description by Burkitt of the occurrence of a particular B-cell lymphoma in East Africa[77] and the detection of the Epstein-Barr virus (EBV) in a cell line from a patient with Burkitt's lymphoma[78], this virus has been implicated in the aetiology of this lymphoma and also of another human cancer, nasopharyngeal carcinoma. Burkitt's lymphoma occurs with a high incidence in children in much of sub-Saharan Africa between 10° north and 10° south of the Equator, and in Papua New Guinea, areas where malaria is holoendemic; it is found at much lower frequencies elsewhere (see[79]). Nasopharyngeal carcinoma also shows a distinctive geographical distribution, affecting particularly populations originating from or living in southern China[80]. The basis for the association with EBV is very similar for both types of tumour, consisting mainly of the early presence and persistence of high antibody titres for EBV in patients with Burkitt's lymphoma or nasopharyngeal carcinoma and the presence of EBV DNA and EBV nuclear antigen in the tumour cells. In addition, EBV is oncogenic in experimentally infected New World primates[81], although the lymphoma induced has important dissimilarities (e.g., polyclonal *versus* monoclonal) from Burkitt's lymphoma[82].

Recent evidence, however, strongly suggests that EBV infection alone cannot be responsible for the aetiology of these tumours. In the case of Burkitt's lymphoma, it was reported recently[83] that repeated attacks of malaria result in alteration of T-cells, leading to an increased proliferation of B-lymphocytes secreting a large amount of immunoglobulins and antibodies; this B-cell sub-population may subsequently be the target of chromosomal translocations particularly relevant to the neoplastic transformation of these cells. Of more than 100 Burkitt's lymphoma cell lines analysed, all showed one of three translocations, t(8;14), t(8;22) and t(2;8), that appear to be relevant to the activation of the c-*myc* proto-oncogene[84]. (See also Chapter 2). It has also been found that markers of EBV infection cannot be detected in malignant cells in 4% of Burkitt's lymphoma cases from a high incidence area and in up to 85% of cases occurring in some low incidence areas (see[84]). These findings point to the limited role of EBV in the aetiology of Burkitt's lymphoma (see[85]).

There is also evidence that nasopharyngeal carcinoma is of multifactorial origin; in fact, it is difficult to reconcile a unique role of EBV with the geographical and ethnic distribution of nasopharyngeal carcinoma and the ubiquity of EBV infection. The habit among Chinese populations of eating salted fish (shown to contain nitrosamines) early in life has been shown[86,87] to be strongly associated with the risk of developing nasopharyngeal carcinoma, and on the basis of the results of a recent study[88], it was estimated that over 90% of nasopharyngeal cancers occurring in young southern Chinese could be attributed to this dietary habit.

Human T-cell leukaemia virus, papillomavirus, herpes simplex virus

At present, the most convincing evidence of an association between a virus and a human cancer is provided by the clinical, epidemiological and experimental studies clearly linking human T-cell leukaemia virus (HTLV) with adult T-cell leukaemia/lymphoma, a type of leukaemia with particular clustering in certain areas of the world (see[89]). Epidemiological, virological and molecular biological studies also support an association between some types of papilloma virus and genital cancer in humans[90,91] whereas the involvement of herpes simplex 2 virus in the aetiology of cervical cancer is not substantiated by more recent molecular and epidemiological studies[91-93].

PROSPECTS FOR PREVENTION

Introduction: the epidemiological approach

A British scientist, R. D. Passey, employed in 1922 a method developed in 1918 in Japan by M. Tsutsui, a pupil of Yamagiwa, for the induction of cancer on the skin of mice, to show the capacity of other extracts of chimney soot to produce cancer. These results were taken as providing experimental proof that the tumours described in 1775 by Pott were, as he claimed, caused by soot. At the time Passey's results were produced, they were received as a very significant scientific achievement which indeed they were, and together with the experiments of Ichikawa and Yamagiwa and of Tsutsui are historical landmarks in experimental carcinogenesis. Since that time, advances in the understanding of the carcinogenesis process, as well as methodologies applied to the testing of chemicals and the development of the epidemiology of non-communicable diseases, has permitted the elaboration of more effective approaches to cancer prevention. Nobody would today, therefore, be ready to accept as an achievement an experimental result which would provide confirmation of an epidemiological observation. Similarly, an epidemiological observation which would provide confirmation in humans of the carcinogenicity of a chemical for which experimental evidence already existed, would not be considered as a remarkable achievement either. The advantages and limitations of experimental and epidemiological studies in cancer prevention are briefly discussed below, as well as their integration in field studies (molecular, biochemical cancer epidemiology).

At present, we are aware of a variety of risk factors, be these defined chemicals, groups of chemicals, complex chemical mixtures or biological agents, for which there is a proven causal relationship with human cancer (Tables 7.3-7.5), and we also know that for another group of chemicals or complex mixtures there is a high probability of a causal relationship with human cancer[94].

Only epidemiological studies can provide the absolute proof that there is a causal relationship between an exposure and the occurrence of cancer in humans. However, this epidemiological approach to the identification of the aetiology of cancer is limited for two main reasons. First, epidemiological methods, due to their lack of sensitivity, can generally only detect an effect in a highly exposed group of the order of a two-fold relative risk. They may therefore miss exposures that entail risks that are of a lower magnitude, although these may be far from negligible, and may in addition concern large sections of the population. The second reason is that epidemiological surveys are based on observation of an effect which is a consequence of an exposure that occurred many years previously: clearly from a public health point of view, this is a totally unsatisfactory approach since the purpose of an effective prevention programme is by definition to intervene before the adverse effects occur, or even before the exposure to a hazardous agent takes place.

Notwithstanding these limitations, the epidemiological approach is certainly of the greatest help in discovering the relationship between cancers that occur today and exposures that have occurred in the past and may still occur today; and it should also not be forgotten that we owe to epidemiologists much of what we know about the long-term adverse effects of environmental agents on humans[95]. Epidemiological surveys may also be of great usefulness in assessing if some new hazard has been let into our environment in spite of screening based on experimental studies. Experimentally-based screening procedures are in fact (together with some obvious *a priori* structure-activity observations) the only way to predict an adverse effect in humans before the effect occurs or, preferably, before the exposure occurs[96]. The epidemiological approach can by definition be of no help in preventing the release into the environment and/or exposure to new man-made risk factors.

Although the experimental approach has undoubted advantages, it has also considerable limitations that it would be unwise to ignore.

Animal carcinogenicity testing

The greatest limitation of epidemiological studies is that they cannot pick up a low risk – that is, they produce false negative results. The major limitation of carcinogenicity tests in experimental models, by contrast, is that they may suggest cancer risks which reflect very high and perhaps unrealistic exposure levels, not at all comparable with the exposures to be expected in man – in other words, they may produce false positive results.

Experimental tests which have as their endpoint the production of tumours are carried out on a limited number of animals. The animals are exposed to generally high dose levels to increase tumour yield and to compensate for the small size of the experimental groups. It is this practice, and also perhaps a tendency to abuse it, which has generated the strongest reaction against accepting data from long-term animal tests to predict human risks. Past experience, however, has shown that such experimental data can indeed predict similar effects in man[96]. In several cases animal test results have preceded, and could have predicted, the evidence later provided by epidemiological studies, as for example in the cases of vinyl chloride, 4-amino-biphenyl and diethylstilbestrol[97]. An analysis of recognised human carcinogens shows that for the majority, if not all, there is experimental evidence of carcinogenicity. Because a fraction of human carcinogens fail to show complete concordance with carcinogenic data obtained in experimental animals, it is often argued that the animal data do not have predictive value. The lack of concordance may, however, merely reflect imperfect experimental design or reporting of the data (as, for example in the case of myleran or arsenic). It may equally well be argued that even limited evidence of carcinogenicity in long-term animal tests represents a sufficient warning that a chemical may represent a carcinogenic risk to humans[98].

The apparent disagreement about the significance of experimental results is highest in relation to chemicals for which there is evidence of human exposure, but for which the only results available are from experimental tests and no epidemiological study has been carried out. As argued above, past experience, as well as the basic similarity in the biological characteristics of mammals, would witness in favour of the value of animal tests to predict qualitatively similar risks to humans. Since, however, no adequate criteria are yet available to extrapolate directly from experimental animals to humans, the predictive value relies heavily on interpretation. If one objects to making an empirical qualitative correlation between animal data and results in man, this objection becomes even stronger when the value of the animal data is attacked from its weakest side, that is the quantitative prediction of risks. A few attempts have been made to support the view that experimental data can provide a reliable basis for quantitative assessment of risks[99]. The potency of chemical carcinogens in inducing cancer in animals varies by a factor of 10^7 (ref. 100), and it is difficult to extrapolate these data to humans without some confidence about the degree of error involved in doing such an exercise. Results from short-term tests, as well as better understanding of the mechanism of action of a given carcinogen, are certainly valuable for the efficient implementation of *ad hoc* public health measures to reduce human exposure to carcinogens; but the present state of our knowledge does not allow an oversimplified approach to this complex issue.

Despite all the possible caveats indicated by the points just made, it would appear that the ensemble of the available evidence indicates that experimental carcinogenicity studies, intelligently used, are very sensitive and effective tools for predicting possible human risks. The situation does, however, become rather confused when results are obtained in experimental animals using doses that are totally unrealistic and these results are then referred to humans as if they had the same value as results obtained in carefully planned dose-response studies.

Measuring individual exposure

In recent years, considerable advances have been made in developing simple methodologies for defining individual exposures which have allowed their use in large numbers of individuals and thus their integration to epidemiological studies. A major limitation of epidemiological studies has in fact been the inability to measure individual exposures to exogenous or endogenous carcinogenic agents, and these exposures have had to be inferred from indirect data obtained from the individuals themselves (e.g., dietary and smoking histories) or from records (e.g., of occupation)). The methods which have been developed include the analytical detection of carcinogens or their metabolites in human tissues or body fluids, the use of specific antibodies to DNA or protein adducts formed by carcinogens, and the presence of biological markers (e.g., mutagenicity in urine, presence of micronuclei or sister chromatid exchanges in peripheral blood cells) that may reflect early responses to carcinogens[101-104]. These methodologies will improve the sensitivity and specificity of epidemiological studies and will also be valuable in providing a more scientific basis for the extrapolation of animal data to humans. In addition, such approaches may facilitate studies of the multifactorial origin of certain cancers or the identification of human carcinogens in complex mixtures.

Assays for carcinogen-DNA adducts

Of these methods, the extremely sensitive immunoassays using antibodies highly specific for carcinogens or carcinogen-DNA adducts appear to be promising for determining individual exposures in large human populations. Application of these methods to humans has so far, however, been limited. One example, aimed at determining the role of nitrosamines in the aetiology of human cancer, will be described briefly.

Nitrosamines are carcinogenic to some 40 animal species. Exposure of humans to these carcinogens occurs either directly or as a result of their formation in vitro[105]. Although nitrosamines may be reasonably expected to represent a carcinogenic risk for humans, however, no causal relationship between any particular type of human cancer and exposure to this group of carcinogens has yet been firmly established. Recently, in England[106], no association was observed between the risk of stomach cancer and levels of nitrate-nitrite in the saliva. In the northern part of China, where the incidences of oesophageal and gastric cancer are particularly high, there is some evidence for exposure to nitrosamines[107,108]. Radioimmunoassays using monoclonal antibodies against O^6-methyl-deoxyguanosine have detected elevated levels of this DNA alkylated base in oesophageal tissue from some people in this area; such elevated levels may be related to exposure to alkylating agents[109]. These studies together with other methodologies for measuring in vivo formation of nitrosamines in the human stomach[110] may provide a solid basis from which to clarify the role of N-nitroso compounds in human cancer.

Practical attempts at prevention

The integration of laboratory with epidemiological studies is essential for the elucidation of components of the diet that might be associated with various forms of human cancer. Although it is clear that dietary patterns affect the incidences of various forms of cancer (e.g. stomach, colon and rectum, breast and prostate), the specific components of the diet responsible for such effects are largely unknown[111,112]. There are now many epidemiological studies investigating the relationship between macronutrients (e.g., fat, fibre, protein) and human cancer, but although some general patterns emerge, the results are by no means clearcut[12,13]. Partly, this is due to the limitations inherent in observational studies; but it has to be admitted that the organizational problems, likely non-compliance, and the timescale involved in any randomized trials of dietary items make this a rather unlikely alternative approach[15]. The situation is somewhat different for micronutrients. A large body of experimental data shows that retinoids can prevent the development of various epithelial tumours induced by chemicals, probably by altering the control mechanism of cell differentiation and/or cell proliferation[113]. Causal epidemiological studies have shown increased risks of cancers at various sites in populations with a low intake of vitamin A or β-carotene[114]; but notable exceptions have been observed. In theory, intervention studies to assess the protective effect of micronutrients are feasible, but the size and logistics of trials which use cancer incidence or mortality as endpoints are still considerable[115]. Conditions which are considered precursors of invasive cancer (for example, dysplasic[116] or micronucleated exfoliated cells[117]) offer a simpler alternative, but extrapolation of these results to the potential protective effects against invasive cancers is less straightforward.

A more difficult situation exists for breast cancer for which the aetiopathogenesis remains even more cloudy, thus undermining the possibility of reducing mortality through preventive or intervention measures. Early age at menarche and late first full-term pregnancy are recognized as major risk factors for breast cancer, indicating that hormone levels (oestrogen and prolactin) play a critical role in the stage of initiation or progression of this cancer[113]. Pike et al[119] have proposed a model in which 'ageing' of breast tissue (starting at the menstrual cycle), which is controlled mainly by levels of oestrogen and prolactin during the sexual life of a woman, is critical in the development of breast cancer. The cell kinetics of breast tissue are closely linked with the 'ageing' of the mammary glands, and experimental studies in rats (see[120]) have shown that susceptibility to cancer induction is dependent on the presence of proliferative components (terminal end buds and terminal ducts) in the breast epithelium. Cairns[121] has proposed that the risk of breast cancer, which increases the longer the interval between puberty and full-term pregnancy, is determined by the number of stem cell generations that have occurred within this time.

Intervention to reduce exposure to an endogenous 'risk factor' – oestrogens – has been proposed recently as a means of preventing breast cancer[122]. Such studies will be less contentious where there is a more clearly defined exogenous risk factor, and where the value of the intervention appears to be justified by public health considerations other than cancer. This is the case for vaccination against hepatitis B virus, a major risk factor for liver cancer in parts of Africa and South-east Asia (see above).

Control of human exposure to carcinogenic agents has increased since 1970. This is particularly true of occupational carcinogens in industrialized countries, even if not to the same degree in every country. An increased control over man-made carcinogens is probably not occurring in developing countries undergoing rapid industrialization. Similarly the consumption of the major human carcinogen, tobacco, is increasing in developing countries while an indication of reduced consumption is appearing in only a few industrialized countries (USA, Finland and UK)[38]. Thus, the effort of implementing primary preventive measures based on the experimental and/or epidemiological evidence of carcinogenicity of various chemicals is still an enormous task.

Classification of carcinogens according to their mechanisms of action could contribute to the prevention of cancer since carcinogens that have different mechanisms of action and exhibit different biological effects might eventually be controlled by different appropriate methods. Although at present such a classification would be neither exhaustive or definitive it may become possible once we know more about the various events preceding the appearance of cancer.

Acknowledgements

We would like to thank Professor R. Sohier for critical reading of the manuscript and B. Ponder for valuable suggestions. We also thank Mrs E. Heseltine for editorial help and Mrs P. Collard-Bianchi for typing the manuscript.

References

1. Morrison, A. S. (1985). *Screening in Chronic Disease*. (New York: Oxford University Press)
2. Cairns, J. (1985). The treatment of diseases and the war against cancer. *Sci. Am.*, **253**, 31-39
3. Parkin, D. M., Stjernswärd, J. and Muir, C. S. (1984). Estimates of the worldwide frequency of twelve major cancers. *Bull. WHO*, **62**, 163-182
4. Haenszel, W. and Kurihara, M. (1968). Studies of Japanese migrants. In: Mortality from cancer and other diseases among Japanese in the United States. *J. Natl. Cancer Inst.*, **40**, 43-68
5. Kmet, J. (1970). The role of migrant populations in studies of selected cancer. *J. Chron. Dis.*, **23**, 305-324
6. U.S. Public Health Service (1980). Populations at low risk of cancer: cancer patterns in ethnic groups. *J. Natl. Cancer Inst.*, **65**, 1127-1159
7. Wynder, E. L. and Gori, G. B. (1977). Contribution of the environment to cancer incidence: an epidemiologic exercise. *J. Natl. Cancer Inst.*, **58**, 825-832
8. Higginson, J. and Muir, C. S. (1979). Environmental carcinogenesis: misconceptions and limitations to cancer control. *J. Natl. Cancer Inst.*, **63**, 1294-1298
9. Doll, R. and Peto, R. (1981). *The Causes of Cancer*. (Oxford: Oxford University Press, Oxford Medical Publications)
10. McMahon, B. and Pugh, T. F. (1970). *Epidemiology, Principles and Methods*. (Boston: Little Brown Co.)
11. Terris, M. (1968). A social policy for health. *Am. J. Public Health*, **58**, 5-12
12. National Research Council (1982). *Diet, Nutrition and Cancer*. (Washington: National Academy Press)
13. Graham, S. (1983). Toward a dietary prevention of cancer. *Epidemiol. Rev.*, **5**, 38-50
14. Willett, W. C. and McMahon, B. (1984). Diet and cancer: An overview. *N. Engl. J. Med.*, **310**, 633-638 and 697-703

15. Zaridze, D. G., Muir, C. S. and McMichael, A. J. (1985). Diet and cancer: Value of different types of epidemiological studies. *Nutr. Cancer*, **7**, 155-166
16. IARC Monographs on the Evaluation of the Carcinogenic Risk of Chemicals to Humans (1972-1985). Vols. 1 to 38. (Lyon: International Agency for Research on Cancer)
17. IARC Monographs on the Evaluation of the Carcinogenic Risk of Chemicals to Humans (1982). *Chemicals, Industrial Processes and Industries Associated with Cancer in Humans.* Supplement 4. (Lyon: International Agency for Research on Cancer)
18. Tomatis, L. (1986). The contribution of the IARC Monographs programme to the identification of cancer risk factors. *N. Y. Acad. Sci.* (In press)
19. Vainio, H., Hemminki, K. and Wilbourn, J. (1985). Data on the carcinogenicity of chemicals in the IARC Monographs programme. *Carcinogenesis*, **6**, 1653-1665
20. Merletti, F., Heseltine, E., Saracci, R., Simonato, L., Vainio, H. and Wilbourn, J. (1984). Target organs for carcinogenicity of chemicals and industrial exposures in humans: A review of results in the IARC Monographs on the Evaluation of the Carcinogenic Risk of Chemicals to Humans. *Cancer Res.*, **44**, 2244-2250
21. IARC Monographs on the Evaluation of the Carcinogenic Risk of Chemicals to Humans (1984). Vol. 33. *Polynuclear Aromatic Compounds, Part 2. Carbon Blacks, Mineral Oils and some Nitroarene Compounds.* (Lyon: International Agency for Research on Cancer)
22. Hunter, D. (ed.) (1975). *The Disease of Occupations.* 5th Edn., pp. 773-783. (London: The English Universities Press Ltd.)
23. Rehn, L. (1985). Blasenbeschwulste bei Fuchs in Arbeitern. *Arch. Klin. Chir.*, **50**, 588-600
24. International Labour Office, Geneva, 23 February 1921, Studies and Reports, Series No. 1
25. Case, R. A. M., Hosker, M. E., McDonald, D. B. and Pearson, J. T. (1954). Tumours of the urinary bladder in workmen engaged in the manufacture and use of certain dyestuff intermediates in the British chemical industry. Part I. The role of aniline, benzidine, α-naphthylamine and β-naphthylamine. *Br. J. Ind. Med.*, **11**, 75
26. Walpole, A. L., Williams, M. H. C. and Roberts, D. C. (1954). Tumours of the urinary bladder in dogs after ingestion of 4-aminodiphenyl. *Br. J. Ind. Med.*, **11**, 105
27. Melick, W. F., Naryka, J. J. and Kelly R. E. (1971). Bladder cancer due to exposure to para-aminobiphenyl: a 17-year fellowship. *J. Urol.*, **106**, 220-226
28. IARC Monographs on the Evaluation of the Carcinogenic Risk of Chemicals to Humans. (1977). Vol. 14. *Asbestos.* (Lyon: International Agency for Research on Cancer)
29. Tomatis, L. (1985). The contribution of epidemiological and experimental data to the control of environmental carcinogens. *Cancer Lett.*, **26**, 5-16
30. Reimer R. R., Hoover, R., Fraumeni, J. F. and Young, R. C. (1977). Acute leukemia after alkylating agent therapy of ovarian cancer. *N. Engl. J. Med.*, **297**, 177-181
31. Boice, J. D., Greene, M. H., Killen, J. Y., Susan, M. D., Ellenberg, S. S., Keehn, R. J., McFadden, E., Chen, T. T. and Fraumeni, J. F. (1984). Leukemia and preleukemia after adjuvant treatment of gastrointestinal cancer with semustine (methyl-CCNU). *N. Engl. J. Med.*, **309**, 1079-1081
32. Rajewsky, M. F. and Huh, N. (1984). Molecular and cellular mechanisms underlying ineffective cancer chemotherapy. *Recent Results Cancer Res.*, **96**, 18-29
33. Gastrointestinal Tumor Study Group (1984). Adjuvant therapy of colon cancer - Results of a prospectively randomized trial. *N. Engl. J. Med.*, **310**, 737-743
34. Gastrointestinal Tumor Study Group (1985). Prolongation of the disease-free interval in surgically treated rectal carcinoma. *N. Engl. J. Med.*, **312**, 1465-1472
35. IARC Monograph on the Evaluation of the Carcinogenic Risk of Chemicals to Humans (1979). Vol. 21. *Sex Hormones.* (Lyon: International Agency for Research on Cancer)
36. IARC Monograph on the Evaluation of the Carcinogenic Risk of Chemicals to Humans (1985). Vol. 37. *Tobacco Habits other than Smoking: Betel-quid and Areca-nut Chewing; and some Related Nitrosamines.* (Lyon; International Agency for Research on Cancer)
37. Hirayama, T. (1966). An epidemiological study of oral and pharyngeal cancer in Central and South East Asia. *Bull WHO*, **34**, 41-69
38. IARC Monograph on the Evaluation of the Carcinogenic Risk of Chemicals to Humans (1985). Vol. 38. *Tobacco Smoking.* (Lyon: International Agency for Research on Cancer)
39. Whittemore, A. S. and MacMillan, A. (1983). Lung cancer mortality among U.S. uranium miners: a reappraisal. *J. Natl. Cancer Inst.*, **71**, 489-499
40. Hammond, E.C., Selikoff, I. J. and Seidman, H. (1979). Asbestos exposure, cigarette smoking and death rates. *Ann. N.Y. Acad. Sci.*, **330**, 473 490

41. Rothman, K. and Keller, R. (1972). The effect of joint exposure of alcohol and tobacco on risk of cancer of the mouth and pharynx. *J. Chron. Dis.*, **25**, 711–716

42. Tuyns, A. J., Pequignot, G. and Jensen, O. M. (1977). Le cancer de l'oesophage en Ille-et-Vilaine en fonction des niveaux de consommation d'alcool et de tabac: des risques qui se multiplient. *Bull. Cancer*, **64**, 45–60

43. US Public Health Service (1982). The health consequences of smoking: cancer. A report of the Surgeon General. (Washington: U.S. Department of Health and Human Services)

44. Ibrahim, A. S. and Elsebai, I. (1983). Epidemiology of bladder cancer. In Elsebai, I. and Hoogstraten, B. (eds.) *Bladder Cancer*. Volume I. *General Review*. CRC Series on Experiences in Clinical Oncology. pp. 17–37. (Boca Raton, Florida: CRC Press, Inc.)

45. El-Aaser, A. A. and El-Merzabani, M. M. (1983). Etiology of bladder cancer. In Elsebai, I. and Hoogstraten, B. (eds.) *Bladder Cancer*. Volume I. *General Review*. CRC Series on Experiences in Clinical Oncology. pp. 39–58. (Boca Raton, Florida: CRC Press, Inc.)

46. Hicks, R. M. (1982). Nitrosamines as possible etiological agents in bilharzial bladder cancer. In Magee, P. N. (ed.) *Nitrosamines and Human Cancer*. Banbury Report 12. pp. 455–471. (New York: Cold Spring Harbor Laboratory)

47. Schwartz, D. A. (1980). Helminths in the induction of cancer: *Opistherchis viverrini, Clonorchis sinersis* and cholangiocarcinoma. *Trop. Geogr. Med.*, **32**, 95–100

48. Land, C. (1980). Estimating cancer risks from low doses of ionising radiation. *Science*, **209**, 1197–1203

49. Kohn, H. I. and Fry, R. J. M. (1984). Radiation carcinogenesis. *N. Engl. J. Med.*, **310**, 504–511

50. Smith, P. G. (1985). Radiation. In Vessey, M. P. and Gray, M. (eds.) *Cancer Risks and Prevention*. (Oxford: Oxford University Press)

51. Kato, H. and Schull, W. J. (1982). Studies of the mortality of A-bomb survivors. 7. Mortality, 1950–1978, Part I: Cancer mortality. *Radiat. Res.*, **90**, 395–432

52. Court Brown, W. M. and Doll, R. (1965). Mortality from cancer and other causes after radiotherapy for ankylosing spondylitis. *Br. Med. J.*, **ii**, 1327–1332

53. Smith, P.G. and Doll, R. (1982). Mortality among patients with ankylosing spondylitis after a single treatment course with X-rays. *Br. Med. J*, **284**, 449–460

54. UNSCEAR (1977). Sources and effects of ionising radiation. United Nations Scientific Committee on the Effects of Atomic Radiation. (New York: United Nations)

55. Jablon, S. and Bailar, J. C. (1980). The contribution of ionising radiation to cancer mortality in the United States. *Prev. Med.*, **9**, 219–226

56. Day, N. E. (1984). Radiation and multistage carcinogenesis. In Boice, J. D. and Fraumeni, J. F. (eds.) *Radiation Carcinogenesis: Epidemiology and Biological Significance*. (New York: Raven Press)

57. Boice, J. D., Land, C. E., Share, R. E., Norman, J. E. and Takunaga, M. (1979). Risk of breast cancer following low dose radiation exposure. *Radiology*, **131**, 559–597

58. Blum, H. (1959). *Carcinogenesis by Ultraviolet Light*. (Princeton: N.J.: Princeton University Press)

59. Muir, C. S. and Nectoux, J. (1982). Time trends: malignant melanoma of skin. In Magnus, K. (ed.) *Trends in Cancer Incidence*. (Washington: Hemisphere)

60. Okuda, K. and MacKay, I. (eds.) (1982). *Hepatocellular Carcinoma, A Series of Workshops on the Biology of Human Cancer*, Report No. 17, UICC Technical Report Series. Vol. 74. (Geneva: Unio International Contra Cancrum)

61. Munoz, N. and Linsell, C. A. (1982). Epidemiology of primary liver cancer. In Correa, P. and Haenszel, W. (eds.) *Epidemiology of Cancer of the Digestive Tract*. pp.161–195. (The Hague, Boston, London: Martinus Nijhoff Publishers)

62. Beasley, R. P., Lin, C. C., Hwang, L. Y. and Chien, C. S. (1981). Hepatocellular carcinoma and hepatitis B virus: a prospective study of 22 707 men in Taiwan. *Lancet*, **ii**, 1129–1132

63. Summers, J., Ogston, C. W., Jonak, G. J., Astrin, S. M., Tyler, G. V. and Snyder, R. L. (1984). Woodchuck hepatitis virus-induced hepatomas contain integrated and closed circular viral DNAs. In Giraldo, G. and Beth, E. (eds.) *The Role of Viruses and Human Cancer*. Volume II, pp. 213–225. (Amsterdam: Elsevier Science Publishers)

64. Mason, W. S., Halpern, M. S. and London, W. T. (1984). Hepatitis B viruses, liver disease and hepatocellular carcinoma. *Cancer Surv.*, **3**, 25–49

65. Blumberg, B. S. and London, W. T. (1985). Hepatitis B virus and the prevention of primary

cancer of the liver. *J. Natl. Cancer Inst.*, **74**, 267-273

66. Shafritz, D. A. (1982). Hepatitis B virus DNA molecules in the liver of HBsAg carriers: mechanistic considerations in the pathogenesis of hepatocellular carcinoma. *Hepatology*, **2**, 35S-41S

67. Ziemes, M., Garcia, P., Shaul, Y. and Rutter, W.J. (1985). Sequence of hepatitis B virus DNA incorporated into the genome of a human hepatoma cell line. *J. Virol.*, **53**, 885-892

68. Shaul, Y, Rutter, W. J. and Laub, O. (1985). A human hepatitis B viral enhancer element. *EMBO J.*, **4**, 427-430

69. Tiollais, P., Pourcel, C. and Dejean, A. (1985). The hepatitis B virus. *Nature*, **317**, 489-495

70. Melbye, M. Skinhøj, P., Nielsen, N. H., Vestergaard, B.F., Ebbesen, P., Hansen, J. P. H. and Biggar, R. J. (1984). Virus-associated cancers in Greenland: frequent hepatitis B virus infection but low primary hepatocellular carcinoma incidence. *J. Natl. Cancer Inst.*, **73**, 1267-1272

71. Szmuness, W. (1978). Hepatocellular carcinoma and hepatitis B virus: evidence for a causal association. *Prog. Med. Virol.*, **24**, 40-69

72. Sun, T.-T. and Chu, Y.-Y. (1984). Carcinogenesis and prevention strategy of liver cancer in areas of prevalence. *J. Cell. Physiol.*, **3**, 39-44

73. Hino, O., Kitagawa, T. and Sugano, H. (1985). Relationship between serum and histochemical markers for hepatitis B virus and rate of viral integration in hepatocellular carcinomas in Japan. *Int. J. Cancer*, **35**, 5-10

74. Busby, W. and Wogan, G. N. (1984). Aflatoxins. In Searle, C. E. (ed.) *Chemical Carcinogens*, ACS Monograph Series. No. 182, pp. 945-1136. (New York: American Cancer Society)

75. Peers, F. G. and Linsell, C. A. (1973). Dietary aflatoxins and liver cancer. A population based study in Kenya. *Br. J. Cancer*, **27**, 473-484

76. Van Rensburg, S. J., Cook-Mozaffari, P., Van Schalkwyk, D. J., Van Der Watt, J. J., Vincent, T. J. and Purchase, I. F. (1985). Hepatocellular carcinoma and dietary aflatoxin in Mozambique and Transkei. *Br. J. Cancer*, **51**, 713-726

77. Burkitt, D. P. (1962). Determining the climatic limitations of a children's cancer common in Africa. *Br. Med. J.*, **ii**, 1019-1023

78. Epstein, M. A., Achong, B. G. and Baor, Y. M. (1964). Virus particles in cultured lymphoblasts from Burkitt's lymphoma. *Lancet*, **i**, 702-703

79. Lenoir, G. M., O'Conor, G. T. and Olweny, C. L. M. (eds.) (1985). *Burkitt's Lymphoma.* IARC Scientific Publications. Vol. 60. (Lyon: International Agency for Research on Cancer)

80. Hirayama, T. (1978). Descriptive and analytical epidemiology of nasopharyngeal cancer. In De-The, G., Ito, Y. and Davis W. (eds.) *Nasopharyngeal Carcinoma: Etiology and Control.* IARC Scientific Publications. Vol. 20, pp. 167-189. (Lyon: International Agency for Research on Cancer)

81. Ernberg, I. and Kallin, B. (1984). Epstein-Barr virus and its association with human malignant diseases. *Cancer Surv.*, **3**, 51-89

82. Thorley-Lawson, D. A., Edson, C. M. and Geilinger, K. (1982). Epstein-Barr virus antigens - a challenge to modern biochemistry. *Adv. Cancer Res.*, **36**, 338-343

83. Whittle, H. C., Brown, J., Marsh, K., Greenwood, B. M., Seidelin, P., Tighe, H. and Wedderburn, L. (1984). T-cell control of Epstein-Barr virus-infected B cells is lost during *P. falciparum* malaria. *Nature*, **312**, 449-450

84. Lenoir, G. and Taub, R. (1986). Chromosomal translocations and oncogenes in Burkitt's lymphoma. In Goldman J. M. and Harnden, D. G. (eds.) *Leukaemia and Lymphoma Research*, 2. *Genetic Rearrangements in Leukaemia and Lymphoma.* pp. 152-172. (Edinburgh: Churchill Livingstone)

85. Smith, P. G. (1985). Rapporteur's report. In Lenoir, G., O'Conor, G. and Olweny, C. I. M. (eds.) *Burkitt's Lymphoma.* IARC Scientific Publications. Vol. 60. (Lyon: International Agency for Research on Cancer)

86. Ho, J. H. C., Huang, D. P. and Fong, Y. Y. (1978). Salted fish and nasopharyngeal carcinoma in Southern Chinese. *Lancet*, **ii**, 626

87. Armstrong, R. W., Armstrong, M. J., Yu, M. C. and Henderson, B. E. (1983). Salted fish and inhalants as risk factors for nasopharyngeal carcinoma in malaysian Chinese. *Cancer Res.*, **43**, 2967-2970

88. Yu, M. C., Ho, J. H. C., Lai, S. H. and Henderson, B. E. (1986). Cantonese-style salted fish

as a cause of nasopharyngeal carcinoma: report of a case-control study in Hong Kong. *Cancer Res.*, **46**, 956-961

89. Gallo, R. C. (1984). Human T-cell leukaemia-lymphoma virus and T cell malignancies in adults. *Cancer Surv.*, **3**, 113-159

90. Gissmann, L. (1984). Papillomaviruses and their association with cancer in animals and man. *Cancer Surv.*, **3**, 161-181

91. Zur Hausen, H. and Schneider, A. (1985). The role of papillomaviruses in human anogenital cancer. In: Howley, P. and Solzman, N. P. (eds.) *Papovaviridae, The Papillomaviruses.* (New York: Plenum Press) (In press)

92. Vonka, V., Kanka, J., Jelinek, J., Subrt, I., Suchanek, A., Havrankova, A. *et al.* (1984). Prospective study on the relationship between cervical neoplasia and herpes simplex type-2 virus. I. Epidemiological characteristics. *Int. J. Cancer*, **33**, 49-60

93. Vonka, V., Kanka, J., Hirsch, I., Zavadova, H., Kromar, M., Suchankova, A. *et al.* (1984). Prospective study on the relationship between cervical neoplasia and herpes simplex type-2 virus. II. Herpes simplex type-2 antibody presence in sera taken at enrolment. *Int. J. Cancer*, **33**, 61-66

94. Tomatis, L. (1984). Exposures associated with cancer in humans. *J. Cancer Res. Clin. Oncol.*, **108**, 6-10

95. Lilienfeld, A. M. (1983). Practical implications of epidemiologic methods. *Environ. Health Perspect.*, **52**, 3-8

96. Tomatis, L., Breslow, N. E. and Bartsch, H. (1982). Experimental studies in the assessment of human risk. In Schottenfeld, D. and Fraumeni, J. F. (eds.) *Cancer Epidemiology and Prevention.* pp. 44-73. (Philadelphia: W. B. Saunders Company)

97. Tomatis, L. (1977). The value of long-term testing for the implementation of primary prevention. In Hiatt, H. H., Watson, J. D. and Winsten, J. A. (eds.) *Origins of Human Cancer.* pp. 1339-1357. (New York: Cold Spring Harbor Laboratory)

98. Tomatis, L. (1985). The contribution of epidemiological and experimental data to the control of environmental carcinogens. *Cancer Lett.*, **26**, 5-16

99. Meselson, M. and Russel, K. (1971). Comparisons of carcinogenic and mutagenic potency. In Hiatt, H. H., Watson, J. D. and Winsten, J. A. (eds.) *Origins of Human Cancer*, Book C: *Human Risk Assessment.* pp. 1473-1481. Cold Spring Harbor Conferences on Cell Proliferation, Vol. 4. (New York: Cold Spring Harbor)

100. Peto, R., Pike, M. C., Berstein, L., Gold, L. S. and Ames, B. N. (1984). The TD50: a proposed general convention for the numerical description of the carcinogenic potency of chemicals in chronic exposure animal experiments. *Environ. Health Perspect.*, **58**, 1-8

101. Berlin, A., Draper, M., Hemminki, K. and Vainio, H. (1984). *Monitoring Human Exposure to Carcinogenic and Mutagenic Agents.* IARC Scientific Publication. Vol. 59. (Lyon: International Agency for Research on Cancer)

102. Perera, F. P. and Weinstein, I. B. (1982). Molecular epidemiology and carcinogen-DNA adduct detection: new approaches to studies of human cancer causation. *J. Chron. Dis.*, **35**, 581-600

103. Kriek, E. Engelse, L. D., Scherer, E. and Westra, J. G. (1984). Formation of DNA modifications by chemical carcinogens identification, localization and quantification. *Biochim. Biophys. Acta*, **738**, 181-201

104. International Agency for Research on Cancer/International Programme on Chemical Safety Working Group Report (1982). Development and possible use of immunological techniques to detect individual exposure to carcinogens. *Cancer Res.*, **42**, 5236-5239

105. Bartsch, H. and Montesano, R. (1984). Relevance of nitrosamines to human cancer. *Carcinogenesis*, **5**, 1381-1393

106. Forman, D., Al-Dabbagh, S. and Doll, R. (1985) Nitrates, nitrites and gastric cancer in Great Britain. *Nature*, **313**, 620-625

107. Yang, C. S. (1980). Research on esophageal cancer in China: a review. *Cancer Res.*, **40**, 2633-2644

108. Lu, S. H., Ohshima, H. and Bartsch, H. (1985). Recent studies on *N*-nitroso compounds as possible etiological factors in oesophageal cancer. In O'Neill, I.L., Von Borstel, R.C., Miller, C.T., Long, J. and Bartsch, H. (eds.) *N-Nitroso Compounds: Occurrence, Biological Effects and Relevance to Human Cancer.* IARC Scientific Publication. Vol. 57, pp. 947-953. (Lyon: International Agency for Research on Cancer)

109. Umbenhauer, D., Wild, C. P., Montesano, R., Saffhill, R., Boyle, J. M., Huh, N., Kirstein, U., Thomale, J., Rajewsky, M. F. and Lu, S. H. (1985). O^6-methyldeoxyguanosine in oesophageal DNA among persons at high risk of oesophageal cancer. *Int. J. Cancer*, **36**, 661-665

110. Ohshima, H. and Bartsch, H. (1981) Quantitative estimation of endogenous nitrosation in humans by monitoring N-nitrosoproline excreted in the urine. *Cancer Res.*, **41**, 3658-3662

111. Sugimura, T. and Sato, S. (1983). Mutagens-carcinogens in foods. *Cancer Res.*, **43**, 2415s-2421s

112. Ames, B. N. (1983). Dietary carcinogens and anticarcinogens. *Science*, **221**, 1256-1264

113. Sporn, M. B. and Roberts, A. B. (1983). Role of retinoids in differentiation and carcinogenesis. *Cancer Res.*, **43**, 3034-3040

114. Peto, R., Doll, R., Buckley, J. D. and Sporn, M. D. (1981). Can dietary beta-carotene materially reduce human cancer rates? *Nature*, **290**, 201-208

115. Hennekens, C. H., Stampfer, M. J. and Willett, W. (1984). Micronutrients and cancer prevention. *Cancer Detect. Prev.*, 7, 147-158

116. Munoz, N., Wahrendorf, J., Lu, J. B., Crespi, M., Thurnham, D. I., Day, N. E., Zheng, H. J., Grassi, A., Li, W. Y., Liu, G. L., Lang, Y. Q., Zhang, C. Y., Zheng, S. F., Li, J. Y., Correa, P., O'Conor, G. T. and Bosch, X. (1985). No effect of riboflavine, retinol, and zinc on prevalence of precancerous lesion of oesophagus. *Lancet*, **ii**, 111-114

117. Stich, H. F., Hornby, P. and Dunn, B. P. (1985). A pilot beta-carotene intervention trial with inuits using smokeless tobacco. *Int. J. Cancer*, **36**, 321-327

118. Miller, A. B. and Bulbrook, R. D. (1980). The epidemiology and etiology of breast cancer. *N. Engl. J. Med.*, **303**, 1246-1248

119. Pike, M. C., Krailo, M. D., Henderson, B. E., Casagrande, J. T. and Hoel, D. G. (1983). 'Hormonal' risk factors, 'breast tissue age' and the age-incidence of breast cancer. *Nature*, **303**, 767-770

120. Nagasawa, H. (1985). Age-related changes in mammary gland DNA synthesis as a limiting factor for mammary tumorigenesis in rats and its implication for human breast cancer. In Likhachev, A., Anisimov, V. and Montesano, R. (eds.) *Age-related Factors in Carcinogenesis*. IARC Scientific Publications. Vol. 58, pp. 105-113. (Lyon: International Agency for Research on Cancer)

121. Cairns, J. (1975). Mutation selection and the natural history of cancer. *Nature*, **255**, 197-200

122. Cuzick, J., Wares, D.Y. and Bulbrook, R.D. (1986). The prevention of breast cancer. *Lancet*, **i**, 33-86

123. IARC Monograph on the Evaluation of the Carcinogenic Risk of Chemicals to Humans. (1984). *Polynuclear Aromatic Compounds. Part 3. Some Complex Industrial Exposures in Aluminium Production, Coal Gasification, Coke Production, and Iron and Steel Founding*. Vol. 34. (Lyon: International Agency for Research on Cancer)

124. IARC Monograph on the Evaluation of the Carcinogenic Risk of Chemicals to Humans (1985). *Polynuclear Aromatic Compounds. Part 4. Bitumens, Coal-tars and Derived Products. Shale-oils and Soots*. Vol. 35. (Lyon: International Agency for Research on Cancer)

125. Silverberg, E. (1985). Cancer Statistics, 1985. *Ca-A Cancer Journal for Clinicians*, **35**, 19-35

8
Genetic determinants of cancer in man

J.M. BIRCH

INTRODUCTION

The clustering of cancers in individual families has long been recognised. In 1866[1] Broca described a family in which breast and gastrointestinal tract cancers occurred over four generations, and a dominant pattern of inheritance was recognised in retinoblastoma as long ago as 1896[2]. However, with the exception of certain rare inherited conditions including retinoblastoma, neurofibromatosis and familial polyposis coli, where susceptibility to malignant disease is marked, genetic factors are generally considered to have much less importance than environmental factors. The study of cancer genetics in man may nevertheless be of considerable importance in understanding the fundamental nature of cancer, in developing cancer control programmes and in advising individual patients and their families. For some patients, possible increased risks of cancer in close relatives may cause considerable anxiety, and reassurances based on misconceptions are of little benefit. The present chapter aims to give a general overview of the more interesting aspects of genetic susceptibility to cancer in man, rather than to provide a detailed review of the literature. This will be used as the basis for a discussion of how a clinical and epidemiological approach to the study of human cancer genetics can be productive and worthwhile for experimentalists, medical practitioners and for patients and their families.

EVIDENCE FOR GENETICALLY DETERMINED SUSCEPTIBILITY TO CANCER IN MAN

It has become clear from the study of heritable syndromes in which excess cancer incidence is a feature that susceptibility to cancer can be inherited in an apparently Mendelian fashion. Other families can be identified which show a pattern of cancers consistent with a genetic aetiology. Heritability of cancers will be considered under the following headings: autosomal recessive syndromes; autosomal dominant syndromes; childhood cancer; and familial cancer.

Autosomal recessive syndromes

A series of conditions including ataxia telangiectasia, Bloom's syndrome and Fanconi anaemia have in common autosomal recessive inheritance, chromosomal fragility (spontaneous or in response to X-ray exposure), and an apparent high incidence of lymphoreticular malignancy.

Ataxia telangiectasia

Ataxia telangiectasia is thought to occur about once in every 40000 births, although higher frequencies have been noted in certain isolated communities[3,4]. The main clinical features of ataxia telangiectasia are progressive cerebellar ataxia with onset during early childhood, and the characteristic oculocutaneous telangiectasis which has a somewhat later onset. Various immunological deficiencies also occur as part of the syndrome, leading to repeated and severe broncho-pulmonary infections. These infections are the most common cause of death in ataxia telangiectasia patients, but where such infections do not prove fatal there is a high frequency of malignant disease, notably Hodgkin's disease, non-Hodgkin's lymphomas and lymphoid leukaemias, although gliomas, germ cell tumours and carcinomas of various sites have also been recorded. The median age at onset for lymphoreticular malignancies is about 8 years, and about 17 years for carcinomas. It appears that approximately one in ten ataxia telangiectasia patients develop a malignant neoplasm[5,6]. Such patients show severe reactions to radio-therapy[7]. It was this clinical observation of radio-sensitivity in the ataxia telangiectasia patient which led to the proposal that a DNA repair defect was present[8]. Ataxia telangiectasia and related research is described in detail by Bridges and Harnden (1982)[9].

Bloom's syndrome

The main features of Bloom's syndrome are growth retardation and photosensitivity, characterised by telangiectatic erythema on the face. Other features include hypogonadism and café-au-lait patches. The syndrome is exceedingly rare. In addition to a high proportion of chromosome aberrations in general, cells from patients affected by Bloom's syndrome display an extremely high frequency of sister chromatid exchanges, which may be diagnostic in the presence of other clinical features. The underlying cellular defect responsible for these characteristics has not yet been identified. As in ataxia telangiectasia, the neoplasms occurring in Bloom's syndrome patients are mainly lymphoreticular in origin and occur at an early age[10].

Fanconi anaemia

The chief clinical manifestations of Fanconi anaemia are a progressive pancytopaenia, which generally becomes apparent during childhood, associated with various congenital anomalies, including genito-urinary defects, ear deformities, skeletal anomalies, retarded growth and hyperpigmentation. *Café-au-lait* spots may also be present[11]. In many patients death can be during childhood[12]. Among young adult patients with Fanconi anaemia, infections. Among those patients who survive the pancytopaenia, acute leukaemia – typically monocytic or myelomonocytic – frequently develops during childhood[12]. Among young adult patients with Fanconi anaemia, carcinomas and hepatic tumours have been observed, the latter possibly associated with long-term androgen therapy[13]. Fibroblast cultures from Fanconi anaemia patients display increased numbers of chromosome aberrations compared with controls. Survival in fibroblast cultures following treatment with mitomycin C also differs significantly between cells from patients with Fanconi anaemia and control cells. Although some evidence exists to support the idea of a DNA repair defect in Fanconi anaemia, this has not been confirmed, and the biochemical basis of the above observations is unknown[13].

Xeroderma pigmentosum

A group of conditions collectively known as xeroderma pigmentosum which also show autosomal recessive inheritance can be included with the chromosomal instability syndromes. The conditions are characterised by a progressive sun-sensitive dermatosis which is manifest in early childhood. In such patients there is a marked tendency for the development of multiple malignant skin tumours. The development of these tumours is related to a defective capacity in the cells of xeroderma pigmentosum patients to repair DNA damage caused by ultraviolet light. In this way predisposition to cancer has directly been linked to an identifiable biochemical defect. For more detailed discussion of xeroderma pigmentosum see Kraemer (1980)[14].

Other autosomal recessive syndromes, which include Werner's syndrome, combined immunodeficiency disease and common variable immunodeficiency, have been reviewed by Swift (1982)[13] and will not be considered here.

Cancer susceptibility in heterozygotes

Ataxia telangiectasia, Bloom's syndrome, Fanconi anaemia, xeroderma pigmentosum and other autosomal recessive cancer-prone syndromes are in themselves extremely rare and make only a small contribution to the total cancer burden. However the possibility that heterozygous carriers for these conditions might also show a predisposition to cancer has aroused considerable interest, since Swift reported an excess of cancer deaths among the families of eight patients with Fanconi anaemia[15]. Since then studies have been carried out on numbers of cancer deaths among blood relatives of a larger series of Fanconi anaemia patients, the families of patients with xeroderma pigmentosum and the families of ataxia telangiectasia patients. The more recent study on the Fanconi anaemia families did not confirm the original findings, and no excess of cancer deaths was found among the xeroderma pigmentosum families[16,17]. However, there was a significant excess of cancer deaths among all blood relatives of ataxia telangiectasia patients included in the study, which was particularly marked at younger ages[18].

The array of cancers seen among the ataxia telangiectasia families included those commonly found among homozygotes, but the data suggest that persons heterozygous for ataxia telangiectasia may also be predisposed to other cancers. This work is reviewed by Swift (1982)[19]. Although ataxia telangiectasia is rare in the homozygous state, heterozygotes may comprise at least one per cent of the general population. Therefore, their possible predisposition to cancer could significantly contribute to cancer incidence in general. It is of considerable importance that this work should be extended and substantiated. A major difficulty is that there is no suitable marker for identifying ataxia telangiectasia heterozygotes in the general population and work is restricted to the study of blood relatives of homozygotes.

Autosomal dominant syndromes

There are a number of syndromes which show a familial pattern consistent with autosomal dominant inheritance in which neoplasia is the main manifestation. These include the naevoid basal cell carcinoma syndrome (Gorlin's syndrome), familial polyposis coli, and the multiple endocrine neoplasia syndromes. In neurofibromatosis, malignant tumours mostly of the central nervous system occur in a significant minority of those affected.

Gorlin's syndrome (the naevoid basal cell carcinoma syndrome)

The principal features of Gorlin's syndrome include multiple basal cell carcinomas, jaw cysts, skeletal deformities, skin pits on palms and soles, soft tissue calcification and, less frequently, mental retardation and other neoplasms (including medulloblastoma and ovarian fibromas). The syndrome was first clearly described by Gorlin and Goltz in 1960[20], but case reports consistent with the syndrome had been published much earlier than this, e.g. Straith (1939)[21], and skeletal anomalies characteristic of the syndrome have been described in skeletons excavated in Egypt which dated from the dynastic period[22]. The pattern of inheritance is that of an autosomal dominant with a high degree of penetrance but variable expressivity. The syndrome is rare, but from a study of the records of more than a thousand patients with one or more of the following diagnoses: basal cell carcinoma, epithelioma adenoides cysticum, multiple benign cystic epithelioma and odontogenic cysts, Anderson estimated that 1%-2% were affected by the syndrome[23].

Although patients may spontaneously develop more than 100 basal cell carcinomas during their lifetime, onset of these lesions may be greatly accelerated following radiotherapy. This effect is seen most dramatically in

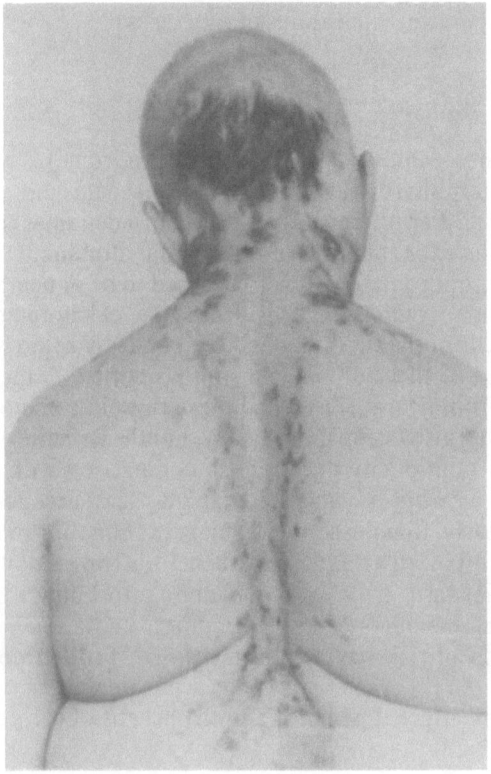

Figure 8.1 Patient with Gorlin's syndrome showing multiple basal cell carcinomata in the field of previous X-ray therapy for medulloblastoma

children with medulloblastoma in whom the syndrome may not have been recognised at the time of diagnosis of their medulloblastoma, and who were treated with craniospinal irradiation (Figure 8.1). Characteristically in these patients, large numbers of basal cell carcinomas develop, sometimes within months of the radiotherapy, throughout the radiation field[24,25].

Familial polyposis of the colon

Patients carrying the gene for familial polyposis of the colon typically develop multiple adenomatous polyps in the colon at an early age. Such patients are strongly predisposed to the development of colorectal carcinoma, and on average half of them will have developed colon cancer by the age of 40 years[26]. Age at onset of the colon cancer has been reported to range from 9 to 70 years. The condition is inherited as an autosomal dominant, and in families with polyposis of the colon regular screening of persons at risk is recommended, with prophylactic colectomy once the diagnosis in an individual has been made. The frequency of carriers of the familial polyposis gene may be one in six or eight thousand[13].

Multiple endocrine neoplasia type 2

Multiple endocrine neoplasia type 2 (Sipple's syndrome) is characterised by multifocal medullary thyroid carcinoma and phaeochromocytoma, which is commonly bilateral. Parathyroid hyperplasia, or adenomas, may also occur. The syndrome shows a pattern of autosomal dominant inheritance. In common with neurofibromatosis it is considered to be of neural crest origin[27]. Medullary thyroid carcinoma arises from the calcitonin-secreting para-follicular or 'C' cells of the thyroid gland, and phaeochromocytoma from the chromaffin cells of the adrenal medulla, both of which are derived embryologically from neural crest. Medullary thyroid carcinoma and phaeo-chromocytoma may also occur sporadically, but the hereditary tumours show early onset and a multiplicity of lesions in comparison with sporadic cases. The tumours of the thyroid and adrenal may be successfully dealt with surgically, and early diagnosis by regular examinations of members of families potentially at risk may be of benefit. However, it is difficult to distinguish familial cases from sporadic, and so to know which families to screen, and among members of known multiple endocrine neoplasia type 2 families the period of risk has not been defined. Furthermore, the natural history of the tumours characteristic of the syndrome may show considerable variability between affected persons, and the benefit of early surgery may be doubtful in some cases[28].

Neurofibromatosis

Two forms of this syndrome have been defined: peripheral neurofibromatosis (von Recklinghausen's disease) and central neurofibromatosis. The peripheral form is more common and occurs about once in every 3000 births. The main characteristics are multiple neurofibromata and *café-au-lait* patches where increased melanin is present in the epidermal basal layer. Neurofibromas arise from the connective tissue sheath surrounding the peripheral nerves and are thought to be derived from Schwann cells, fibroblasts and occasionally perineurial cells. Schwann cells usually predominate. The majority of neurofibromas arise subcutaneously, but less commonly deeper tumours resulting in diffuse tortuous enlargement of peripheral nerves, designated plexiform neurofibromas, may develop. Sarcomatous change may occur in one or more of the neurofibromas in about 10% of patients, although estimates of frequency vary between 2 and 30 per cent[29]. Malignant trans-formation occurs particularly in tumours affecting large nerve trunks of the neck or extremities and is rare in peripheral superficial neurofibromas[30]. Central nervous system tumours are frequent among patients with peripheral neurofibromatosis, typically optic nerve gliomas, but other intracranial or intraspinal neoplasms may also occur. In the central form of neurofi-bromatosis *café-au-lait* spots and multiple peripheral neurofibromas are less common, and when present occur in smaller numbers than in the peripheral form, but they may nevertheless be found in 60% of the cases[31]. The main features of central neurofibromatosis are multiple tumours of the central nervous system and meninges, and acoustic Schwannomas (tumours of the Schwann cells of the VIIIth cranial nerve), often bilateral, are also typical. For a more detailed description of the various forms of neurofibromatosis see Moots and Rubinstein (1984)[32].

Numerous other autosomal dominant conditions associated with neoplasia have been described, and many of these are listed in Mulvihill (1977)[33]. The contribution of these syndromes to the total cancer burden of man is difficult to assess. One problem is that in many cancer patients there may be a failure to diagnose an underlying genetic condition. For example, phenotypic expression of the neurofibromatosis gene is very variable, and a number of malignant conditions have been associated with neurofibromatosis in addition to the neurofibrosarcomas and gliomas, typically of the optic nerve, which are characteristic of the syndrome. Among these are leukaemia[34], Wilms' tumour[35], rhabdomyosarcoma[36], and malignant Triton tumour[37]. Signs and symptoms other than malignant disease attributable to neurofibromatosis, for example café-au-lait patches, may be minimal. Unless cancer patients and their families are examined by clinicians familiar with the stigmata of the various syndromes which may be associated with neoplasia, under-diagnosis of these heritable cancer-prone conditions will be inevitable.

Childhood cancer

Malignant disease in children is of particular interest to the cancer geneticist. Many childhood cancers are typically diagnosed under 5 years of age, e.g. acute lymphoid leukaemia, Wilms' tumour, neuroblastoma, and examples of congenital malignant neoplasms and tumours diagnosed within the first few months of life are seen. These observations, together with their frequent embryonal nature, would suggest a pre-natal origin for perhaps the majority of cancers occurring in children. The prognosis of many types of childhood cancer has improved dramatically in recent years, and survivors present an interesting group in which to study the effect of putative cancer genes, both from the point of view of vertical transmission, i.e. the development of tumours in the offspring of survivors, and a general susceptibility to cancer in the individual, i.e. the development of second and subsequent primary neoplasms in the survivors. Such studies, however, may be complicated by the fact that the treatment itself may to some extent be carcinogenic and, furthermore, may result in infertility in some survivors.

Retinoblastoma

Perhaps the best known example of a heritable tumour is retinoblastoma which occurs approximately once in every 20000 live births, although estimates vary[38-40]. In contrast to the majority of childhood cancers retinoblastoma has had a good prognosis for a considerable time.

The possibility that retinoblastoma may be vertically transmitted was first reported in 1892[6], and subsequently in 1910 when de Gouvea[41] described a family in which three out of seven children whose father had had an enucleation for retinoblastoma during infancy were also affected by retinoblastoma. As pedigree data accumulated it became apparent that retinoblastoma could occur in two forms, sporadic and hereditary. Among hereditary cases a dominant pattern was seen and the disease tended to be bilateral. It was subsequently shown that bilaterality, even in the absence of a family history, was indicative of the hereditary form of the disease[42]. However, unilateral disease can occur among hereditary cases, especially in the first generation. Smith[43] states that two factors favour reduced bilaterality in the first generation: better survival among unilateral cases and undiagnosed spontaneously arrested tumours in first generation 'unilateral' cases and their relatives. It cannot be assumed that unilateral cases without a family history are necessarily sporadic.

From his observations on a population-based series of retinoblastoma from North West England, Smith (1976)[43] concluded that, of new cases not associated with a family history, 40% would be hereditary and 60% sporadic. This accords well with other estimates[44]. In addition to bilateral disease, patients with familial retinoblastoma may also show multiple primary tumours within one eye. Conversely a small number (of the order of 5%) of carriers of familial retinoblastoma may be completely unaffected by the disease. The number of tumours developing in carriers of familial retinoblastoma follows a Poisson distribution with a mean number of three to four tumours per individual[45]. Assuming an incidence of approximately 5 per 100 000 children, on average three of these children will have solitary unilateral lesions attributable to the sporadic form of retinoblastoma, and two will have three to four tumours each, attributable to hereditary disease. The relative risk for carriers of familial retinoblastoma of developing tumours is therefore approximately 100 000. Furthermore, ectopic retinoblastoma, especially in the pineal, representing independent primary lesions rather than metastases, has been described in a small proportion of patients with bilateral disease, and the term 'trilateral retinoblastoma' has been coined to describe this condition[46].

Retinoblastoma has long been considered the classic example of a dominantly inherited neoplasm, but recent advances in cytogenetics and molecular biology have demonstrated that at the cellular level the retinoblastoma gene is recessive, and must achieve homozygosity or hemizygosity, resulting from deletion of the corresponding normal allele for tumour development to proceed. Tumour development may also occur as the result of total loss of the gene, i.e. deletion on both chromosomes. (These issues are discussed in detail in Chapter 2).

Wilms' tumour

The pattern of disease seen in retinoblastoma may be paralleled in Wilms' tumour. It is probable that Wilms' tumour occurs in both hereditary and non-hereditary forms, and that the hereditary form of tumour may be bilateral and/or multifocal, and shows an autosomal dominant pattern of inheritance. It has been estimated that the hereditary form of the disease may account for approximately 40% of all cases, but that the penetrance is about 63%, in contrast to retinoblastoma, where penetrance appears to be 80% or more[47,24]. Evidence for the hereditary nature of a proportion of Wilms' tumours rests mainly on observation of sibling pairs or cousin pairs, but apparent vertical transmission of Wilms' tumour has also occasionally been reported, for example, Brown *et al.* (1972)[48] and Kaufman *et al.* (1973)[49].

In contrast to retinoblastoma, Wilms' tumour had a relatively poor prognosis until fairly recent times, and this would account for the small number of families showing vertical transmission. With modern combination therapy, the majority of affected children survive. However, many of the current survivors received abdominal irradiation as part of their treatment

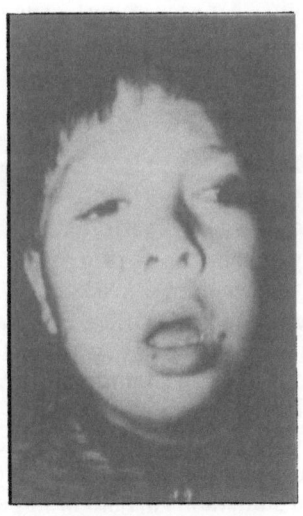

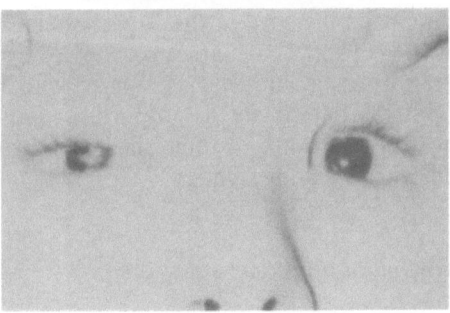

Figure 8.2 Patient with 11p⁻ syndrome: bilateral congenital aniridia, Wilms' tumour and mental retardation

and as a consequence are infertile. The present trend is away from the more aggressive treatment protocols, and the elimination of radiotherapy from the treatment of children with early stage disease and favourable histology has been recommended[50]. It is possible that in the future more examples of Wilms' tumour in successive generations will be seen. A further similarity with retinoblastoma has recently been demonstrated. It seems that although clinically a dominant pattern of inheritance is seen in Wilms' tumour, at the cellular level the Wilms' tumour gene may be recessive, and achievement of homozygosity or hemizygosity is associated with tumour development (see Chapter 2).

Wilms' tumour occurs with increased frequency in patients with certain congenital anomalies, notably aniridia, hemihypertrophy and Beckwith-Wiedemann syndrome[51]. The aniridia-Wilms' tumour syndrome is associated with a deletion on the short arm of chromosome 11, which includes the Wilms' tumour gene (Figure 8.2). Beckwith-Wiedemann syndrome is also associated with increased frequency of rhabdomyosarcoma, hepatoblastoma and adrenal cortical tumours. A recent report[52] suggests that these tumours may share a common pathogenetic pathway with Wilms' tumour, involving the same locus on chromosome 11.

Childhood cancer among siblings

Families in which more than one child is affected by cancer occur more often than would be expected by chance[53,54]. A proportion of childhood cancer is associated with known cancer-prone syndromes, for example neuro-fibromatosis, Gorlin's syndrome, and ataxia telangiectasia, but after elimination of those families with known genetic disease, Draper et al.[54] estimated that the risk to siblings of children with malignant disease of themselves developing a cancer is approximately 1 in 300, that is, double the normal risk of childhood cancer. Both Draper[54] and Miller[53] reported an excess of childhood central nervous system tumours among sibships, comparing with population statistics. This might in part be accounted for by under-diagnosis of cancer-prone syndromes, for example neurofibromatosis, and associations with other cancer family syndromes.

The series of sibling-pairs included in the Manchester Children's Tumour Registry shows an excess of soft tissue sarcomas: 29% of the tumours among the sibling-pairs were soft tissue sarcomas, compared with 5% in the registry as a whole. It is not possible to estimate the proportion of soft tissue sarcomas in other series, since these are not distinguished as a group in published reports of childhood cancers among siblings.

Second primaries in childhood cancer survivors

With improvements in the prognosis of many childhood cancers in recent years, it has become apparent that some survivors are at increased risk of developing second and subsequent neoplasms. This problem was first highlighted among survivors of retinoblastoma, when Kitchin and Elsworth (1974)[55] reported an excess of cancers among survivors which was confined almost exclusively to the hereditary form of the disease. Bone and soft tissue sarcomas were the most common malignancies among their series. Although many of the tumours developed within previous fields of radiotherapy, some were distant from treatment fields, and Kitchin and Elsworth proposed a pleiotropic effect of the retinoblastoma gene. Farwell and Flannery (1984)[56] reported an excess of second malignant neoplasms in survivors of childhood central nervous system tumours. There was also an excess of cancers among the parents and siblings of the patients with multiple tumours, and they concluded that the occurrence of multiple tumours in such children may be part of a familial cluster of cancers.

Meadows et al. (1985)[25], reporting a large multi-centre study of second malignant neoplasms in the survivors of childhood cancer, showed that the majority of the second and subsequent malignancies appeared to be associated with previous radiation therapy and a number developed in children with known predisposing conditions, notably retinoblastoma and neurofibromatosis. Tucker et al. (1986)[57], reporting for the same multi-centre study, have demonstrated that leukaemia occurring subsequent to a previous cancer in childhood can be almost entirely attributed to previous treatment with alkylating agents.

However, multiple primary neoplasms apparently unassociated with previous therapy or known cancer-prone syndromes also occur[25]. It is possible – perhaps even probable – that genetic factors play a role in the development of second malignant neoplasms in survivors of childhood cancer, and that perhaps these children are particularly susceptible to the carcinogenic effects of treatment of their primary neoplasms.

Familial cancer

The clustering of cancer in certain families is a well-known phenomenon and reports of such families date back at least to the 17th century[58]. More recently, studies of cancer among the relatives of affected probands have consistently shown a significant two to four-fold excess of cancer. This applies to many of the common cancer sites, for example breast, colon, uterus and lung[59]. To what extent this excess of cancer is due to shared environmental exposures within families, and how much can be attributed to genetic factors, has long been a matter of some controversy.

Familial cancer is generally considered under two headings: first, site or tumour-specific familial aggregations, exemplified by breast cancer, and, second, the clustering of dissimilar types of cancer within individual families, or 'cancer family syndromes'.

Site-specific familial breast cancer

Breast cancer is extremely common in the western developed countries, and represents the most common type of cancer in women[60]. Many families in which more than one member develops breast cancer would therefore be expected to occur by chance. In considering the possibility of inherited susceptibility, a number of questions have to be answered. Firstly, do the number of examples of 'familial' breast cancer exceed chance expectation? Secondly, can truly familial examples be distinguished from chance familial aggregations? And thirdly, is there a genetic basis for at least some of the familial clusters?

The first systematic large-scale study of familiality showed that the families of the breast cancer patients were, on average, at higher risk of developing the disease than the families of patients with other cancers, or patients with no history of cancer[61]. However, this and subsequent studies failed to demonstrate whether these average elevated risks applied uniformly to all families or were the result of a subset of families at exceptionally high risk. Some clarification of this situation and evidence for the involvement of genetic factors in at least some examples of familial breast cancer was provided by the work of Anderson[62-65]. By considering laterality of the breast cancer, whether the disease was diagnosed pre-menopausally or post-menopausally, and classifying the families of breast cancer patients according to which members were affected, Anderson was able to demonstrate considerable variation in relative risks to unaffected members of the families.

Thus, the highest risks of breast cancer were found in the sisters and daughters of patients whose mother also had breast cancer. Furthermore, if the disease was pre-menopausal in onset in the affected members of a family, and was bilateral in at least one case, then the lifetime probability of breast cancer developing in other close members was about 50%. An example of this type of pedigree is shown in Figure 8.3.

Anderson has proposed that breast cancer may be classified into two main types: that with post-menopausal onset, in which extrinsic or environmental

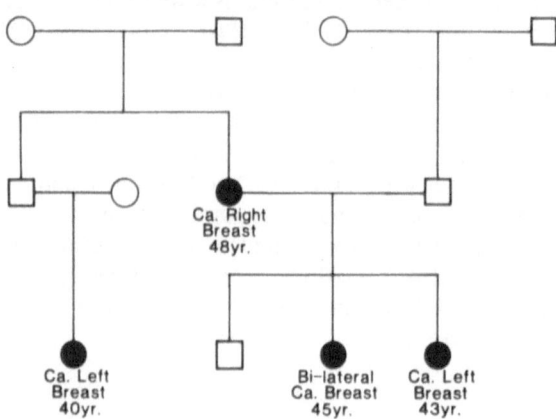

Figure 8.3 Familial pre-menopausal breast cancer

factors are of prime importance in aetiology; and pre-menopausal disease, in which genetic factors are important, the genetic subset being characterised by a relatively high frequency of bilaterality. These findings and conclusions have gained wide acceptance.

However, recent reports on other large series have cast some doubt on Anderson's original findings. In a case-control study of familial breast cancer, Adami et al. (1981)[66] found an overall excess of breast cancer in first degree relatives of patients compared with that in unaffected controls. However, no association of familial disease with bilaterality or early onset could be demonstrated. Ottman et al. (1983)[67], in a population-based series, found the greatest risk of breast cancer among the relatives of probands with bilateral disease diagnosed below the age of 41 years but, among the relatives of patients with unilateral disease, age at onset in the probands was not important in determining breast cancer risk.

Applying the methods for risk estimation described by Ottman et al. (1983) to the sisters of patients from three pedigree groups previously defined by him in the work referred to above, Anderson (1985)[68] found that the type of pedigree and laterality of disease in the proband were important in determining breast cancer risk among the sisters of probands, but that age at diagnosis in the proband was of no importance. Thus the highest lifetime risks to their sisters were found among patients with bilateral disease who also had an affected mother or sister, and lowest risks were found among the sisters of probands with unilateral disease and an affected second-degree relative.

Inconsistencies in the results of these various studies on familial breast cancer may be due to differences in study design, for example means of ascertaining the cases (hospital-based or population-based series), methods used in obtaining family histories (personal interview or postal questionnaire), and the extent to which these familial data are verified by reference to medical records and by special histological review.

Empirical risk estimates currently available in the literature must be viewed with caution and regarded as approximations only (see p. 183).

Cancer family syndromes

The great majority of studies of the risk of breast cancer in relatives of patients with the disease and of discussions on the role of genetic factors in breast cancer aetiology have centred on site specific familial breast cancer. During the past 15 years data have accumulated from the detailed study of selected cancer patients with respect to all types of cancer within individual pedigrees. It has become clear that cancers of specific types cluster within certain families in a pattern consistent with dominant inheritance. Various combinations of cancers are seen within families, representing different cancer family syndromes. Patterns of disease seen in these cancer-prone families are summarised by Fraumeni (1977)[69]. Breast cancer is consistently involved in many familial tumour aggregations, and Lynch has defined several breast cancer-prone genotypes. These include breast cancer in association with: cancer of the gastrointestinal tract; ovarian carcinoma;

malignant melanoma; and sarcomas in the children and other young relatives of the breast cancer proband. Other cancers are found within these families in addition to the principal tumour associations. These include neoplasms of prostate, lung, endometrium, skin, brain, cervix and reticuloendothelial system. The features of such cancer families are described in detail by Lynch (1981)[70].

Perhaps the most interesting of these cancer family syndromes is that characterized by early onset breast cancer and sarcomas, where the tumour spectrum seen also includes brain tumours, leukaemia, carcinomas of the larynx and lung, and adrenal cortical tumours, designated the SBLA syndrome by Lynch[70], and also known as the Li-Fraumeni syndrome. The interest in this particular syndrome lies in the different histogenesis of the tumours involved.

A family of this type was first reported by Bottomley and Condit (1968)[71] and subsequently Li and Fraumeni described four other families showing the association of breast cancer with sarcomas, and proposed that this may represent a cancer family syndrome[72,73]. An example of this type of family is shown in Figure 8.4.

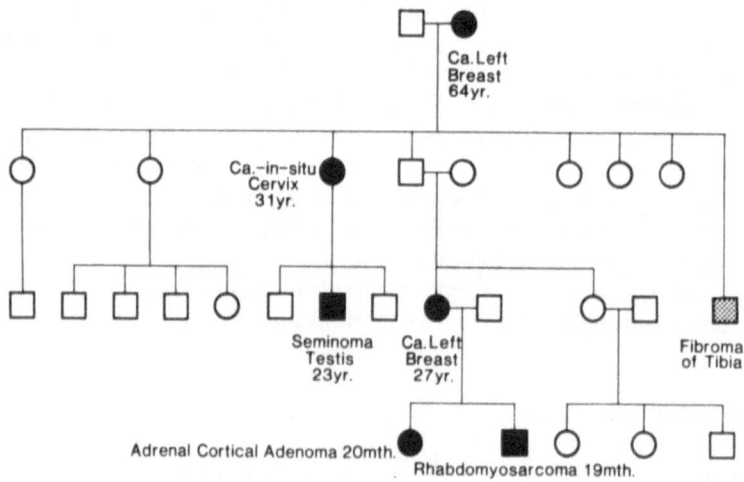

Figure 8.4 An example of the SBLA (Li-Fraumeni) syndrome showing pre-menopausal breast cancer, rhabdomyosarcoma and adrenal cortical tumour in a mother and two children

The apparent rarity of Li-Fraumeni type families suggested by the literature probably leads to an under-estimate of the proportion of childhood sarcomas in which familial associations of this nature can be found. The majority of reported families have been ascertained because of the close proximity in time of diagnosis of sarcoma in the child and of breast cancer in the mother, or because of the identification of pairs of childhood sarcomas in siblings or cousins. Childhood soft tissue sarcomas had a very poor prognosis until relatively recently. Once a child has died, contact between the family and clinicians is usually lost.

A recent study traced the mothers of all children with soft tissue sarcomas included in the Manchester Children's Tumour Registry. A significant excess of breast cancer was found among these mothers. The breast cancers found were pre-menopausal in onset, and two mothers had histologically proven bilateral disease. Furthermore, the risk of breast cancer was not evenly distributed, and a group of mothers at particularly high risk could be defined, depending on the clinical characteristics of their child's sarcoma[74].

A genetic basis in familial cancer

Specific types of cancer do appear to cluster in excess of expectation in some families. Although cancer is very common, especially in western developed countries, it has been stated that allowing for family size, only 1.5–6% of individuals will have in excess of two relatives with cancer[75]. Evidence that these familial clusters have a genetic basis includes: occurrence of cancers in multiple generations (Figure 8.5), where it seems unlikely that successive generations will have been exposed to exactly the same dietary and environmental influences; the occurrence of tumours in extended pedigrees within the same generation, where different sibships living distant from each other are involved (for example, the breast cancer family shown in Figure 8.3); the onset of cancer at an unusually early age, which is characteristic of these families; and the occurrence of multiple tumours within an individual, which may also be seen as distinct primaries in separate individuals within a

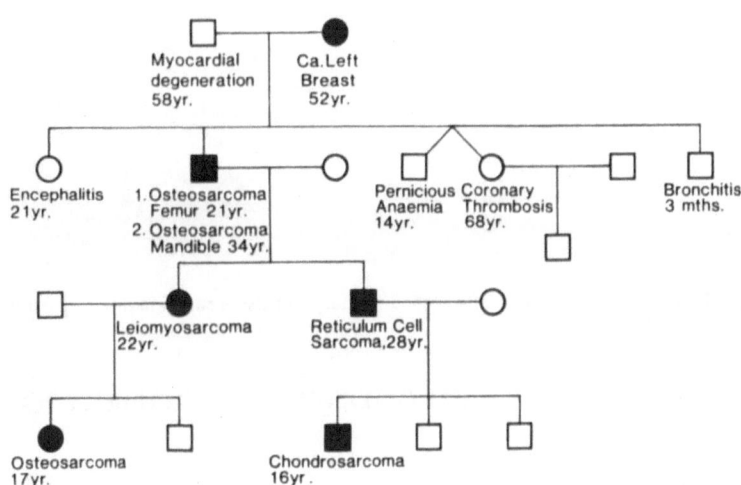

Figure 8.5 Familial bone and soft tissue sarcoma

family. An example of the latter is the association of carcinomas of the breast and ovary as multiple primaries within an individual[76], and breast and ovarian cancer clustering within families. Multiple primaries of similar types may also occur in familial cancer, for example, in paired organs (breast, ovary) or in the same type of tissue at distant sites in the body. An example of this is shown in Figure 8.5, where a double primary osteosarcoma is seen in a family showing bone and soft tissue sarcomas, breast cancer and reticulum cell sarcoma.

Evidence supporting genetic factors in familial cancer may also be found from the study of the general epidemiology of cancers involved in familial clusters, for example the huge world-wide variations in incidence seen in most adult cancers are not found among childhood cancers[77,78], suggesting that environmental influences are relatively unimportant in the aetiology of cancer in children. In breast cancer, although large differences in overall incidence are seen between countries, for example, Western Europe and the white population of the USA, compared with Japan, variation in the incidence of pre-menopausal breast cancer is considerably less marked[79].

The variety of cancers seen within these families has been used as an argument against a genetic aetiology. However, it is clear from the study of retinoblastoma, which is unequivocally accepted as a genetically determined disease, that tumours of quite different histological types can occur, i.e. the development of bone and soft tissue sarcomas in retinoblastoma survivors (Figure 8.6.), and the occurrence of sarcomas in members of retinoblastoma families who are themselves unaffected by retinoblastoma, e.g. Gordon (1974)[80].

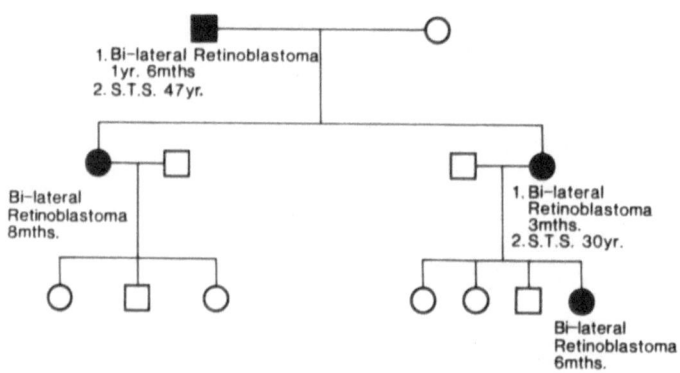

Figure 8.6 Familial retinoblastoma with second primary soft tissue sarcoma in two generations

IMPLICATIONS OF GENETICALLY DETERMINED SUSCEPTIBILITY TO CANCER

Observations on the incidence of cancers among patients with the autosomal dominant and autosomal recessive syndromes described above clearly demonstrate that predisposition to cancer can be inherited. Although less clear, the evidence for a genetic aetiology in the cancer family syndromes is mounting, and recent work in certain childhood tumours at the cellular and molecular level supports earlier clinical and epidemiological studies. The proportion of cancers which can be unequivocally attributed to genetic disease, given the present state of knowledge, is small. Nevertheless, at the cellular level it is self-evident that cancer is heritable, since a cancer cell will give rise to other cancer cells, and it is probable that heritable factors play an aetiological role in most if not all cancers at the level of the whole organism, including man.

The extent of the genetic contribution to the aetiology of human cancers

The genetic contribution to the aetiology of human cancers is likely to vary considerably between different types of malignant disease and individual patients. Knudson (1985) has defined four 'oncodemes' in which expectations of cancer differ, depending on hereditary and environmental variables[81]. The first 'oncodeme' would be represented by a group of the population among whom spontaneous mutations produce a 'background' level of cancer. A population group exposed to agents which can produce changes in the host genome, such that this 'background' incidence is increased, forms the second oncodeme. Individuals having inherited abnormalities favouring either spontaneous or induced mutations which result in an increased risk of cancer form the third, and those individuals in whom there is inheritance of an initiating mutation which is part of the multi-step sequence leading to cancer represent the fourth.

Knudson hypothesizes that the first group may represent the 20 per cent of the world's cancer which would remain after elimination of the estimated 80 per cent environmentally induced cancer. In the second group, industrial or other environmental chemicals, radiation or viruses could act as mutagenic agents. The third group would include conditions such as ataxia telangiectasia, and xeroderma pigmentosum, and the 'hereditary cancers,' for example retinoblastoma, would form the fourth group.

In the second and third groups the probability that one or more of the steps in the pathway to tumour development will occur is increased, but the number of steps remains the same, whereas in the fourth group the number is reduced by one, and this group may be at very high risk of cancer if the number of steps involved in the development of any particular cancer is small.

The notion that 80 per cent of the world's cancer is 'environmentally induced' would perhaps lead to the supposition that the majority of these would fall in the second group. However, under-diagnosis of such conditions as neurofibromatosis, the finding that heterozygosity for ataxia telangiectasia (and perhaps other cancer-prone conditions) may increase cancer risk, and the possibility that there are genetically determined variations in the ability of individuals to activate or inactivate mutagens (see p. 184) may considerably increase the proportion of cancers suspected to fall into the third group. Examples of genetically determined variation in susceptibility to environmental carcinogens include the sensitivity of xeroderma pigmentosum patients to ultraviolet light resulting from the defective DNA repair mechanism in their cells, and the comparative sensitivity of the white races to the induction of skin cancers by ultraviolet light. The absorption of ultraviolet light by melanin granules present as a perinuclear cap in the skin cells of the black races protects the nucleus from damage[82]. Thus, although skin cancers could be cited as examples of environmentally induced cancers, it can be seen that induction is also to some extent under genetic control. Furthermore, the fourth group, exemplified by retinoblastoma, may also be considerably larger than is at present suspected.

It has been demonstrated that the relative risk for retinoblastoma gene carriers of acquiring a tumour is about 100000[45], and most carriers develop carriers of genes predisposing to cancer, compared with that in non-carriers, is 1000-fold or more, a clear pattern of inherited susceptibility is likely to emerge. However, it cannot be assumed that genetic factors are unimportant where no definite familial pattern is seen.

Peto (1980)[83] has demonstrated theoretically that in individuals where genetic predisposition increases the incidence of a particular cancer by a factor of 10 to 100 times compared with non-predisposed individuals, such a genetic effect would be difficult to detect by familial clustering, but could nevertheless contribute substantially to the total incidence of that cancer in the population. A two- to four-fold increased risk of cancer in relatives of patients with many of the common cancers has been found, which would perhaps not be suggestive of a strong genetic effect. In this type of study, however, 'relative risk' implies the observed risk in relatives of *all* cancer patients (whether genetically predisposed or not), compared with the risk in the general population, rather than the risk among individuals known to be predisposed to cancer compared with that among non-predisposed individuals. Peto argues that the cancer risk in predisposed versus non-predisposed individuals will usually be more than an order of magnitude higher than that for relatives of cancer patients versus the general population for the following three reasons: first, not all cancer patients are predisposed; second, fewer of their relatives will be predisposed; and third, the general population comprises both predisposed individuals and non-predisposed.

By assuming that predisposition to cancer is determined by a single gene which increases the age-specific incidence of the disease by a constant factor, and applying a Mendelian dominant or recessive model of inheritance, Peto demonstrates that it is necessary for the gene to increase the incidence of the cancer at least ten-fold for the dominant, or 20-fold for the recessive model, to produce a relative risk of 2 for the cancer in siblings of patients. Peto gives several more theoretical examples of relative risks in twins, other siblings and children of cancer patients, assuming various gene frequencies and increases in incidence for both dominant and recessive models. In most situations the relative risk is less than 5. Simple Mendelian inheritance of a single gene was assumed in order to derive these estimates, but in practice inheritance of susceptibility to many cancers may be controlled by polygenic mechanisms which may also involve interaction with environmental factors for their expression.

It might appear, therefore, that unless the increase in risk imposed by such genes is so high that most carriers develop the disease, the study of families of individual cancer patients would contribute little to the understanding of underlying mechanisms of inherited susceptibility to cancer. However, such studies are important in the establishment of empirical risks, and the identification of high risk groups in the absence of genetic markers, for the purposes of genetic counselling and identifying sub-groups worthy of study in the laboratory.

Genetic counselling

Where the diagnosis of a heritable cancer or cancer-prone condition, for example retinoblastoma or polyposis coli, is made, genetic counselling and/or screening should be offered as appropriate, ideally at a centre specializing in the care of patients with that disease.

In both retinoblastoma and polyposis coli a clear pattern of inheritance is apparent, and there are very definite benefits to the patient from early diagnosis and appropriate treatment. For many cancers in which there is evidence of genetic susceptibility, however, patterns of inheritance may be less clear. The identification of families, and individuals within those families, who are at high risk is far from easy. Furthermore, an appropriate screening programme may not be available. In the case of cancer family syndromes, although it may be possible to identify an individual at high risk of cancer, the increased risk may apply to any of several types of malignancy. For example, a member of a family with the SBLA syndrome might be at high risk for sarcomas – which could occur virtually anywhere in the body – pre-menopausal breast cancer and brain tumours, as well as several other cancers, and an effective screening programme for such a person is difficult to envisage.

The issue of genetic counselling and what sort of advice should be given to patients who are anxious about their relatives presents many difficulties. A number of situations may occur in clinical practice: a patient with a strong family history of cancer, compatible with a cancer family syndrome, may request advice; a patient without a family history but who is worried about heritability of the disease may express anxiety about risks to relatives; a mother of a child with cancer may be deeply concerned about her other children or future children; and finally a patient may have a disease with the characteristics of heritable cancer, e.g. bilateral premenopausal breast cancer in a woman whose mother also had breast cancer, but be unaware that her sisters and daughters may be at risk.

At present there are few reliable data on risk estimates, and such data as do exist generally apply to site-specific familial cancers. Perhaps the most extensive data are available for breast cancer and, although a number of reports attempt to stratify risk to relatives in terms of clinical characteristics in the proband, there is no absolute agreement between the various reports. The available estimates of risk to siblings of patients with paediatric cancer do not adequately take into account the detailed morphology and other clinical characteristics of the various tumours. It is likely that there is considerable variation in risk to siblings, depending on such variables in the proband.

Furthermore, existing estimates do not take cancers in adult members of the families into account and these may also influence risk to siblings[84].

Until more extensive and reliable data have been published, present estimates of risks to relatives of cancer probands should be interpreted with caution. If counselling is contemplated the following points should be taken into account before advice is offered: the level of anxiety in the patient and relatives; the possible benefits or otherwise likely to be derived from available screening programmes; the benefits and acceptability of prophylactic surgery in a patient at risk if this is an option; whether adequate psychosocial support will be available to a family at risk, and the accuracy with which a particular syndrome can be diagnosed.

Approaches to the identification of individuals at high risk in the general population

Differences in cancer susceptibility may result from variation among individuals with respect to their ability to metabolise or activate carcinogens. Such polymorphisms would only be manifest among populations exposed to the appropriate carcinogen. An example of this type of mechanism has been reported in relation to susceptibility to lung cancer among cigarette smokers[85]. The frequency of metabolic oxidation phenotypes among patients with histologically verified bronchial carcinoma was compared with that among control patients matched for smoking history, age, ethnic origin and sex. Among the cancer patients there was a high proportion (approximately 79%) of individuals conforming to a homozygous dominant 'extensive metabolizer' phenotype with respect to debrisoquine 4-hydroxylation compared with a low proportion (approximately 29%) among non-cancer control patients. Furthermore only four out of 245 cancer patients conformed to the recessive 'poor metabolizer' phenotype. The authors conclude that among cigarette smokers homozygous dominants for debrisoquine 4-hydroxylation appear to be at high risk for lung cancer.

It is probable that comparable situations exist for a variety of other environmental agents. If such markers could be identified for specific agents, especially industrial carcinogens, the question of screening exposed populations, e.g. a workforce, so that susceptible individuals could be protected or advised to seek alternative employment, is raised. These issues could have far-reaching implications with respect to industrial legislation and payments of compensation for industrial diseases. The institution of screening programmes to identify susceptible and non-susceptible individuals may also lead to the erroneous assumption that certain individuals are 'safe' from the effects of a particular carcinogen, or that it is 'safe' for some people to smoke.

APPROACHES TO CLINICAL AND EPIDEMIOLOGICAL STUDIES OF THE HERITABILITY OF CANCER

Available data on patterns of familial cancer have largely been derived from two main sources, firstly the study of large cancer pedigrees which have been randomly ascertained or ascertained because a particular association has been sought, and secondly the systematic study of patient populations with respect to frequency of familial occurrences of particular cancers.

The former approach has led to the identification of cancer family syndromes, but fails to give any indication of the proportion of total cancers which might be largely genetically determined. Although risks to individuals within identified pedigrees might be estimated, risks to relatives of patients in the general population with particular cancers cannot, using this approach.

The latter approach has generally been applied to site-specific cancers and although estimates of risk to relatives of patients have been made, there have often been inconsistencies between the results of various studies. These inconsistencies may have been the result of selection bias in the populations under study. Most studies using this approach do not take all cancers in the families into account but concentrate on cancers at particular sites.

Published work utilising both approaches has in general failed adequately to take into account clinical and histopathological features in the probands and their relatives when stratifying the study populations in terms of risk and in defining the populations to be studied.

In order to estimate the magnitude of the genetic component in the aetiology of any particular cancer the population under study should be carefully defined in terms of clinical characteristics and morphological criteria of the cancers concerned, and the patient population should be, as far as possible, unselected and preferably derived from a geographically defined population. Special histological review of cancers in the probands and their relatives would ensure consistency in their classification. Patients and, if possible, their close relatives should be examined, by a clinician participating in the study, for features of known cancer-prone conditions and any other features of interest, e.g. congenital anomalies. Details of relevant environmental exposures and previous medical history should be recorded. All these data would contribute to a more accurate definition of heritable cancer and more reliable estimates of risk to individual members of families.

Studies of this kind are of importance in counselling families at high risk and in reassuring those individuals who may be at no greater risk than the population in general. However, no individual can be identified with certainty as being at high risk in the absence of a biological marker. Such markers may be clinical – for example, a characteristic congenital anomaly – or may be at the cellular or molecular level, e.g. chromosomal deletions. While it would seem reasonable to concentrate on large cancer pedigrees, in which there are multiple affected members over at least three generations, in the search for biological markers, such families are extremely rare. Furthermore, when such a family is identified, the majority of affected members may be dead or unavailable for study for other reasons.

The systematic study of patient populations as outlined above would enable 'high risk' families, worthy of study in the laboratory, to be identified at the time of diagnosis of the proband, regardless of the number of relatives affected at that time. Such families could be followed up on a regular basis to test the predictive value of clinical, cytological and molecular characteristics thought to be indicative of a high cancer risk.

In conclusion, the clinical and epidemiological study of the heritability of cancer is important not only from the medical point of view, but also in contributing to the scientific understanding of the fundamental basis of cancer genetics.

Acknowledgement

The Manchester Children's Tumour Registry and associated epidemiological research is supported by the Cancer Research Campaign.

References

1. Broca, P. (1866). Traite des tumours. *Des Tumeurs en General.* Vol. I. (Paris: Anselin, Becket et Labe)
2. de Gouvea, H. (1896). *Bull. Soc. Med. Chir.*, **8**, 25
3. Sedgwick, R. P. and Boder, E. S. (1972). Ataxia-telangiectasia. In Vinken, P. J. and Breyer, G. W. (eds.) *Handbook of Clinical Neurology.* pp. 317-318. (Amsterdam: North Holland)
4. Hecht, F. and Kaiser-McCaw, B. (1982). Ataxia-telangiectasia: genetics and heterogeneity. In Bridges, B. A. and Harnden, D. G. (eds.) *Ataxia-telangiectasia. A Cellular and Molecular Link between Cancer, Neuropathology, and Immune Deficiency.* pp. 197-201. (Chichester: John Wiley & Sons)
5. Filipovich, A. H., Spector, B. D. and Kersey, J. H. (1980). Immunodeficiency in humans as a risk factor in the development of malignancy. *Prev. Med.*, **9**, 252-259
6. Spector, B. D., Filipovich, A. H., Perry, G. S. III and Kersey, J. H. (1982). Epidemiology of cancer in ataxia-telangiectasia. In Bridges, B. A. and Harnden, D. G. (eds.) *Ataxia-Telangiectasia. A Cellular and Molecular Link between Cancer, Neuropathology, and Immune Deficiency.* pp. 103-138. (Chichester: John Wiley & Sons)
7. Cunliffe, P. N., Mann, J. R., Cameron, A. H., Roberts, K. D. and Ward, H. W. C. (1975). Radiosensitivity in ataxia-telangiectasia. *Br. J. Radiol.*, **48**, 374-376
8. Taylor, A. M. R., Metcalfe, J., Oxford, J. M. and Harnden, D. G. (1976). Is chromatid-type damage in ataxia-telangiectasia after irradiation at G_0 a consequence of defective repair. *Nature*, **260**, 441-443
9. Bridges, B. A. and Harnden, D. G. (eds.) (1982). *Ataxia-telangiectasia. A Cellular and Molecular Link between Cancer, Neuropathology, and Immune Deficiency.* (Chichester: John Wiley & Sons)
10. German, J., Bloom, D. and Passarge, E. (1979). Bloom's syndrome. VII. Progress report for 1978. *Clin. Genet.*, **15**, 361-367
11. Schroeder, T. M., Tilgen, D., Kruger, J. and Vogel, F. (1976). Formal genetics of Fanconi's anaemia. *Hum. Genet.*, **32**, 257-288
12. Schroeder, T. M., Pohler, E. and Hufnagl, H. D. (1979). Fanconi's anaemia: terminal leukaemia and *"forme fruste"* in one family. *Clin. Genet.*, **16**, 260-268
13. Swift, M. (1982). Single gene syndromes. In Schottenfeld, D and Fraumeni, J. F. Jr. (eds.) *Cancer Epidemiology and Prevention.* Ch. 25, pp. 475-482. (Philadelphia: W. B. Saunders Co.)
14. Kraemer, K. H. (1980). Xeroderma pigmentosum. In Demis, D. J., Robson, R. L. and McGuire, M. (eds.) *Clinical Dermatology.* pp. 1-33. (New York: Harper & Row)
15. Swift, M. (1971). Fanconi's anaemia in the genetics of neoplasia. *Nature*, **230**, 370-373
16. Swift, M., Caldwell, R. J. and Chase, C. (1980). Reassessment of cancer predisposition of Fanconi anaemia heterozygotes. *J. Natl. Cancer Inst.*, **65**, 863-867
17. Swift, M. and Chase, C. (1979). Cancer in xeroderma pigmentosum families. *J. Natl. Cancer Inst.*, **62**, 1415-1421
18. Swift, M., Sholman, L., Perry, M. and Chase, C. (1975). Malignant neoplasms in the families of patients with ataxia-telangiectasia. *Cancer Res.*, **36**, 209-215

19. Swift, M. (1982). Disease predisposition of ataxia-telangiectasia heterozygotes. In Bridges, B. A. and Harnden, D. G. (eds.) *Ataxia-telangiectasia. A Cellular and Molecular Link between Cancer, Neuropathology, and Immune Deficiency*. pp. 355-361. (Chichester: John Wiley & Sons)

20. Gorlin, R. J. and Goltz, R. W. (1960). Multiple naevoid basal cell epithelioma, jaw cysts and bifid ribs: a syndrome. *N. Engl. J. Med.*, **262**, 908-912

21. Straith, F. E. (1939). Hereditary epidermoid cyst of the jaws. *Am. J. Orthodont. Oral Surg.*, **25**, 673-691

22. Satinoff, M. I. and Wells, C. (1969). Multiple basal cell naevus syndrome in ancient Egypt. *Med. Hist.*, **13**, 294-297

23. Knudson, A. G. Jr., Strong, L. C. and Anderson, D. E. (1973). Heredity and cancer in man. *Prog. Med. Genet.*, **9**, 113-157

24. Strong, L. C. (1977). Genetic considerations in pediatric oncology. In Sutow, W. W., Vietti, T. J. and Fernbach, D. J. (eds.) *Clinical Pediatric Oncology*. 2nd Edn., Ch. 2, pp. 16-32. (St Louis: The C.V. Mosby Co.)

25. Meadows, A. T., Baum, E., Fassati-Bellani, F., Green, D., Jenkin, R. D. T., Marsden, B., Nesbit, M., Newton, W., Oberlin, O., Sallan, S. G., Siegel, S., Strong, L. C., and Voute, P. A. (1985). Second malignant neoplasms in children: an update from the Late Effects Study Group. *J. Clin. Oncol.*, **3**, 532-538

26. Bussey, H. J. R. (1975). *Familial Polyposis Coli*. (Baltimore and London: The Johns Hopkins University Press)

27. Schimke, R. N. (1977). Tumors of the neural crest system. In Mulvihill, J. J., Miller, R. W. and Fraumeni, J. F. Jr. (eds.) *Genetics of Human Cancer*. Ch. 14, pp. 179-198. (New York: Raven Press)

28. Ponder, B. A. J. (1984). Role of genetic and familial factors. In Stoll, B. A. (ed.) *Risk Factors and Multiple Cancer. New Horizons in Oncology*. Vol. 3. (Chichester: John Wiley & Sons)

29. Hope, D. G. and Mulvihill, J. F. (1981). Malignancy in neurofibromatosis. *Adv. Neurol.*, **29**, 33-56

30. Rosai, J. (1981). *Ackerman's Surgical Pathology*. Vol. Two, Ch. 24. 6th Edn. (St. Louis: The C. V. Mosby Co.)

31. Eldridge, R. (1981). Central neurofibromatosis with bilateral acoustic neuroma. *Adv. Neurol.*, **29**, 57-65

32. Moots, P. L. and Rubinstein, L. J. (1984). Multiple neoplasms of the nervous system. In Stoll, B. A. (ed.) *New Horizons in Oncology*. Vol. 3. (Chichester: John Wiley & Sons)

33. Mulvihill, J. J. (1977). Genetic repertory of human neoplasia. In Mulvihill, J. J., Miller, R. W. and Fraumeni, J. F. Jr. (eds.) *Genetics of Human Cancer*. Ch. 11, pp. 137-143. (New York: Raven Press)

34. Bader, J. L. and Miller, R. W. (1978). Neurofibromatosis and childhood leukemia. *J. Pediatr.*, **92**, 925-929

35. Stay, E. J. and Vawter, G. (1977). The relationship between nephroblastoma and neurofibromatosis (von Recklinghausen's disease). *Cancer*, **39**, 2550-2555

36. McKeen, E. A., Bodurtha, J, Meadows, A. T., Douglass, E. C. and Mulvihill, J. J. (1978). Rhabdomyosarcoma complicating multiple neurofibromatosis. *J. Pediatr.*, **93**, 922-993

37. Brooks, J. S. J., Freeman, M. and Enterline, H. T. (1985). Malignant "Triton" tumors. Natural history and immunohistochemistry of nine new cases with literature review. *Cancer*, **55**, 2543-2549

38. Elsworth, R. M. (1969). The practical management of retinoblastoma. *Trans. Am. Ophthalmol. Soc.*, **67**, 462-534

39. Falls, H. F. and Neel, J. V. (1951). Genetics of retinoblastoma. *Arch. Opthalmol.*, **46**, 367-389

40. Devesa, S. S. (1975). The incidence of retinoblastoma. *Am. J. Opthalmol.*, **80**, 263-265

41. de Gouvea, H. (1910). L'hérédité des gliomes de la rétine *Ann. Ocul.*, **CXLIII**, 32-35

42. Sorsby, A. (1972). Bilateral retinoblastoma: A dominantly inherited affection. *Br. Med. J.*, **2**, 580-583

43. Smith, J. L. S. and Bedford, M. A. (1976). Retinoblastomas. In Marsden, H. B. and Steward, J. K. (eds.) *Tumours in Children*. 2nd Edn. *Recent Results in Cancer Research*. Vol. 13, pp. 245-281 (Berlin: Springer-Verlag)

44. Knudson, A. G. Jr. (1971). Mutation and cancer: Statistical study of retinoblastoma. *Proc. Natl. Acad. Sci. USA.*, **68**, 820–823

45. Knudson, A. G. Jr. (1978). Retinoblastoma: a prototypic hereditary neoplasm. *Semin. Oncol.*, **5**, 57–60

46. Kingston, J., Plowman, P. N. and Hungerford, J. R. (1985). Ectopic intracranial retinoblastoma in childhood. *Br. J. Ophthalmol.*, **69**, 742–749

47. Knudson, A. G. Jr. and Strong, L. C. (1972). Mutation and cancer: A model for Wilms' tumor of the kidney. *J. Natl. Cancer Inst.*, **48**, 313–324

48. Brown, T., Puranik, R., Altman, H. and Hardin, H. C. (1972). Wilms' tumor in three successive generations. *Surgery*, **72**, 756–761

49. Kaufman, R. L., Vietti, T. J. and Wabner, C. I. (1973). Wilms' tumour in father and son. *Lancet*, **i**, 43

50. Green, D. (1985). The Diagnosis and management of Wilms' tumour. In A. J. Altman (Guest Ed.) *The Pediatrics Clinics of North America*. Vol. 32, No. 3, June 1985. pp. 735–754. *Symposium on Pediatric Oncology*. (Philadelphia: W. B. Saunders Co.)

51. Breslow, N. E. and Beckwith, J. B. (1982). Epidemiological features of Wilms' tumour. Results of the National Wilms' Tumor Study. *J. Natl. Cancer Inst.*, **68**, 429–436

52. Koufos, A., Hansen, M. F., Copeland, N. G., Jenkins, N. A., Lampkin, B. C. and Cavenee, W. K. (1985). Loss of heterozygosity in three embryonal tumours suggests a common pathogenetic mechanism. *Nature*, **316**, 330–334

53. Miller, R. W. (1971). Deaths from childhood leukaemia and solid tumors among twins and other sibs in the United States 1960-67. *J. Natl. Cancer Inst.*, **46**, 203–209

54. Draper, G. J., Heaf, M. M. and Wilson, L. M. K. (1977). Occurrence of childhood cancers among sibs. and estimation of familial risks. *J. Med. Genet.*, **14**, 81–90

55. Kitchin, F. D. and Ellsworth, R. M. (1974). Pleiotropic effects of the gene for retinoblastoma. *J. Med. Genet.*, **11**, 244–246

56. Farwell, J. and Flannery, J. T. (1984). Second primaries in children with central nervous sytem tumors. *J. Neuro-Oncol.*, **2**, 371–375

57. Tucker, M. A., Meadows, A. T., Boice, J. D., Stovall, M., Oberlin, O., Stone, B. J., Birch, J., Voute, P. A., Hoover, R. N., and Fraumeni, J. F. Jr. (1986). Leukaemia after therapy with alkylating agents for childhood cancer. Submitted for publication

58. Lynch, H. T. (1967). In Lynch, H. T. (ed.) *Hereditary Factors in Carcinoma. Recent Results in Cancer Research.* Vol. 12, pp. 1–184. (New York: Springer)

59. Anderson, D. E. (1975). Familial susceptibility. In Fraumeni, J. F. Jr. (ed.) *Persons at High Risk of Cancer. An Approach to Cancer Etiology and Control.* Ch. 2, pp. 39–54. (New York: Academic Press)

60. Waterhouse, J., Muir, C., Shanmugaratnam, K. and Powell, J. (eds.) (1982). *Cancer Incidence in Five Continents.* Vol. IV. IARC Scientific Publications No. 42. World Health Organisation. (Lyon: International Agency for Research on Cancer)

61. Macklin, M. T. (1959). Comparison of the number of breast cancer deaths observed in relatives of breast cancer patients, and the number expected on the basis of mortality rates. *J. Natl. Cancer Inst.*, **22**, 927–951

62. Anderson, D. E. (1972). A genetic study of human breast cancer. *J. Natl. Cancer Inst.*, **48**, 1029–1034

63. Anderson, D. E. (1974). Genetic study of breast cancer. Identification of a high risk group. *Cancer*, **34**, 1090–1097

64. Anderson, D. E. (1977) Genetic predisposition to breast cancer. In Arneault, G. and Israel I. L. (eds.) *Breast Cancer: A Multidisciplinary Approach.* p. 10. (Berlin: Springer-Verlag)

65. Anderson, D. E. (1977). Breast cancer in families. *Cancer*, **40**, 1855–1860

66. Adami, H.-O., Hansen, J., Jung, B and Rimsten, A. (1981). Characteristics of familial breast cancer in Sweden. Absence of relation to age and unilateral versus bilateral disease. *Cancer*, **48**, 1688–1695

67. Ottman, R, Pike, M. C., King, M.-C., and Henderson, B. E. (1983). Practical guide for estimating risk for familial breast cancer. *Lancet*, **ii**, 556–558

68. Anderson, D. E., and Badzioch, M. D. (1985). Risk of familial breast cancer. *Cancer*, **56**, 383–387

69. Fraumeni, J. F. Jr. (1977). Clinical patterns of familial cancer. In Mulvihill, J. J., Miller, R. W. and Fraumeni, J. F. Jr. (eds.) *Genetics of Human Cancer.* Ch. 19, pp. 223–233. (New York: Raven Press)

70. Lynch, H. T. (1981). Genetic heterogeneity and breast cancer: variable tumor spectra. In Lynch, H. T. (ed.) *Genetics and Breast Cancer.* Ch. 6, pp. 134-170. (New York: van Nostrand Reinhold Co.)

71. Bottomley, R. D. and Condit, P. T. (1968). Cancer families. *Cancer Bull.*, **20**, 22-24

72. Li, F. P. and Fraumeni, J. F. Jr. (1969). Soft-tissue sarcomas, breast cancer and other neoplasms. A familial syndrome? *Ann. Intern. Med.*, **71**, 747-752

73. Li, F. P. and Fraumeni, J. F. Jr. (1982). Prospective study of a family cancer syndrome *J. Am. Med. Assoc.*, **247**, 2692-2694

74. Birch, J. M., Hartley, A. L., Marsden, H. B., Harris, M. and Swindell, R. (1984). Excess risk of breast cancer in the mothers of children with soft tissue sarcomas. *Br. J. Cancer*, **49**, 325-331

75. Mulvihill, J. (1984). Clinical ecogenetics of human cancer. In Bishop, J. M., Rowley, J. D. and Greaves, M. (eds.) *Genes and Cancer.* pp. 19-36. UCLA Symposia on Molecular and Cellular Biology, New Series, Vol. 17. (New York: Alan R. Liss)

76. Prior, P. and Waterhouse, J. A. H. (1981). Multiple primary cancers of the breast and ovary. *Br. J. Cancer*, **44**, 628-636

77. Birch, J. M. (1983). Epidemiology of paediatric cancer. In Duncan, W. (ed.) *Paediatric Oncology. Recent Results in Cancer Research.* Vol. 88, pp. 1-10. (Berlin: Springer-Verlag)

78. Breslow, N. E. and Langholz, B. (1983). Childhood cancer incidence: geographical and temporal variations. *Int. J. Cancer*, **32**, 703-716

79. Hirayama, T., Waterhouse, J. A. H., and Fraumeni, J. F. Jr. (1980). *Cancer Risks by Site.* UICC Technical Report Series, Vol. 41. (Geneva: UICC)

80. Gordon, H. (1974). Family studies in retinoblastoma. *Birth Defects*, Vol. X, No. 10, pp. 185-190

81. Knudson, A. G. Jr. (1985). Hereditary cancer, oncogenes and antioncogenes. *Cancer Res.*, **45**, 1437 1443

82. Harnden, D. G. (1984). The Nature of inherited susceptibility to cancer. *Carcinogenesis*, **5**, 1535-1537

83. Peto, J. (1980). Genetic predisposition to cancer. In Cairns, J., Lyon, J. L. and Skolnick, M. (eds.) *Cancer Incidence in Defined Populations.* Banbury Report 4. pp. 203-213. (New York: Cold Spring Harbor Laboratory)

84. Lynch, H. T., Katz, D. A., Bogard, P. J. and Lynch, J. F. (1985). The sarcoma, breast cancer, lung cancer, and adrenocortical carcinoma syndrome revisited. Childhood cancer. *Am. J. Dis. Child.*, **139**, 134-136

85. Ayesh, R., Idle, J. R., Ritchie, J. C., Crothers, M. J. and Hetzel, M. R. (1984). Metabolic oxidation phenotypes as markers for susceptibility to lung cancer. *Nature*, **312**, 169-170

9
The role of the host in facilitating and controlling the development and spread of cancer

P. ALEXANDER

INTRODUCTION AND SUMMARY

The capacity of cells to multiply, to spread from one site in the body to another and to invade adjacent tissues, though inherent in cancer is not unique to cancer. The failure to do so under control by the body is the critical difference between normal and malignant cells. Yet the complexities of the natural history of malignant disease tell us that cancer cells cannot be considered as completely autonomous parasites within the host which merely plays a role as incubator and provider of nutrients. This chapter aims to document the concept that host–tumour interaction can be decisive for the development and spread of cancer in general; not only for the subset of mammary and prostatic cancer that require steroid or pituitary hormones for growth. The dependence on endocrine hormones, which has been effectively exploited for therapy of certain tumours, will not be discussed in this chapter. Apart from such hormonal effects the major emphasis on the role of the host in the development of cancer has in the past been on the elimination of cancer cells. Facilitation of the growth of cancer by host processes must not, however, be forgotten.

Antitumour action of host

The concept of surveillance evolved to accommodate the hypothesis that the occurrence in an animal of a single cell having a fully transformed phenotype is sufficient to initiate a malignant lesion. Even if transformation required several independent mutations, Burnet[1] calculated from the known somatic mutation rate that the appearance of transformed cells ought to be very much greater than the occurrence of cancer when allowance is made for the very large number of cells which are at risk in an adult organism. Even more compelling are the data from *in vitro* transformation of mammalian cells into a phenotype capable of growing as malignant tumours when transplanted into animals. This occurs remarkably readily and in tissue culture the transformation of normal cells to a form which exhibits malignant characteristics is far from being very rare or infrequent. Because of the ease of dosimetry this is most readily demonstrated for the carcinogenic effect of ionising radiations[2] although the same applies to chemical carcinogens or indeed to 'spontaneous' transformation. One Gray (= 100 rad) X-rays given to embryonic cells in tissue culture causes about one cell in 10^4 to be transformed, and after clonal expansion such a transformed cell will grow *in vivo* into a tumour. Yet clearly the carcinogenicity of X-rays for intact animals is many orders of magnitude less than would result from induction (at the rate observed *in vitro*) of a single malignant cell if one considers the number of cells capable of being transformed. To resolve the discrepancy between the rate of induction of cancer in animals and the rates of somatic mutation and transformation of cells *in vitro*, the existence in animals of a mechanism which results in the selective destruction of cells exhibiting a transformed phenotype was postulated. Burnet[1] was a most persuasive advocate of the hypothesis that specific T-cell acquired immunity was responsible for surveillance of potentially malignant cells. But experience in animals and man failed to reveal a major increase in cancer incidence following immunosuppression, except when the cancers would be attributed to DNA-containing viruses, when the surveillance was that of the viral infection and not of the transformed cells. The role of eliminating transformed cells has therefore been allocated to so-called non-specific immune processes mediated by leukocytes. However, as with surveillance by T-cells direct experimental data fails to support this concept. Control (or surveillance) by the host, however, is an important factor once a tumour has arisen, in its subsequent dissemination and spread.

A way out of the conflict between the ease of cell transformation *in vitro* and the rarity of tumours *in vivo* is to abandon the concept that tumours arise from single cells[3]. Such an hypothesis would imply that an isolated and discrete cancer cell is not capable of autonomous growth. Support for this idea comes from studies which suggest that the host plays a major role in facilitating rather than impeding the development of cancer. The finding that cancer cells are capable of clonal growth from a single cell *in vitro* is not inconsistent with lack of autonomy of a single cancer cell *in vivo* because the tissue culture medium does not reflect the normal *in vivo* environment. Thus only at sites of injury where blood coagulation has occurred will the tissue fluids contain the platelet derived factors present in serum. It is relevant that for radiation carcinogenesis, where dose–response relationships have been studied very precisely, the effect on cancer incidence of both total dose and of dose rate is incompatible with events involving only one cell.

One of the most striking aspects of blood-borne metastasis is its inefficiency, which stems from intravascular death of circulating cancer cells before they have succeeded in extravasating. Post-mortem studies indicate that invasion of veins is common and that the shedding of cancer cells and their arrest in small blood vessels, either singly or as clusters, is much more frequent than the incidence of progressively growing metastases. There have been several reports of circulating tumour cells being detected in patients without metastases. Massive destruction of blood-borne cancer cells is also indicated in patients from whom malignant ascites were drained by a surgically introduced peritoneal venous shunt. As a result of this procedure, millions of cancer cells were delivered to the lung, yet no lung metastases developed[4].

In experimental animals direct evidence for intravascular cell death comes from three types of experiment:

(1) identification with an antiserum of large numbers of cancer cells in the efferent blood from a tumour that rarely metastasises[5];

(2) the presence of viable tumour cells in cell suspensions prepared from the lungs of animals bearing subcutaneous tumours that, if left undisturbed, would not develop metastases[6]. The cancer cells are detected by a bioassay in which cells from the lung are transplanted into another animal. Frequently this test does not reveal cancer cells within the blood since they are trapped in the first passage through the lung and, as a result, the number in the circulation will represent less than one minute's output of cancer emboli;

(3) the rapid autolysis of cancer cells arrested in the lung. This has been demonstrated by injecting intravenously cancer cells, the DNA of which had been radioactively labelled. More than 90% of cancer cells introduced in this way autolyse completely within 24 h, in mice. That the cancer cells have died and have been broken down in the lung is proved by the disappearance of DNA-associated radioactivity in the lung and its eventual appearance in the urine as low molecular weight breakdown products[7,8].

Specific immunity contributes to the destruction of cancer emboli from immunogenic tumours, but metastatic inefficiency is also very evident with tumours that do not evoke an immune response as well as in immunosuppressed hosts. Mechanical trauma on entering capillary beds and toxicity of dissolved oxygen have been identified as possible mechanisms for the destruction of cancer cells once they have entered the blood. Killing of blood-borne metastases by leukocytes in an immunologically non-specific manner may also occur, but it is unlikely to be a major contributor to metastatic inefficiency as this is not significantly affected by leukopenia.

Promotion of tumour growth by the host

Tumours with the exception of haemangiomas derive their blood supply from surrounding normal tissues and angiogenesis is therefore an essential accompaniment of tumour growth. The host can however also facilitate tumour growth by providing mitogenic stimuli for the cancer cells. For a long time the idea held sway that proliferation is the natural state for all well-nourished cells and that in vivo this mitotic exuberance was suppressed by some form of negative feedback (e.g. by chalones). Cancer was consequently regarded as a state in which control over proliferation had been lost; an absence of, or unresponsiveness to hypothetical suppression mechanisms. In recent years overwhelming evidence has accumulated for the alternative view which states that normal cells proliferate as an adaptive response to a sequence of external signals. However, the corollary that cancer can be regarded as a gain of function, namely the ability to undergo division without the need for triggering stimuli from the environment, is not wholly true.

The simplest hypothesis, that the malignant phenotype differs from the normal phenotype in not requiring mitogenic stimuli from polypeptide growth factors, is difficult to sustain in view of a large body of evidence which shows that many cancer cells, human as well as animal, synthesise (and frequently release into culture media) polypeptides which are closely related to (if not chemically identical with) mitogens produced by normal cells, notably platelets, macrophages and fetal tissues. From these findings it seems much more likely that cancer cells, like normal cells, relying upon mitogens made by other and probably neighbouring cells, require a mitogenic stimulus by a polypeptide, but the distinction lies in normal cells relying upon mitogens made by other and probably neighbouring cells, whereas malignant cells make their own growth factors. When this autocrine stimulation hypothesis was proposed[9] the view was that the growth factors made by the cancer cells for their own use differed from those made by normal cells. We now know that this is not true and that at least some of the cancer-derived growth factors are also produced by normal cells. We[10] have therefore suggested that an essential component of malignant transformation is that the same cell constitutively synthesises both the mitogen and the receptor for the mitogen, whereas normal cells in general express only one of the two components required for cell division. However, the simultaneous expression of ligand and receptor need not render a single isolated cell autonomous because the concentration of the factor in the microenvironment of a single cell may not be adequate for mitogenesis. Only in a cluster of cancer cells will the concentration needed for continuous proliferation be attained. In other words, a single cancer cell is not autonomous but a cluster of cells may be. Support for this model comes both from *in vitro* studies, which indicate that in serum-free medium cancer cells require high cell densities to proliferate, and from the growth pattern *in vivo* of blood-borne cancer cells[11]. These data suggest that for an isolated cancer cell to grow *in vivo* it requires host-derived mitogens which can replace or augment the autocrine growth factors.

Stimulation of host by factors stemming from the tumour

An effect of the tumour on the tissues of the host must also be recognised in the tumour-host relationship. It has long been known that certain cancers produce endocrine hormones which affect normal organs of the host. ACTH is perhaps the best studied example because of the well-defined symptoms produced, but it represents the tip of an iceberg. The synthesis and release of polypeptide growth factors by many if not all malignant cells raises the possibility of paracrine-mediated changes in tissues adjacent to cancer. Thus sarcomas release one of the forms of platelet derived growth factor (PDGF) at sites of platelet aggregation such as wounds. PDGFs induce fibroblasts to proliferate. PDGF release from sarcomas raises the possibility that normal fibroblasts in the stroma of such tumours may be induced to divide in the same way as in wounds where the PDGF comes from the platelets in a blood clot. Is hyperplasia of normal cells a common adjunct of tumours? This is certainly the case for angiogenesis where it seems clear that the stimulation of normal endothelial cells is signalled at least in part by growth factors originating from the tumour. The techniques are at hand to determine which of the dividing cells in a tumour are malignant and which normal.

SURVEILLANCE

Regulation by specific T-cell dependent effector mechanisms

The proposition (cf. ref. 1) has frequently been echoed that cells which have undergone a transformation to malignancy are eliminated immunologically by the specific effector mechanisms which are known to come into play in the rejection of homografts. These processes include T-cells which bind to the target cells via immunologically unique receptors. Some T-cells when bound to the specific target kill the cells directly by a mechanism similar to complement-induced lysis. Another class of T-cells on contacting the antigen release lymphokines which may induce other leukocytes to become cytotoxic. Antibodies which require T-cells for their induction can kill cancer cells either in conjunction with complement or by linking the target cell to leukocytes which release locally acting toxins such as OH radicals.

While there is a great diversity of mechanisms by which antigenic tumour cells could be rejected by the host, the first requirement for any such process to come into play is that the tumour must mimic a homograft in displaying antigens in its membrane against which the host reacts. While there is evidence for the existence of such antigens in some chemically and virally induced tumours[12,13] in experimental animals, there are no convincing data that man responds immunologically via a T-cell dependent immunological response to the majority of malignancies. Also frequently, no immune reaction against 'spontaneous' cancers that arise in experimental animals can be observed[14]. That specific immune mechanisms do not in general determine the incidence of malignant disease is indicated by observations in immune deprived hosts. Until relatively recently it was difficult to maintain immunosuppressed experimental animals alive for long periods because of their susceptibility to infection, but isolation procedures have now been perfected so that animals with an inherited defect in immunity (e.g. the 'nude' rodent which has no thymus), or animals treated with immunosuppressive agents, can enjoy a normal life span. Such experimental animals[15-17], in which T-cell dependent immunity is effectively absent as indicated by their ability to accept foreign organs such as skin or kidneys, do not have a markedly higher incidence of malignant disease, except for an increase in lymphoma at old age[18]. Oncogenic DNA viruses which are carcinogenic in neonates but not in immunologically competent adult animals will induce tumours in adults if they are immunosuppressed. Extensive proliferation of such viruses is necessary for tumour induction and, since viral infection is controlled by T-cell dependent immunity, the condition for this type of viral carcinogenesis only exists in the murine or rat neonate which has not yet developed its immune machinery to the full, or in immuno-deprived adults. Here we are dealing with an effect of the immune system on the virus and not on the cancer.

Rather unexpectedly the appearance of chemically induced cancers is, like the occurrence of spontaneous tumours, not significantly hastened nor increased by immunosuppression, despite the fact that the tumours induced will frequently be immunogenic. This indicates that even when there is the capacity for a host response this is not a rate-determining step for carcinogenesis. However, the subsequent growth and above all the dissemination and metastasis of an immunogenic tumour can be markedly altered by immunosuppression. Thus antigenic chemically induced sarcomas (see Figure 9.1) and lymphomas (Figure 9.2) which in immunologically normal hosts do not readily metastasise through blood or lymph will do so if the host is immunosuppressed[19-21]. Consequently, a cancer which in a normal

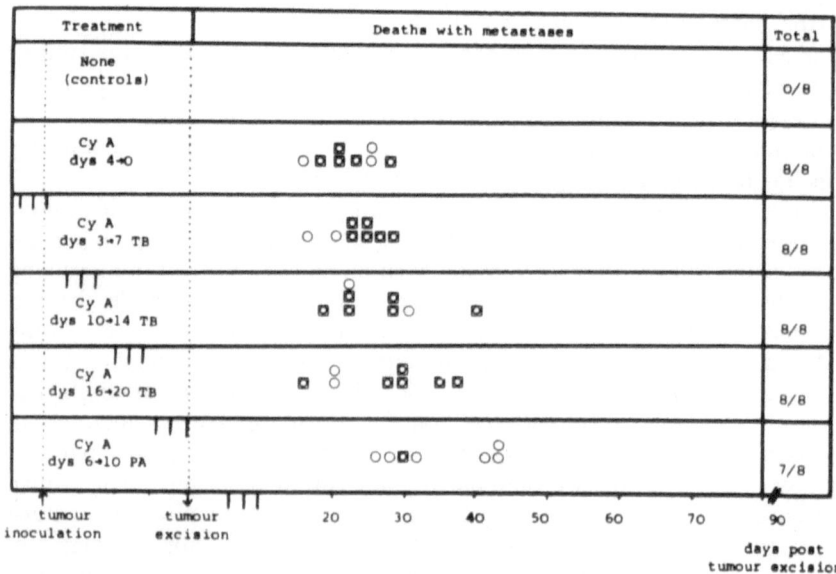

Figure 9.1 Effect of the immunosuppressive agent Cyclosporin A (Cy A) on the occurrence of distant metastases in rats into which a syngeneic fibrosarcoma (MC24) was implanted by intramuscular inoculation on day 0 and then surgically excised together with its draining node on day 14. Cy A was administered by intramuscular injection, 40 mg/kg in oil, on three occasions at two-day intervals as indicated (|||). Metastases to the lung (□) and lymph nodes (O) were recorded. Cy A promoted metastasis formation when given prior to implanation of the tumour, during the growth of the tumour and even six days after surgical excision of the tumour[20]

host could be cured by local surgery becomes incurable in an immunosuppressed host because of widespread dissemination. It must be stressed that in man promotion of metastasis by immunosuppression is likely to be rare because human cancers do not in general appear to be antigenic. A parallel to the animal data has been found in a few cases in patients who received a kidney or liver transplant from a donor who - unbeknownst - had cancer. Cancer cells were transplanted unwittingly with the replacement organ and the immunosuppressed recipient grew the cancer. When immunosuppression was stopped both the cancer regressed and the organ transplant was rejected. The paradox that immunosuppression has no effect on the *de novo* induction of an antigenic tumour but is capable of controlling its metastasis has not been resolved.

Experience with immunosuppression and cancer in man comes from different groups of patients. Those that had been thymectomised; those given immunosuppressive drugs, usually in connection with organ transplantation but also for auto-immune diseases[22,23]; those with a genetic T-cell defect (mostly children with combined immunodeficiency); and those with AIDS. The findings are clear (see Table 9.1): in none of these groups is there a significant increase in the common carcinomas. The most striking change in the pattern of malignant disease, which has been documented most precisely in the transplant patients, is a marked increase in the incidence of B-cell

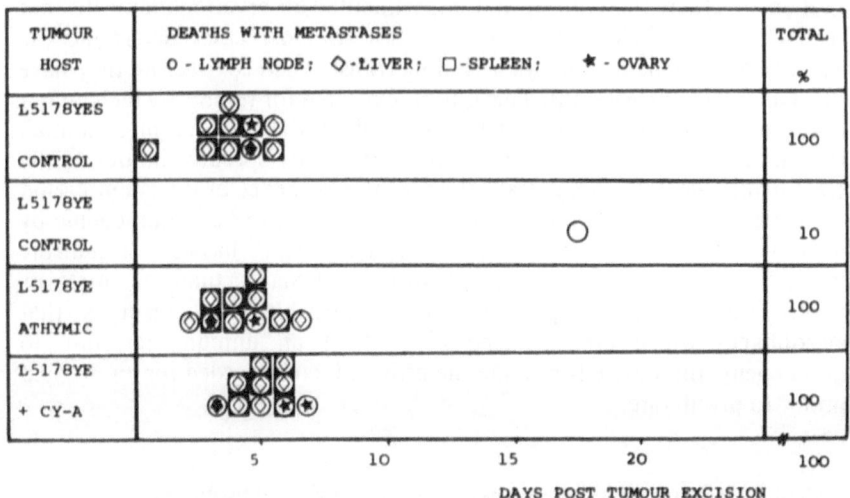

Figure 9.2 The transplantable murine lymphoma L5178YE when inoculated subcutaneously into normal immunocompetent syngeneic mice metastasises only very rarely, and if the local tumour is surgically removed when approximately 0.5 cm in diameter 90% of the mice remain tumour free. If this lymphoma is transplanted into immunosuppressed mice (either by treatment with Cyclosporin A (Cy-A) or because they were congenitally athymic - 'nude mice') all of the mice die from widespread metastases. L5178YE is immunogenic. A non-immunogenic variant, L5178YES, metastasises widely in normal mice in which it disseminates in the same way as the parent line does in immunosuppressed hosts[21]

lymphomas. These transplantation-associated B-cell lymphomas are characterised by the presence within the genome of EB virus DNA, and their aetiology involves infection with EB virus which is not limited by the normal immune response of the host. EB virus is mitogenic for B-cells and when there is no host surveillance of the virus a brisk proliferation of B-cells results. B-cell lymphomas are thought to arise from rapidly dividing normal B-cells as a result of a 'spontaneous' karyotypic change which endows the cell with a truly malignant phenotype. The pattern with EB virus in man closely resembles that with the oncogenic DNA viruses in immunosuppressed adult rodents. The principal malignant disease in patients with AIDS is Kaposi's sarcoma, although the incidence of EB virus-related lymphomas is also increased. Kaposi's sarcoma also has a higher than expected incidence in transplant patients in whom, however, it does not approach the frequency of the B-cell lymphoma. The reason for this inverse relationship of Kaposi's sarcoma and B-cell lymphoma in the two groups of immunosuppressed individuals is not known, nor is it clear as yet whether a virus plays some role in the causation of Kaposi's sarcoma. There is evidence from registries of transplant patients, particularly in Australia, of a meaningful increase in skin cancer associated with transplantation and there have also been suggestions that *in situ* cervical cancer is more frequent. The proper interpretation of such findings is difficult, however, since such relatively benign conditions may be picked up earlier in transplant patients, who are under continued medical supervision, than in the general population.

Taken together, the clinical and experimental observations indicate that T-cell dependent host immunity does not in most cases determine the incidence of malignant tumours by killing transformed cells before they have grown into detectable lesions. This is to be expected for tumours which do not evoke an immune response and it may well be the case for most human cancers. However, it remains a mystery that specific immunity in experimental animals does not affect either the incidence or the latent period of chemically induced tumours which can be shown to be immunogenic by the conventional transplantation tests. Indeed, Prehn[24] has data to indicate that an immune response to a transformed cell may actually facilitate its growth into a macroscopic tumour. A possible mechanism is that macrophages which are attracted as part of an immune response to immunogenic tumour cells provide the growth factors needed for an isolated tumour to proliferate.

Control by immunologically non-specific tumoricidal leukocytes

While the original concept of immune control of cancer incidence is untenable, the idea that cancer results from a mutation (or sequence of mutations) involving a single cell has for many become an article of faith. It is therefore almost dogmatic that there has to be a mechanism to resolve the discrepancy that such a transformation event occurs *in vitro* much more frequently than do tumours *in vivo*. The suggestion has gained ground that the majority of cancer cells are eradicated as and when they arise *in vivo* by

Table 9.1 UK · Australasia study of cancer incidence (no. of cases expected and no. observed) in patients immunosuppressed because of kidney transplantation or as therapy for auto-immune and other conditions[23]

Type of cancer	UK transplants (3671 patients)		Australasian transplants (1542 patients)		Non-transplant (1634 patients)	
	Observed	Expected	Observed	Expected	Observed	Expected
Non-Hodgkins-lymphoma*	23*	0.49	19	(0.36)	6	0.55
Skin Basal	11	1.85	—	—	2	2.87
Squamous	8	0.29	—	—	3	0.60
Melanoma	2	0.32	—	—	0	0.30
Other	30**	21.42	15	(8.31)	54	36.17

*Less than 2 years after transplant, 12 cases (0.20 expected); after 2 years, 6 cases (0.12 expected); after 4 years, 5 cases (0.17 expected).
**Includes one case of Kaposi's sarcoma.

leukocytes which selectively recognise and kill cells that have been transformed, by a mechanism which does not involve specific immunity. *In vitro*, leukocytes will kill nucleated mammalian cells. The relative susceptibility of a range of target cells depends on the nature of the effector. Table 9.2 shows that the ranking order of sensitivity among a series of mouse tumours is quite different for killing by macrophages, NK cells, granulocytes or the toxin released from an activated T-cell[25]. If such *in vitro* studies have a counterpart *in vivo*, then macrophages would seem to be the most promising candidate since after activation by, for example, endotoxin[26] or a T-cell lymphokine[27] they are more cytotoxic to cells that have been transformed. The decisive experiment to test whether macrophages influence susceptibility to cancer would be, as in the case of T-cells, to deplete the host of macrophages. Since the *in vitro* data have shown that macrophages are only cytotoxic after activation, there should be little or no surveillance in germ-free mice or the fetus as in such hosts the principal stimuli for activation are absent. A high susceptibility to cancer is not, however, observed in these situations. In any case, it is questionable whether *in vivo* activated macrophages are able to kill nucleated cells without the intervention of antibodies[28].

A heterogenous group of mononuclear leukocytes referred to as NK cells[29] will kill some but by no means all tumour cells *in vitro*. *In vivo* NK cells have been shown to provide a major effector mechanism in the rejection of bone-marrow allografts[30], but the cell killing requires the presence of specific antibody directed against the foreign marrow. However, no amount of negative evidence seems to dim the enthusiasm of those who advocate a tumour surveillance role for these cells by a non-immunological process. The level of NK activity found in the blood of different mice varies widely between strains, in mutants with bone-marrow defects and with age, being very low in neonates as well as in mice older than one year[31]. Yet the measured NK activity does not correlate with the susceptibility of such animals to the induction of tumours or to the growth of transplanted tumours. Even *in vitro* NK cells do not kill all tumour cells; in general susceptibility to NK cytotoxicity only becomes pronounced after tumour explants have been grown in culture for long periods[32].

In vitro, neutrophils (especially after activation) are the most cytotoxic of all leukocytes (see Table 9.2). Again, however, there is no evidence that neutrophils kill cancer cells *in vivo*[33]. If neutrophils directly influence susceptibility to cancer, then mutants with neutrophil defects or hosts with prolonged myelosuppression should be significantly more cancer prone. No such correlation has been found.

Conclusion

The available data fail to provide any support for surveillance against cancer induction either by specific (T-cell dependent) immunity or so-called 'natural' immunity, which I have preferred to call leukocyte cytotoxicity. Without evoking surveillance, two possibilities which are not mutally exclusive can be

Table 9.2 Susceptibility in vitro of tumours to immunologically non-specific leukocyte effectors[25]

Tumour cells used	Percentage lysis by:				
	NK cells	MAF activated macrophages	Stimulated granulocytes	'Lymphotoxin'* diluted 1:64	1:256
Sarcoma (C57/BL) FS6	15	21	9	100	95
Sarcoma (CBA) FS29	27	26	13	65	47
Melanoma (C57/BL) B16	20	12	11	8	4
Lymphoma (DBA/2) L5178Y	19	50	28	6	0
Lymphoma (57/BL) TLX9	4	62	18	0	0

*Supernatant from cultures containing T-cells obtained from mice immunised with BCG plus the soluble tuberculosis antigen PPD.

considered to resolve the discrepancy between the relatively high rate of transformation *in vitro* and the rarity of cancer *in vivo*. Cancer is a clonal disease starting from a transformation event which may be very much less frequent than *in vitro* experiments suggest. Or, *in vivo* tumour growth requires the participation of several independently transformed cells at the same site whereas the ability of a single transformed cell to grow clonally occurs only *in vitro*[3]. In the latter case the resulting cancer may still exhibit a predominantly monoclonal phenotype as a result of selective pressure during outgrowth of an originally polyclonal population.

DESTRUCTION OF CIRCULATING CANCER CELLS IN THE HOST

That it is necessary to distinguish between host control in the genesis of cancer as opposed to the spread and dissemination of an established tumour is clear from experiments where immunosuppression facilitated the metastasis of immunogenic tumours but did not accelerate their *de novo* genesis (Figures 9.1 and 9.2). Cancer cells, once they have detached from the tumour and, as a result of invasion of a vessel, have entered the vascular system are extremely vulnerable (see Table 9.3). If the tumour evokes a specific immune response to an antigen in its membrane then antibody to this antigen will contribute to the destruction of the cancer embolus probably before it has had an opportunity to extravasate[34]. Antibody-coated tumour cells can be killed either by lysis with complement or in conjunction with macrophages or B-cells. For cells which are not trapped in the first capillary bed they encounter but which can pass through capillaries (e.g. lymphomas and leukaemias), immuno-phagocytosis in spleen and liver is a very effective means of elimination[35]. Specific immunity is, however, only one mechanism which destroys circulating cancer cells and the phenomenon of metastatic inefficiency is also very marked for non-immunogenic tumours[36]. The suggestion has frequently been made that intravascular destruction of circulating cancer cells is caused

Table 9.3 Vulnerability of tumour emboli arrested in microvasculature. Probability of causing a metastasis determined by both (a) rate of cell death while intravascular and (b) rate of extravasation

a) *Mechanisms responsible for intravascular cell death:*
Mechanical damage from shearing forces in capillaries
Toxicity of oxygen at arterial concentrations
Thrombus formation
Specific immunity (especially via antibody) for immunogenic tumours
?? Non-specific destruction by leukocytes

b) *Mechanisms determining rate of extravasation:*
Extent of exposure of basement membrane
Attachment to basement membrane
Penetration

by NK cells or macrophages. However, the same arguments which render it improbable that these leukocytes control tumour induction also apply to their role in controlling metastases.

Mechanical damage

Two mechanisms are known which contribute to intravascular death of cancer emboli. Using rat ascites cells Sato and Suzuki and Weiss and his colleagues[37] demonstrated that cancer cells sustained irreversible mechanical damage from the shearing forces to which they are exposed in narrow capillaries. The same phenomenon has been demonstrated *in vitro* by passing cancer cells through large-pore membrane filters. Mechanical damage also contributes to the death of carcinoma and sarcoma cells in the blood. If carcinoma and sarcoma cells are injected into the arterial circulation via the left heart, about a third of the cells that are carried to the skeletal muscle are not trapped in the capillary bed of the muscle but pass through the large capillaries – the so called preferred channels – into the venous circulation which brings them to the lung in which they are completely arrested. We[11] were able to show that sarcoma and carcinoma cells that had reached the lung by this indirect route were irreversibly damaged and could not develop into tumours. This we attribute to the mechanical damage consequent on passing through the large capillaries in the muscle.

Oxygen toxicity

The oxygen concentration in arterial blood is three to four times higher than that in extra-cellular fluid which is the normal milieu for mammalian cells other than those lining blood vessels. We have tested the hypothesis[36] that toxicity of oxygen at concentrations attained by equilibration with air contributes to the death of tumour cells trapped in the microvasculature. While many long-established cell lines are not inhibited by oxygen at normal concentrations and grow readily *in vitro* from low cell numbers, the evaluation of the optimum oxygen concentration for growth in culture of cells taken from the animal and not adapted to *in vitro* conditions is complicated, since such cells normally only grow from large inocula when the actual oxygen concentration to which the cells are exposed is much lower than that which corresponds to atmospheric pressure. In dense cultures the consumption of oxygen is greater than the rate of diffusion of oxygen into the culture vessel. The magnitude of this effect obviously depends on the seeding density and the metabolic rate of the cells. Indeed, at high cell densities the oxygen concentration may fall below that needed for optimum growth even when the culture is exposed to the atmosphere. To determine the effect of oxygen tension on growth, therefore, cells need to be seeded at low densities so as to minimize depletion of oxygen. There have been several reports that normal cells isolated directly from animals grow better in cultures exposed to a gas phase containing 5% oxygen than to air.

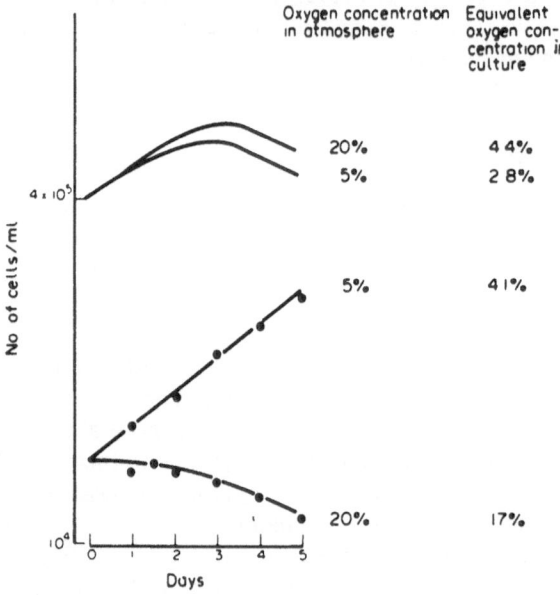

Figure 9.3 Facilitation of growth *in vitro* at low seeding densities of freshly explanted cancer cells by lowering the oxygen concentration in the surrounding atmosphere to 5%. FS19 murine sarcoma cells derived directly from a tumour were plated at two different cell densities in an atmosphere of either 20% or 5% oxygen. The oxygen concentration in the culture at the level of the cells (the steady-state concentration) was determined with an oxygen micro-electrode 16 h after plating and expressed as the equivalent atmospheric oxygen concentration with which it would be in equilibrium[1k]

We have investigated the effect of oxygen concentration on the rate of proliferation of sarcoma and carcinoma cells taken from mice and rats with cancer[11,38]. Most of the tumours studied conform to the pattern illustrated in Figure 9.3. That is, at low seeding densities the cells grow only in atmospheres having a low oxygen concentration, but this toxic effect of atmosphere rich in oxygen is lost if the initial seeding density is high. We have noted that cancer cells rapidly adapt to oxygen when grown *in vitro* and that sometimes after as few as two passages in culture (and usually after five passages) the cells grow equally as well at 18% as at 5% oxygen, even at low densities. Sometimes when cells that have 'adapted' to oxygen are grown *in vivo* they recover their sensitivity to oxygen on return to culture.

We have attempted to study more directly whether changing the oxygen concentration breathed by mice and rats following intravenous injection of cancer cells changes the number of lung tumours produced or the rate of autolysis of the trapped cancer cells. In initial experiments exposure of mice to hyperbaric (2.5 atmospheres) oxygen reduced the incidence of lung tumours, but in repeated experiments the results were extremely variable and we were unable to reach any conclusions. Others[39] had similar experience in that only occasionally was hyperbaric oxygen effective in reducing the capacity of cancer cells to grow in the lung. One reason for the variability could be that the physiological response to hyperbaric oxygen is complex and the actual change in blood oxygen concentration difficult to evaluate. We[40] therefore decided to approach the question of the role of oxygen concentration on tumour growth *in vivo* from an opposite angle by studying it in mice and rats breathing a low concentration of oxygen. We found that 8% is the lowest oxygen concentration under which mice and rats can survive for six hours. There is a dramatic increase in the number of lung tumours produced by syngeneic sarcomas in both species if they are kept for six hours in such an atmosphere compared with air. The trapping in the lung of sarcoma cells injected intravenously is essentially complete (i.e. greater than 95%) under both conditions, but the rate at which they suffer autolysis after inoculation is markedly slowed for rodents breathing 8% oxygen. These experiments suggest that the toxicity of oxygen observed *in vitro* may well have a counterpart *in vivo*.

CONTRIBUTION OF HOST-DERIVED GROWTH FACTORS TO METASTASIS AND CARCINOGENESIS

In 1978 DeLarco and Todaro[41] observed that the supernatant of tissue cultures of transformed cells (but not from cultures of non-transformed cells) contained a mitogenic polypeptide(s) which promoted the growth of normal cells. When this was found to be a general property of malignant cells, Sporn and Todaro[9] advanced the autocrine stimulation hypothesis for malignancy which states that malignant cells require mitogenic signals in order to divide, but that they have acquired the capacity to synthesise the necessary factors constitutively. The discoverers of the mitogenic polypeptides made by cancer cells considered that their biological properties were qualitatively distinct from those of the then known normal growth factors like epidermal growth factor (EGF) and platelet derived growth factor (PDGF) since they caused normal cells to proliferate *in vitro* with a malignant phenotype expressed in morphology and pattern of growth. Moreover, polypeptides present in culture supernatants from malignant cells enabled normal cells to grow as colonies in soft agar which hitherto had been thought to be a characteristic of transformed cells. Extracts from cancer cells – usually prepared employing acidified ethanol – produced the same effect. These properties led Todaro to designate the mitogenic polypeptides from cancer cells as transforming growth factors (TGFs). Sporn and Todaro's autocrine hypothesis stated that an essential feature of malignant transformation was the acquisition by cells of the capacity to synthesise TGFs which then led to autonomous growth. TGF activity is now known to result from the interaction of two polypeptides. Alpha-TGFs show close structural homology with epidermal growth factor (EGF) and bind to EGF receptors. Beta-TGF is a larger molecule made up of two chains linked by disulphide bonds and does not bind to EGF receptors. However, the hypothesis that production of TGFs is a correlate or consequence of malignancy cannot be sustained because acid ethanol extracts of normal tissues (in particular kidney and placenta) yield polypeptides which mimic in every respect the TGF activity of polypeptides from cancer cells and appear to be chemically identical. On degranulation, platelets release beta-TGF in addition to EGF and PDGF. Also cDNA coding for one of the TGFs hybridises with an mRNA in normal cells although the amount of message made is greatly increased after the cells have been virally transformed[42].

All this suggests that the essential difference between normal and malignant cells is not the synthesis by cancer cells of a special type of mitogenic polypeptide. The original autocrine stimulation hypothesis may have to be modified. A key factor in malignancy is not the production of novel (or untimely) mitogens, but the constitutive synthesis of both polypeptide growth factors and the receptors for them. According to our hypothesis[10] autocrine stimulation can arise in one of two ways: on becoming transformed, a cell that normally makes a particular growth factor starts to express the membrane receptor for it; or a cell that normally expresses the receptor acquires the capacity to synthesise the growth factor. Parallels in normal tissue are the synthesis by T-cells of their growth factor interleukin-2, when activated by the specific antigen to which the T-cells have become responsive. In this way clonal expansion of antigen-specific T-cells occurs during an immune response. This clonal growth is however, limited to the period of antigenic stimulation. The autocrine driven growth ceases with the elimination of antigen, unlike production of growth factors by tumours which does not need a stimulus. Another example[43] where rapid proliferation coincides with the simultaneous expression of a growth factor and its receptor occurs during a restricted period in fetal development when embryonic fibroblasts acquire the capacity to synthesise platelet derived growth factor (PDGF), for which fibroblasts have a receptor. This results in rapid growth, which is however limited as the capacity of fibroblasts to make PDGF is phase-specific. Many sarcomas and carcinomas[44,45] constitutively produce a growth factor which is indistinguishable from one type of PDGF. Whether this tumour-derived PDGF leads to autocrine-led proliferation remains to be demonstrated[46].

Can autocrine stimulation be interrupted?

We[11] have speculated that autocrine stimulation resulting in self sustaining neoplasia with the presence of exogenous mitogenic factors may not occur at the level of an isolated cell, but is a phenomenon of a cluster of cancer cells. There has to be a minimum local concentration of growth factors at the periphery of the cancer cells to ensure binding to the surface receptor. The constitutively produced growth factor will diffuse away from the cancer cell before the minimum concentration to achieve binding has been attained. However, if there are several cancer cells within a defined volume then an adequate local concentration can be attained for autocrine mitogenesis. In other words, tight coupling between the growth factor produced by a cancer cell and its association with the receptor on its membrane cannot occur at the level of an isolated cell (Figure 9.4) and true autonomy becomes a property of a cluster of malignant cells. Evidence that there is a lack of tight coupling comes from both *in vitro* and *in vivo* studies. *In vitro* the concentration of TGF sufficient for proliferation in the absence of serum is only attained in cultures at high cell densities. Growth in serum-free medium from low cell inocula requires the addition of growth factors such as TGFs, either extracted from cancer cells or found in the supernatants from dense cultures of tumour cells. In the presence of serum, clonal growth is possible because co-operation between a number of transformed cells is not required; here the need to establish an adequate concentration of TGF has been by-passed by the release of TGFs from platelets into the serum used for culture.

TIGHTLY LINKED

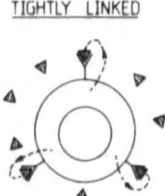

TGF immediately binds to receptors Single cell capable of autonomous replication

LOOSELY LINKED

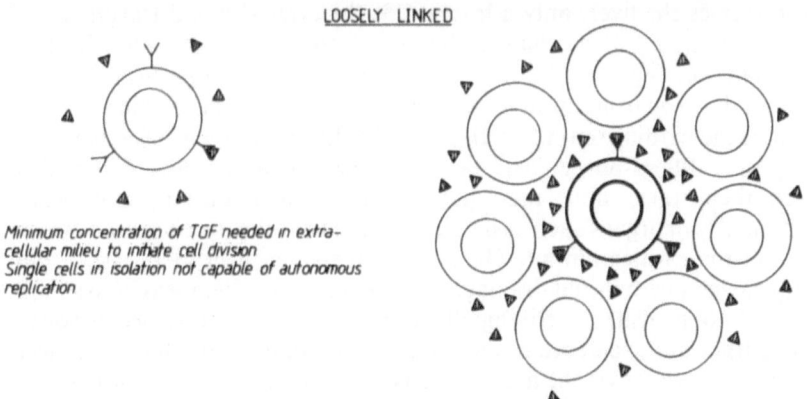

Minimum concentration of TGF needed in extra-cellular milieu to initiate cell division
Single cells in isolation not capable of autonomous replication

Local TGF concentration in cluster of cells adequate to activate receptors and initiate cell division

Figure 9.4 Diagrammatic representation of autocrine stimulation by a growth factor (TGF) with receptors on the same cell that produces the TGF. To induce mitogenesis the concentration of TGF in the immediate vicinity of the tumour cell must exceed a minimum value. Two situations can therefore be envisaged: (1) 'Tightly coupled': The concentration of TGF produced by an isolated cancer cell is sufficient in spite of diffusion. When this occurs a single isolated cancer cell is capable of autonomous growth, i.e. does not need growth factors either from serum (for growth *in vitro*) or tissues (for growth *in vivo*). (2) 'Loosely coupled': A concentration of TGF adequate for mitogenesis is not produced around an isolated cancer cell, but is only attained when there is a cluster of cancer cells so that loss by diffusion is reduced. In this case an isolated cancer cell requires growth factors in the medium for growth *in vitro* or from surrounding normal tissues for growth *in vivo*[1]

207

Organ preference of blood-borne metastasis

The concept that single cancer cells, which have not undergone powerful
selection by prolonged passage, are incapable of giving rise to a tumour and
that true autonomy of cancer requires a cluster of malignant cells which have
to create a micro-environment adequate for proliferation, would at first sight
appear to be in conflict with blood-borne metastasis where single cells are
capable of initiating tumour growth. However, one of the most striking
features of the metastatic process is the peculiarity of its relative frequency in
different organs which a century ago led Paget[47] to postulate in 1889
that the soil has to be right if the seed is to grow. It is unquestionable that
organ preference of blood-borne metastasis is in part determined by blood
flow, and that the organ which an embolus first encounters has the highest
incidence of metastases. Careful analyses of post-mortems on a large series of
cancer patients have consistently shown that when the blood of the primary
carcinoma drains into the vena caval system lung metastases are the most
common, whereas for tumours draining into the portal system liver
metastases predominate[48,49]. For emboli that have gained access to the arterial
circulation organ preference is not dependent on haemodynamic considerations, and the seed and soil phenomenon is very evident. While the
whole of the venous blood traverses the lung and the whole of the portal
blood traverses the liver, only a fraction of the arterial blood traverses any
one organ or tissue. If mechanical factors of the circulation were the sole
determinant of the distribution of metastases, then the incidence of
metastases deriving from the arterial circulation should be proportional to the
fraction of the cardiac output received by the different organs. The facts are
the opposite. Blood-borne metastases are rare in muscle and gut, which
between them take more than half of the cardiac output, and occur
predominantly in organs such as liver and adrenals which receive a very small
fraction of the cardiac output. The high frequency of liver metastases from
primary cancers with initial drainage into the venous system was considered
by Willis[49] to provide a striking illustration of the discordance between
cardiac output and incidence of metastases, since in this situation the cancer
emboli reach the liver via the hepatic artery which receives only a few per cent
of the arterial blood.

The remarkable site selectivity of metastases stemming from cells in the
arterial circulation can be investigated experimentally by inoculating tumour
cells directly into the left side of the heart. When this is done the relative
incidence of metastases in different organs bears no relationship to cardiac
output. In a detailed study[50,51] we have inoculated histologically distinct rat
cancer cells into the left heart of syngeneic rats via a cannula introduced into
the carotid. The distribution of cardiac output to the various organs was
determined by the injection of radioactive plastic microspheres with a
diameter of $15\,\mu m$ which ensures complete trapping in capillary beds. The
proportion of cancer cells arrested at different sites was determined by
injecting radiolabelled cancer cells and then measuring the radioactivity of the
different organs. From these experiments there was no indication that for the

tumours employed the cells re-distributed after the initial arrest*. The radioactivity in all of the organs except the liver fell progressively and to the same extent in the 24 h after injection. This fall is the result of intravascular autolysis of the arrested cells. The increase in the radioactivity in the liver is caused by reticulo-endothelial clearance of the cell debris. Table 9.4 summarises the results obtained with the three rat cancers studied in greatest detail. Similar results have been obtained with three other syngeneic rat sarcomas and two human xenografts (a melanoma and a pancreatic carcinoma) which were injected into the hearts of immune deprived rats (both genetically athymic *nu/nu* rats and cyclosporin A treated rats were used). The metastatic pattern of the syngeneic rat tumours was the same in normal as in immune deprived rats, which shows that immune reactions did not contribute to the site selectivity observed.

Clearly there is a very pronounced 'soil' effect and the incidence of metastasis in the various organs is unrelated to the blood flow to the organ, or to the number of cancer cells trapped in the organ, which closely parallels the blood flow. The organ preference can best be described quantitatively as the probability of a single arrested cell causing a metastasis. Since the blood-borne cancer cells are distributed within the different capillary beds as single isolated cells there can be no question of a co-operative effect between the trapped cancer cells. We are therefore dealing with the probability of a single cell developing into a metastasis, and this can be estimated from the observed proportion of cells arrested in a particular organ compared with the number of metastatic lesions detected at post-mortem. The values thus obtained are imprecise, but as they differ for different organs by orders of magnitude, their significance is real. Thus 10 to 30 sarcoma cells deposited in the microvasculature of an adrenal sufficed to produce a metastatic deposit, whereas a metastasis in muscle occurred only when more than 10^6 sarcoma cells had been arrested in the skeletal muscles of the animal. The number of cells needed to produce a tumour in lung or liver following intravenous or intraportal injection, respectively, lay for this tumour between 1000 and 10 000 cells. With each of the four tumours studied (one carcinoma, two sarcomas and a hepatoma) the adrenal was always the organ which was most susceptible to metastasis from arterial emboli, and other organs in which tumours developed with comparable probability were the ovary and bone. Two organs which received a high proportion of the total cardiac output but were refractory to all of the tumours studied were gut and skeletal muscle. There is a third category of tissues which constitute a good soil for some, but not all, of the tumours studied: the most striking example is brown fat for the sarcoma. Lung is preferred for the carcinoma (for cells coming via the bronchial arteries). A 'soil effect' for blood-borne metastasis is not in doubt, but its mechanism remains to be established. As long ago as 1934 Haddow (cf. ref. 49) proposed that growth promoting substances from the host tissue

---

*All tumour cells do not behave in this way. Certainly leukaemias and lymphomas and possibly even some other tumours redistribute after initial arrest and there is no correlation between their organ distribution and blood flow to the organ.

Table 9.4   Sites of metastases after left ventricular injection of 10^6 cancer cells into syngeneic rats[50]

Organ	% Cells trapped*	Per cent incidence of metastasis		
		Sarcoma (n = 31)+	Mammary carcinoma (n = 27)	Hepatoma (n = 12)
Adrenals	0.2±1	100	100	100
Ovaries	0.2±0.2	74	89	100
Bone and muscle	24±7	65	44	33
Lung	17±6	22	67	8
Brown fat	5.8±2	87	7	0
Gastrointestinal tract	12.1±5	0	0	0
Kidney	9.0±3	0	0	0

*5 min after intracardiac injection of [^{125}I]iododeoxyuridine labelled sarcoma cells.

†Number of animals per group.

were responsible. The alternative explanation of selective trapping is definitively excluded by the clear demonstration (at least with the carcinomas and sarcomas studied by us) that cells are arrested in the first capillary bed they encounter and that therefore the cells go where the blood goes. Variations in the rate of intravascular cell death would be expected to affect the probability of cells initiating a metastasis, but our data on the rate of autolysis of radiolabelled cells in different organs provided no support for such an hypothesis. Similarly, there is no evidence to support the view that the dramatic organ preferences stem from differences in the structure of blood vessels leading to variation in the rate of extravasation.

The hypothesis which I favour is that following extravasation an isolated cancer cell can only proliferate if the environment supplies factors that can augment the TGFs produced by the cancer cell itself, as their concentration around a single cell is inadequate for mitogenesis. This host help could stem from locally produced polypeptide growth factors with biological activity similar to TGFs or from substances such as cortisone which potentiate the activity of growth factors by inducing an increase in receptors. Direct support for this view comes from an experiment[50] in which dexamethasone was given to rats *following* intracardiac injection of sarcoma cells. Metastases appeared in the liver and the kidney, organs which are not involved in the absence of dexamethasone. Since an effect of dexamethasone could still be observed even when administered 2 and 4 days after injection of the sarcoma cells, we are led to conclude that at least some of the sarcoma cells remained quiescent (or grew only very slowly) in kidney and were stimulated into active division by the dexamethasone. This effect of dexamethasone was not dependent on its immunosuppressive action nor on its effect on prostaglandins since administration of the powerful immunosuppressive agent, cyclosporin A, or of a non-steroidal anti-inflammatory agent does not modify the pattern of metastases following intracardiac injection of these cancer cells.

Dormant metastases

The phenomenon of metastases that lie dormant for many years after successful removal of the primary lesion is well documented clinically[52]. In animal models[6] the presence in the lung of dormant cancer cells, which stemmed via blood-borne spread from a distant primary tumour, that did not give rise to macroscopic lung metastasis could be shown by transplantation. In the lung the cells do not grow, but when a cell suspension was prepared from the lungs of animals from which the 'primary' had been surgically removed a week previously and was injected into the peritoneal cavity, tumours indistinguishable from the 'primary' grew out within the cavity (see Table 9.5). Dormant tumour cells can also be demonstrated in organs other than the lung following intracardiac injection[50]. Despite the fact that 15% of the injected cells are trapped in kidney, we have never observed macroscopic metastases in the kidneys of rats that had received the MC28 sarcoma intra-aortically. Yet when the kidneys were transplanted as long as 7 days after the injection of tumour cells into the peritoneal cavity of another syngeneic rat, tumours grew in the peritoneal cavity (see Table 9.5). We conclude that these cancer cells when deposited from blood-borne emboli as single and discrete cells lack growth stimuli and remain dormant within the kidney. On transfer to the peritoneal cavity they are in an environment in which they receive stimuli and hence grow out. The phenomenon that isolated tumour cells remain dormant in some tissues but grow out in others is fully consistent with the hypothesis that single isolated cancer cells are not truly autonomous, but require locally-produced growth factors to divide.

GROWTH PROMOTING ACTION OF TISSUE MACROPHAGES

Intratumoral macrophages

The tumoricidal action of macrophages activated *in vitro* by a variety of procedures (e.g. lymphokines or endotoxins) or when acting in conjunction with antibody has been discussed in earlier sections. The observation that macrophages can actually facilitate the growth of some, but by no means all, chemically induced sarcomas in rodents was made by Evans[52,53] who noted that certain murine sarcomas which were highly immunogenic grew more slowly when transplanted into an irradiated as compared to a normal syngeneic host. Macrophage infiltration of tumours is in part associated with an immune response to the tumour[54] and this increases with an increase in the immunogenicity of the tumour but falls if the host is immunosuppressed. The slower growth in the irradiated host found by Evans was associated with a fall in the proportion of macrophages in the tumour. A mixed inoculum of tumour cells and macrophages grew more rapidly in the irradiated recipient. Subsequently, accelerated growth as a result of adding macrophages to the tumour inoculum was also observed with some sarcomas in normal hosts[55]. It is even possible that macrophages promote carcinogenesis. Prehn, who discovered that chemically-induced rodent tumours possess tumour specific

Table 9.5 Demonstration of dormant metastases by transplantation of lung or kidney tissue into peritoneal cavity.[6,50]

(a) Dormant metastases in lung derived from intra-muscular sarcomas

Experimental protocol				FS12 *syngeneic mouse sarcoma*	MC1 *syngeneic rat sarcoma*
Day 0	*Day 16*	*Day 20*	*Day 90*		
10^5 sarcoma cells (i.m., leg)	Surgically remove tumour (0.5cm dia.)		Kill animals Autopsy	0% with metastases	2.5% with metastases
10^5 sarcoma cells (i.m., leg)	Surgically remove tumour	Kill animals Remove lung and implant[a]		67% with large i.p. sarcoma	70% with large i.p. sarcoma

(b) Dormant metastases in kidney derived from 10^6 rat sarcoma cells injected intra-arterially via the left ventricle

Experimental protocol					
Day 0	*Day 1 or Day 5 or Day 12*	*Day 18*	*Day 26*		
Intracardiac injection	—	Rats killed Autopsy	—	Macroscopic metastases in many organs but none in kidney	
Intracardiac injection	Rats killed, kidney removed and implanted[a] into normal rats	—	Recipient rats killed Autopsy	All had large tumour masses in peritoneum	

i.m. = intramuscular; i.p. = intraperitoneal.
[a]Tissue finely chopped and implanted i.p.

212

transplantation antigens against which the host can mount an immune response, subsequently observed[24] that the induction of sarcomas by methylcholanthrene occurred less readily (i.e. with lower incidence and longer latent period) in immunosuppressed as opposed to normal mice. This immunostimulation of carcinogenesis may well be associated with the infiltrating properties of macrophages since the proportion of macrophages to tumour cells decreases sharply when the host is immunosuppressed.

Intraperitoneal macrophages and the omentum

Reference has already been made to the fact that blood-borne metastases can lie dormant in some tissues and their presence can be revealed by transplanting a cell suspension from such tissues into the peritoneal cavity. Thus carcinoma and sarcoma cells which had failed to grow when deposited in the kidney or the lung on transfer to the peritoneum grew rapidly as solid deposits on the omentum from which the tumours subsequently spread to other organs. The omentum is a tissue which is particularly rich in macrophages and on intraperitoneally (i.p.) injecting the branched chain hydrocarbon pristane (2,6,10,14-tetramethylpentadecane) the omentum becomes dramatically enlarged mainly because of a proliferation of macrophages[56]. Transplantation of tumour, i.p., is dramatically facilitated by pretreatment of rodents with pristane and, in our hands (see Table 9.6), tumours which grew only from inocula in excess of 1000 cells when injected subcutaneously, intramuscularly or intravenously, developed from less than 50 cells, given i.p., on the omentum of pristane treated mice and rats (Table 9.6). Consequent upon the enlargement of the macrophage-rich white spots, pristane causes the appearance of a cellular exudate containing predominantly macrophages which are not activated (i.e. which are not cytotoxic) unlike those evoked by immunologically induced inflammatory stimuli. Stimulation with pristane is therefore highly suitable for studying the growth promoting properties of macrophages without the complication of induced cytotoxicity.

Wound healing

Sites of tissue injury and trauma facilitate the growth of many experimentally transplanted tumours. This phenomenon was first observed by Fisher and Fisher[57] who found that cancer cells injected directly into the liver via the portal vein grew more readily if the liver was damaged mechanically or chemically. A similar phenomenon can be strikingly demonstrated in the muscle at the site of a laparotomy incision following intracardiac injection. Blood-borne cancer emboli only grow extremely rarely in skeletal muscle. In spite of the fact that 30% of cancer cells injected intra-arterially via the left ventricle are arrested in such muscle, only one or two muscle metastases occur in the whole animal following a dose of 10^6 cells. Yet in the muscle of a scar produced prior to the injection of the tumour cells, multiple metastases arise

Table 9.6 Oil (pristane) induced macrophages facilitate tumour growth in the peritoneal cavity

Tumour type	No. cells injected	Animal strain	Killed (day)	Tumour incidence*	
				Control	Pristane**
MT1 mammary carcinoma	500	CBA mice	30	1/5 (small)	5/5 (large) Mice moribund
B16 melanoma	500	C57/B1 mice	34	0/3	5/5 (large) Mice moribund
MC28 sarcoma	50	Ho-Lister rats	22	2/5 (small)	5/5 (large) Rats moribund

*Macroscopic solid tumours predominantly involving omentum.
**Given 15 days prior to tumour cells: 0.5 ml i.p. for mice; 2.5 ml i.p. for rats.

even though only about 3% of the total muscle mass is involved. A possible involvement of tissue macrophages in this phenomenon is suggested by an experiment (unpublished) which shows that facilitation of tumour growth arises some 4 to 5 days after wounding. Wound healing is initially associated with the release of growth factors from platelets which have degranulated at the site of a blood clot. As healing progresses, macrophages enter the lesion usually between the third and fifth days, i.e. at the time when the growth of blood-borne cancer cells is maximally facilitated at the site of a wound.

Promotion of carcinogenesis

Tissue trauma also potentiates carcinogenesis and the term 'promoter' was coined by Peyton Rous[59] for the phenomenon by which tumours could be induced by low doses of carcinogens in the ears of rabbits which had a hole punched through them. Even before these studies Lacassagne[60] reported that doses of X-rays which were not sufficient to induce tumours in intact skin of rabbits did so when applied at sites of ulceration. This finding was confirmed by Burrows et al.[61] and subsequently extended to other aspects of radiation carcinogenesis[62]. These studies provide additional evidence for the view that host factors are frequently necessary to permit a cell (or cells) that have undergone a malignant transformation to grow into a tumour. While the evidence is not conclusive it seems likely that macrophages play an important role in promotion of carcinogenesis, probably by releasing growth factors into the immediate environment. Macrophages have been shown to produce growth factors for epithelial and endothelial cells as well as for fibroblasts[58,63]. Supernatants from cultures of macrophages which are not activated (i.e. which do not produce cytotoxins such as tumour necrosis factor) powerfully promote the clonal growth of cancer cells in soft agar. The available facts are fully consistent with the following hypothesis, developed in relation to the preferential growth of blood-borne cancer cells at specific sites and organs, viz. that isolated cancer cells require tissue derived growth factors to start their growth into a tumour and that the lesion only becomes autonomous after attaining a minimum size. Macrophages seem capable of producing the growth factors needed by at least some cancer cells and this can explain not only the preferential growth of metastases in wounds but the promotion of carcinogenesis by wounding.

ANTERIOR PREFERENCE – THE AUERBACH EFFECT

While several investigators commented independently that the growth of tumours transplanted subcutaneously or intramuscularly varied with the anatomical site of the inoculation, the generality of this phenomenon was highlighted by Auerbach. In 1978 his group[64] showed that tumour cells injected anteriorly into the dorsal or lateral trunk grew at more than twice the rate of an equivalent number of tumour cells administered more posteriorly, and also grew with a higher frequency (i.e. the minimum number of cells required to cause a tumour was lower by a factor of four). 'Anterior preference' was found with all of a wide range of tumours studied, including sarcomas, lymphomas, adenocarcinomas and a mastocytoma. The effect was independent of sex, the genetic strain of the mouse or the immunogenicity of the tumour. Moreover, it was fully demonstrable in mice that were immunosuppressed by irradiation or congenital absence of a thymus. Auerbach, as well as other investigators who confirmed this phenomenon, attempted to find the biological basis for the regional differences in tumour growth. The first presumption was that an effect of such magnitude was caused by major differences in the local physiology of the host, but none have been identified[65]. No anterior/posterior differences were found as regards a variety of aspects of the vascular supply, including the microcirculation, angiogenesis or temperature. There were no differences in lymphatic drainage, or in clearance or retention of dead cells and debris. Auerbach was forced to conclude[66]:

> given the broad range of systems that demonstrate the differential pattern of growth and development it would seem reasonable to believe that the underlying mechanism should be readily apparent as well as of major significance. Why the identification of that mechanism has been so elusive is not clear to us. We simply have no ready explanation for the biological basis underlying the observed regional differences.

In view of findings summarised in the previous section, it would be interesting to know if there are regional differences in wound healing comparable to those of tumour growth.

ANGIOGENESIS

A network of capillary blood vessels supplies the nutritional needs of every tissue and organ in the body. The same applies to tumours. In the initial stages of tumorigenesis the multiplying tumour cells can receive nutrients and oxygen by diffusion. However, growth beyond a nodule with diameter in the range 0.1 to 1mm requires the ingrowth of capillaries. If this process of angiogenesis does not occur the size of the tumour will remain static as cell loss by 'starvation' is compensated by cell division on the outside of the tumour nodule. Indeed, for rapidly dividing malignant cells *in vivo*, the speed of tumour growth may be determined by the rate at which neovascularisation takes place. As the new blood vessels are of host origin (except for the rare endothelial cancers) tumour development may be controlled by the proliferation of normal cells. Angiogenesis in the adult organism is not, of course, confined to tumours but is an essential component of wound healing, inflammation and many types of immune pathology. Capillary ingrowth into tumours is a complex process involving several sequential steps[67] starting with the local degradation of the basement membrane of the parent vessel (e.g. a small vein) and the extension of endothelial cells through the hole formed. Degradative enzymes must play a part and these could come from tumour cells. The endothelial cells migrate to the tumour in response to a chemotactic signal, form a sprout and then elongate and extend by cell division. There are clearly many factors involved in angiogenesis and the widely used term 'Angiogenesis Factor' is now seen to apply in general – though not always – to growth factors that cause endothelial cells to divide. It must be emphasised that the availability of an endothelial growth factor is not sufficient for angiogenesis to occur, but it may well be rate limiting.

The endothelial cells that line capillaries perform a variety of metabolic, immunological and above all haemostatic functions. Endothelial cells are usually out of cycle, 'resting' cells with turnover times measured in years, but growth factors can quickly induce cell proliferation. It was shown 50 years ago that tumour extracts can induce the formation of new blood vessels, and for 25 years Folkman has been an articulate and innovative exponent of the view that interference with angiogenesis might be used for the medical control of tumour growth[67]. Protamine, heparin, chondroitin sulphates and some steroids[68] inhibit angiogenesis but initial claims[69] that they can control tumour growth *in vivo* have not been substantiated. In 1985 Vallee's group isolated and then gene cloned a polypeptide derived from a colonic tumour which is angiogenic *in vivo* and a potent endothelial growth factor *in vitro*[70-72] The material (called angiogenin) has a molecular weight of 14 100 and shows a striking sequence homology with human ribonuclease but does not exhibit ribonuclease activity. Expression of the angiogenin gene is probably not limited to tumour cells but it may be over-expressed by them. Angiogenin is not the only polypeptide growth factor for endothelial cells and the recent literature is burgeoning with endothelial growth factors extracted from numerous different tissues[73-75]. One class of endothelial growth factors is characterised by powerful binding to heparin yet some of them are anionic proteins whereas others are cationic[76,77]. The potent interaction of an anionic polypeptide with strongly negatively charged heparin indicates the existence of some very strong interactions between polysaccharide and peptide. A material described as fibroblast growth factor, the subject of a voluminous literature[78,79] is now known to be in reality an endothelial growth factor whose apparent effect on fibroblasts was caused by contamination of the extracts.

Of particular interest is the finding that macrophages amongst several other growth factors also produce polypeptides which are potent endothelial mitogens[80]. This could contribute to the tumour promoting activity of macrophages discussed previously. Investigators studying the role of macrophages in wound healing found that the production of endothelial growth factor is greatly enhanced if the macrophages are hypoxic[81]. A process dependent on anoxia would provide effective feed-back control for angiogenesis in wound healing since new blood vessels are only required so long as the lesion is hypoxic. There are obvious implications for tumours which frequently outgrow their blood supply and in consequence develop hypoxic rims surrounding necrotic centres. This process may be counterbalanced to some extent by infiltrating macrophages[82].

Finally, it must be stressed that angiogenesis can be induced *in vivo* by a variety of chemical substances[83] which include copper ions, prostaglandin E_2 and low molecular weight materials extracted from tumours. At what stage in the chain of events leading to neovascularisation these 'angiogenic factors' are active remains to be elucidated.

References

1. Burnet, M. (1970). *Immunological Surveillance*. (Oxford: Pergamon Press)
2. Borek, C. (1985). The induction and control of radiogenic transformation *in vitro*: Cellular and molecular mechanisms. *Pharmacol. Ther.*, **27**, 99-142
3. Alexander, P. (1985). Do cancers arise from a single transformed cell or is monoclonality of tumours a late event in carcinogenesis? *Br. J. Cancer*, **51**, 452-457
4. Tarin, D., Price, J., Kettlewell, M., Souter, R., Vass, A. and Crossley, B. (1984). Clinicopathological observations on metastasis in man studied in patients treated with peritoneovenous shunts. *Br. Med. J.*, **288**, 749-751
5. Alexander, P. and Eccles, S. (1984). Host-mediated mechanisms in the elimination of circulating cancer cells. In Nicolson, L. and Milas, L. (eds.) *Cancer Invasion and Metastasis: Biologic & Therapeutic Aspects*. pp. 293-308 (New York: Raven Press)
6. Alexander, P. (1983). Dormant metastases - studies in experimental animals. *J. Pathol.*, **141**, 379-383
7. Hofer, K. G. (1970). Radiation effects on death and migration of tumor cells in mice. *Radiat. Res.*, **43**, 663-667
8. Fidler, I. J. (1970). Metastasis: Quantitative analyses of distribution and fate of tumour emboli labelled with ^{125}I-5-iodo-2-deoxyridine. *J. Natl. Cancer Inst.*, **45**, 773-782
9. Sporn, M. and Todaro, G. (1980). Autocrine secretion and malignant transformation of cells. *N. Engl. J. Med.*, **303**, 878-880
10. Alexander, P. and Currie, G. (1984). Concomitant synthesis of growth factors and their receptors an aspect of malignant transformation. *Biochem. Pharmacol.*, **33**, 941-943
11. Alexander, P., Senior, P., Murphy, P. and Clarke, R. (1985). Role of growth stimulatory factors in determining the sites of metastasis. In Honn, D., Powers, W. and Sloane, B. (eds.) *Mechanisms of Cancer Metastasis*. pp. 173-191. (Boston: Martinus Nijhoff Publishing).
12. Prehn, R. and Main, J. (1957). Immunity to methylcholanthrene-induced sarcomas. *J. Natl. Cancer Inst.*, **18**, 769-774
13. Klein, G. and Klein, E. (1977). Rejectability of virus-induced tumors and non-rejectability of spontaneous tumors: A lesson in contrasts. *Trans. Proc.*, **9**, 1095
14. Hewitt, H., Blake, E. and Walder, A. (1976). A critique of the evidence for active host defense against cancer, based on personal studies of 27 murine tumours of spontaneous origin. *Br. J. Cancer*, **33**, 241-251
15. Sanford, B., Kohn, H., Daly, J. and Soo, S. (1973). Long-term spontaneous tumor incidence in neonatally thymectomized mice. *J. Immunol.*, **110**, 1437-1441
16. Rygaard, J. and Povlsen, C. (1976). The nude mouse vs. hypothesis of immunological surveillance. *Transplant. Rev.*, **28**, 43-45
17. Stutman, O. (1974). Tumor development after 3-methylcholanthrene in immunologically deficient athymic-nude mice. *Science*, **183**, 534-536
18. Outzen, H., Custer, R., Eaton, G. and Prehn, R. (1975). Spontaneous and induced tumor incidence in germ-free nude mice. *J. Reticuloendothel. Soc.*, **17**, 1-18
19. Eccles, S. and Alexander P. (1974). Macrophage content of tumours in relation to metastatic spread and host immune reaction. *Nature*, **250**, 667
20. Eccles, S., Heckford, S. and Alexander, P. (1980). Effect of cyclosporin A on the growth and spontaneous metastasis of syngeneic animal tumours. *Br. J. Cancer*, **42**, 252-259
21. Davey, G., Currie, G. and Alexander, P. (1979). Immunity is the predominant factor determining metastases by murine lymphomas. *Br. J. Cancer*, **40**, 590-596
22. Souadjian, J., Silverstein, M. and Titus, J. (1968). Thymoma and cancer. *Cancer*, **22**, 1221
23. Kinlen, J., Shere, A., Peto, J. and Doll, R. (1979). Collaborative United Kingdom-Australasian study of cancer in patients treated with immunosuppressive drugs. *Br. Med. J.*, ii, 1461-1466

24. Prehn, R. (1977). Immunostimulation of chemical oncogenesis in the mouse. *Int. J. Cancer*, **20**, 918-922

25. Parr, I., Jackson, L. and Alexander, P. (1983). Role of "lymphotoxin" in the local anti-tumour action associated with inflammation caused by delayed hypersensitivity responses or intralesional BCG. I. Variations in response of different syngeneic mouse tumours. *Br. J. Cancer*, **48**, 395-403

26. Alexander, P. and Evans, R. (1971). Endotoxin and double stranded RNA render macrophages cytotoxic. *Nature New Biol.*, **232**, 76-78

27. Evans, R. and Alexander, P. (1971). Rendering macrophages cytotoxic by a factor released from immune lymphoid cells. *Transplantation*, **12**, 227-229

28. Parr, I., Wheeler, E. and Alexander, P. (1973). Similarities of the anti-tumour actions of endotoxin, lipid A and double stranded RNA. *Br. J. Cancer*, **27**, 370-389

29. Kimber, I. and Moore, M. (1985). Mechanism and regulation of natural cytotoxicity. *Exp. Cell Biol.*, **53**, 69-84

30. Warner, J. and Dennert, G. (1985). Bone marrow graft rejection as a function of antibody-directed natural killer cells. *J. Exp. Med.*, **161**, 563-576

31. Foodstat, O., Hansen, C., Cannon, G., Statham, C., Lictenstein, G. and Boyd, M. (1984). Lack of correlation between natural killer activity and tumour growth control in nude mice with different immune defects. *Cancer Res.*, **44**, 4403-4408

32. Vanky, F., Argov, S., Einhorn, S. and Klein, E. (1980). Role of alloantigens in natural killing: Allogeneic but not autologous tumor biopsy cells are sensitive for interferon induced cytotoxicity of human blood lymphocytes. *J. Exp. Med.*, **151**, 1151

33. Dallegri, F., Frumento, G. and Patrone, F. (1982). Mechanisms of tumour cell destruction by PMA-activated human neutrophils. *Immunology*, **48**, 273-279

34. Proctor, J., Rudenstam, C. and Alexander, P. (1973). A factor preventing the development of lung metastases in rats with sarcomas. *Nature*, **242**, 29

35. Denham, S., Hooton, J., Barfoot, R., Alexander, P., Mayol, R. and Wrathmell A. (1980). Mechanism by which antibodies to non-AgB antigens mediate rejection of rat leukaemia cells. *Br. J. Cancer*, **42**, 408-415

36. Alexander, P. and Eccles, S. (1984). Host mediated mechanisms in the elimination of circulating cancer cells. In Nicolson, G. and Milas, L. (eds.) *Cancer Invasion & Metastasis: Biologic & Therapeutic Aspects*. pp. 293-308. (New York: Raven Press)

37. Sato, H. and Suzuki, M. (1976). Deformability and viability of tumour cells by metastasis in cancer. In Weiss, L. (ed.) *Fundamental Aspects of Metastasis*. pp. 311-317. (Amsterdam: North Holland)

38. Alexander, P. and Senior, P. (1986). Toxicity of oxygen at atmospheric concentration for newly explanted cancer cells. *Biochem. Pharmacol.*, **35**, 91-92

39. Shewell, J. and Thompson, S. (1980). The effect of hyperbaric oxygen treatment on pulmonary metastasis in the C3H mouse. *Eur. J. Cancer*, **16**, 253-259

40. Clarke, R., Senior, P. and Alexander, P. (1985). In Hellman, K. and Eccles, S. (eds.) *Treatment of Metastasis: Problems and Prospects*, pp. 223 - 226. (London: Taylor & Francis).

41. DeLarco, J. and Todaro, S. (1978). *Proc. Natl. Acad. Sci. USA*, **75**, 4001-4005

42. Lu, D., Rose, T., Webb, N. and Todaro, S. (1985). Cloning and sequence analysis of a c-DNA for rat alpha TGF. *Nature*, **313**, 489

43. Seifert, R., Schwartz, S. and Bowen-Pope, D. (1984). Developmentally regulated production of platelet-derived growth factor-like molecules. *Nature*, **311**, 669-671

44. Leal, F., Williams, L., Robbins, K. and Aaronson, S. (1985). Evidence that the v-*sis* gene product transforms by interaction with the receptor for platelet-derived growth factor. *Science*, **230**, 327-330

45. Rozengurt, E., Sinnett-Smith, J. and Taylor-Papadimitriou, J. (1985). Production of PDGF-like growth factor by breast cancer cell lines. *Int. J. Cancer*, **36**, 247-252

46. Betsholtz, C., Westermark, B., Ek, B. and Heldin, C. (1984). Coexpression of a PDGF-like growth factor and PDGF receptors in a human osteosarcoma cell line: Implications for autocrine receptor activation. *Cell*, **39**, 447-457

47. Paget, S. (1889). The distribution of secondary growths in the cancer of the breast. *Lancet*, i, 571-573

48. Weiss, L., Haydock, K., Pickren, J. and Lane, W. (1980). Organ vascularity and metastatic frequency. *Am. J. Pathol.*, **101**, 101-113

49. Willis, R. (1964). *Pathology of Tumours*. 4th Edn., pp. 174-176. (London: Butterworth)
50. Murphy, P., Taylor, I. and Alexander, P. (1985). Organ distribution of metastases following injection of syngeneic rate tumour cells into the arterial circulation via the left ventricle. In Hellman, K. and Eccles, S. (eds) *Treatment of Metastasis: Problems and Prospects*. pp. 191-194. (London: Taylor & Francis)
51. Murphy, P., Alexander, P., Kirkham, N., Fleming, J. and Taylor, I. (1986). The pattern of spread of blood-borne tumour. *Br. J. Surg.*, (In press)
52. Evans, R. (1978). Macrophage requirement for growth of a murine fibrosarcoma. *Br. J. Cancer*, 37, 1086-1089
53. Evans, R. (1977). Effect of X-irradiation on host-cell infiltration and growth of a murine fibrosarcoma. *Br. J. Cancer*, 35, 557-565
54. Eccles, S. and Alexander, P. (1974). Macrophage content of tumours in relation to metastatic spread and host immune reaction. *Nature*, 250, 667-669
55. Kadhim, S. and Rees, R. (1984). Enhancement of tumor growth in mice: Evidence for the involvement of host macrophages. *Cell. Immunol.*, 87, 259-269
56. Leak, L., Potter, M. and Mayfield, W. (1985). Response of the peritoneal mesothelium to the mineral oil, pristane. *Curr. Topics Microbiol. Immunol.*, 122, 221-233
57. Fisher, B. and Fisher, E. (1959). Experimental support of the dormant tumour cell. *Science*, 130, 918-919
58. Leibovich, S. and Ross, R. (1975). The role of the macrophage in wound repair. *Am. J. Pathol.*, 78, 71-99
59. Friedewald, W. and Rous, P. (1944). The initiating and promoting elements in tumor production. *J. Exp. Med.*, 80, 101-126
60. Lacassagne, A. and Vinzent, R. (1929). Sarcomes provoques chez des lapins par l'irradiation d'abges a *Streptobacillus caviae*. *Soc. Biol.*, 100, 249-251
61. Burrows, H., Mayneord, W. and Roberts, J. (1937). Neoplasia following the application of X-rays to inflammatory lesions. *Proc. R. Soc. B.*, 123, 213-217
62. Warren, S. and Brown, C. (1978). Mammary and other tumors as a response to radiation and multiple stresses. *Arch. Pathol. Lab. Med.*, 102, 224-226
63. Martinet, Y., Bitterman, P., Mornex, J., Grotendorst, G., Martin, G., and Crystal R. (1986). Activated human monocytes express the c-*sis* proto-oncogene and release a mediator showing PDGF-like activity. *Nature*, 319, 158-160
64. Auerbach, R., Morrissey, L. and Sidky, Y. (1978). Regional differences in the incidence and growth of mouse tumors following intradermal or subcutaneous inoculation. *Cancer Res.*, 38, 1739-1744
65. Auerbach, R., Morrissey, L., Kubai, L. and Sidky, Y. (1978). Regional differences in tumor growth: Studies of the vascular system. *Int. J. Cancer*, 22, 40-46
66. Auerbach, R. (1980). Regional differences in tumor growth. *Cancer Res.*, 40, 2197
67. Folkman, J. (1986). How is blood vessel growth regulated in normal and neoplastic tissue? *Cancer Res.*, 46, 467-473
68. Crum, R., Szabo, S. and Folkman, J. (1985). A new class of steroids inhibits angiogenesis in the presence of heparin or a heparin fragment. *Science*, 230, 1375-1378
69. Folkman, J., Langer, R., Linhardt, R., Haudenschild, C. and Taylor, S. (1983). Angiogenesis inhibition and tumor regression caused by heparin or a heparin fragment in the presence of cortisone. *Science*, 221, 719-725
70. Fett, J., Strydom, D., Lobb R., Alderman, E., Bethune, J., Riordan, J. and Vallee, B. (1985). Isolation and characterization of angiogenin, and angiogenic protein from human carcinoma cells. *Biochemistry*, 24, 5480-5486
71. Strydom, D., Fett, J., Lobb, R., Alderman, E., Bethune, J., Riordan, J. and Vallee, B. (1985). Amino acid sequence of human tumor derived angiogenin. *Biochemistry*, 24, 5486-5494
72. Kurachi, K., Davies, E., Strydom, D., Riordan, J. and Vallee, B. (1985). Sequence of the cDNA and gene for angiogenin, a human angiogenesis factor. *Biochemistry*, 24, 5494-5499
73. McAuslan, B., Bender, V., Reilly, W. and Moss, B. (1985). New functions of epidermal growth factor: Stimulation of capillary endothelial cell migration and matrix dependent proliferation. *Cell Biol. Int. Rep.*, 9, 175 182
74. Burgess, W., Mehlman, T., Friesel, R., Johnson, W. and Macaig, T. (1985). Multiple forms of endothelial cell growth factor. *J. Biol. Chem.*, 260, 11389-11392

75. Sullivan, R. and Klagsbrun, M. (1985). Purification of cartilage-derived growth factor by heparin affinity chromatography. *J. Biol. Chem.*, **260**, 2399-2403
76. Schreiber, A., Kenney, J., Kowalski, W., Friesel, R., Mehlman, T. and Macaig, T. (1985). Interaction of endothelial cells growth factor with heparin: Characterization by receptor and antibody recognition. *Proc. Natl. Acad. Sci. USA*, **82**, 6138-6142
77. Klagsburn, M. and Shing, Y. (1985). Heparin affinity of anionic and cationic capillary endothelial cell growth factors: Analysis of hypothalamus-derived growth factors and fibroblast growth factors. *Proc. Natl. Acad. Sci. USA*, **82**, 805-809
78. Schreiber, A., Kenney, J., Kowalski, J., Thomas, K., Gallego, G., Candelore, M., Di Salvo, J., Barritault, D., Courty, J., Courtois, Y., Moenner, M., Loret, C., Burgess, W., Mehlman, T., Friesel, R., Johnson, W. and Macaig, T. (1985). A unique family of endothelial cell polypeptide mitogens: The antigenic and receptor cross-reactivity of bovine endothelial cell growth factor, brain-derived acidic fibroblast growth factor, and eye-derived growth factor II. *J. Cell Biol.*, **101**, 1623-1626
79. Bohlen, P., Esch, F., Baird, A. and Gospodarowicz, D. (1985). Acidic fibroblast growth factor (FGF) from bovine brain: amino-terminal sequence and comparison with basic FGF. *EMBO. J.*, **4**, 1951-1956
80. Polverini, P., Cotran, R., Gimbrone, M. and Unanue, E. (1977). Activated macrophages induced vascular proliferation. *Nature*, **269**, 804
81. Knighton, D., Hunt, T., Scheuenstuhl, H. and Halliday, B. (1983). Oxygen tension regulates the expression of angiogenesis factor by macrophages. *Science*, **221**, 1283
82. Polverini, P. and Leibovich, S. (1984). Induction of neovascularization *in vivo* and endothelial proliferation *in vitro* by tumor-associated macrophages. *Lab. Invest.*, **51**, 635
83. Form, D. and Auerbach, R. (1983). PGE$_2$ and angiogenesis (41548). *Proc. Soc. Expt. Biol. Med.*, **172**, 2214-2218

Index